Textbook of *Nuclear medicine technology*

Textbook of *Nuclear medicine technology*

Paul J. Early, B.S.

Physicist, Nuclear Medicine Institute,
Cleveland, Ohio

Muhammad Abdel Razzak, M.B.B.Ch., D.M., M.D.

Assistant Professor, Medical Unit and Division of Nuclear
Medicine, Faculty of Medicine, Cairo University,
Cairo, U.A.R.

D. Bruce Sodee, M.D., F.A.C.P.

Associate Professor of Radiology (Nuclear Medicine),
George Washington University, Washington, D.C.;
Director, Nuclear Medicine Institute, Cleveland, Ohio;
Director, Nuclear Medicine Department, Hillcrest Hospital,
Cleveland, Ohio

With 241 illustrations

Saint Louis

The C. V. Mosby Company

1969

Printed in the United States of America.
Standard Book Number 8016-1490-2
Library of Congress Catalog Card Number 79-95016
Distributed in Great Britain by Henry Kimpton, London

Preface

The training program for technologists offered at the Nuclear Medicine Institute, Cleveland, Ohio, began as an outgrowth of its physicians' introductory training program. It became apparent early in that teaching endeavor that there was an intense need for trained nuclear medicine technologists. Because few institutions were involved in this type of training, it seemed a logical extension of the N.M.I. facilities to include such a program.

Since the inception of our technologists' training program, an unrelenting search has yielded no applicable text. Although comprehensive texts and other supplementary literature were available for physician training, none of these was found to be suitable for technologists. Several approaches have been used in an attempt to compensate for this void, but all have proved unsuccessful. They have lacked the continuity necessary for class supplements, a necessity that could be supplied by an appropriate text.

Since N.M.I. has been in the process of training nuclear medicine technologists for the past three years, it seemed plausible that we effect a text primarily for the education of the nuclear medicine technologist.

The text is divided into two portions: nuclear science and clinical theory. The clinical section is a systems approach rather than the usual organ approach, so as to better correlate all bodily functions. Because both sections represent the works of a large variety of authors compiled over a long period of time, no attempt has been made to document statements with precise references. A list of references will be found immediately following each section. In this way a partial supplement to the preceding material, as well as credits to the various authors, is provided. Wherever possible, the content has been simplified to make highly theoretical principles more easily understood.

Acknowledgements are extended to the following: Marshall Brucer, M.D., St. Mary's Hospital, Tucson, Arizona, for his contribution of the Trilinear Chart of the Nuclides and accompanying text to be found in Part I; Mallinckrodt Nuclear, Division of Mallinckrodt Chemical Works, St. Louis, Missouri, who, by their continuing grant-in-aid, has allowed the inception and continuation of our physician and technologist educational programs in the field of nuclear medicine; Renner Clinic Foundation, Cleveland, Ohio, under whose organization the Nuclear Medicine Institute functions; all the faculty members of N.M.I., whose advice and suggestions determined the content of the technologist course from which grew this text; the reviewers, William W. Stanbro, M.D., George Washington University, Washington, D.C., George W. Callendine, Jr., Ph.D., Riverside Meth-

v

odist Hospital, Columbus, Ohio, and A. Stone Freedberg, M.D., Harvard Medical School and Beth Israel Hospital, Boston, Massachusetts, whose critiques of the manuscript were greatly appreciated; the illustrator, Susan Nicolet, whose tireless efforts make the material content of the text more meaningful; the secretaries, Georgene Field and Susan Nicolet, for their long hours of aid in the production of the manuscript; and our students, who helped us recognize the depth to which this text should progress.

Paul J. Early
Muhammad Abdel Razzak
D. Bruce Sodee

Contents

Appendixes

Part I Nuclear science

Anatomy of the atom

In any treatise of the basic sciences a detailed discussion of the structure of matter, molecules, and the constituent atoms must first be presented. In any treatise of the basic *nuclear* sciences, the above must also be included. In addition, a discussion of the constituent parts of the atom should be presented, since these parts play such an important role in the understanding of the nuclear sciences. In the following all the parts of the atom that are important to the nuclear sciences, particularly to nuclear medicine, are presented.

MATTER AND MOLECULES
Reducing matter to simplest fraction

Anything that possesses mass and inertia and that occupies any amount of space is composed of matter. Any type of matter must be reduced to its simplest fractions before the fundamental structure can be studied. Salt can be used to illustrate such a reduction (Fig. 1-1). The contents of a dispenser of salt are spoken of as *visible matter.* If one were to take just one granule of table salt, it would still fall into the realm of visible matter. However, if it were possible to halve this granule of salt again and again, a particle would eventually be obtained which, if it were halved again, would no longer be salt. Such a particle is called a *molecule*

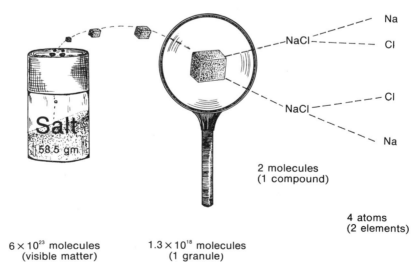

2 molecules
(1 compound)

4 atoms
(2 elements)

6×10^{23} molecules
(visible matter)

1.3×10^{18} molecules
(1 granule)

Fig. 1-1. Diagram showing the components of all matter, beginning with visible matter and proceeding to its smallest unit, the atom.

or a *compound.* (At some point previous to this, human visibility would have been surpassed. Even though it can no longer be seen by the naked eye, the basic character of salt is still retained.) A molecule of table salt is known to be composed of two *elements,* sodium (Na) and chlorine (Cl), which are radically different from each other. Should the molecule of salt be halved, the result would be 2 totally unrelated atoms—one of sodium and one of chlorine. Table salt as such would no longer exist. Each atom would be completely independent of the other and each would exhibit its own physical and chemical properties. All substances, whether they are liquids, solids, or gases, are made up of molecules composed of independent atoms.

The discussion above reveals a number of important concepts regarding matter: (1) All matter is composed of molecules. Some molecules can exist as a single atom and are, therefore, identical with the atom itself. (2) A molecule, by definition, is the smallest unit of any substance which can freely exist and still retain the chemical properties of the original substance. (3) All molecules are composed of atoms. (4) An atom, by definition, is the smallest unit of matter that exhibits the chemical properties of an element.

Dalton's hypothesis. The idea that all matter is composed of atoms dates back more than 2,000 years to the ancient Greeks. It was merely a theory, however, since they had no experimental basis for such a statement. Many centuries passed before it was proved that their basic concepts of matter were correct. It was not until the eighteenth century that John Dalton, an English school teacher, proposed a theory to explain the interrelationships of matter and its constituent parts. Among other things, Dalton hypothesized that:

1. A pure substance (a chemical element) is composed of atoms. These are all exactly alike in mass, size, and shape.
2. The atoms of same or different elements can combine to form molecules (compounds).
3. Each molecule of a particular substance contains the same combination of atoms.
4. Chemical reactions represent one of three possibilities:
   a. The combination of atoms to form molecules ($Na + Cl \rightarrow NaCl$)
   b. The splitting of molecules to form atoms ($NaCl \rightarrow Na + Cl$)
   c. The rearranging of atoms of two different molecules to form new molecules ($NaCl + H_2O \rightarrow NaOH + HCl$).

In chemical reactions, the individual atoms are unchanged. Only their combinations are altered. Since more than 100 elements have been identified, it is conceivable that there are millions of possible combinations. Examples used here are very simple; however, others are exceedingly complex. Today, Dalton's hypothesis is recognized as the beginning of modern chemistry and man is still reaping the benefits of his scientific revelations.

Modification of Dalton's hypothesis. Although Dalton was noted for his knowledge and foresight, it was later proved that his hypothesis was not entirely correct. The basic idea of atomic structure was correct, but he was unable to extend his hypothesis beyond that of the atom. He was unable to discern that the atoms themselves are composed of even smaller and more fundamental particles. He also said that the atoms were unchanged in their physical and chemical characteristics in a chemical reaction. He was unable to know that if, in some cases, sufficient energy was applied to the atom, one atom could be changed into another atom. This phenomenon was not to be learned until 200 years after Dalton's initial work.

The principles of Dalton's hypothesis did not entirely explain phenomena that were observed during later experiments. Scientists found it necessary to explore the interior of the atom for possible answers. As a result, there were further modifications to Dalton's original hypothesis. One modification had to be made since the distinction between mass and pure energy had become clouded. In fact, according to later theories, the two were interchangeable. Another change had to be made to explain the fact that sometimes electromagnetic radiation behaved more like a particle than a wave.

NATURE OF MATTER

Scientists continued to explore the interior of the atom. As a result, a number of subdivisions were revealed. It appears that the atom is composed of a central positively charged core known as a *nucleus*. Traveling in a circular path around the nucleus are one or more smaller negatively charged particles of mass, called *electrons*. Bohr compared this arrangement to a miniature solar system—the nucleus representing the sun, and the electrons representing the planets circling the sun.

The electron

Definition and description. The electron is a high velocity extranuclear particle that has a more or less fixed elliptical path around the nucleus. The electron possesses a known mass that remains constant for electrons of all atoms. The number of electrons that are circling the nucleus is a variable, and that number in an electrically neutral atom is dictated by the constituents of the nucleus. Two criteria may be used to differentiate the electron particle from other particles in the atom; they are *mass* and *electrical charge* (see Table 1-1). Using the electron as a reference point, the electron has a relative mass of 1 and a negative charge. This negative charge apparently cannot be separated from the electron. Possessing a negative charge, the electron exhibits forces of attraction or repulsion to other charged particles. These forces were first noticed by Coulomb and the principle is now an accepted principle of physics. Coulomb's law states in part that *like charges repel; unlike charges attract.*

The mystery of the electron. Because of Coulomb's law and the fact that negative electrons circle the positive nucleus, the question of what effect all this has in the atom may well be asked. A repulsion effect between electrons is exhibited as a distribution in space as they circle the nucleus. The mystery arises from the lack of attraction of the electrons to the nucleus. What prevents the electron from being attracted to the nucleus?

The attraction is prevented through the action of two phenomena working simultaneously. (1) Since the electron is a particle circling the nucleus at high velocities, the electron counteracts the attraction by the nucleus to a certain degree

5

by centrifugal force, the force of inertia which tends to make rotating bodies move away from the center of rotation. (2) A certain amount of energy from the atom known as binding energy is expended for no other reason than to retain the electron in its preordained orbit.

The nucleus

Upon learning of the existence of the nucleus, scientists became intrigued with the fact that the nucleus contained almost all of the weight attributed to the atom. The nucleus, therefore, became a primary target of research. The effort to discover the composition and function of the nucleus still continues. Many aspects of the nucleus are known; others are unknown but theories have been formulated about them. One fact that is considered indisputable is that the nucleus itself is made up of small particles. The two particles most important to students of nuclear medicine are the *proton* and the *neutron.* These particles are normal constituents of the nucleus and are commonly referred to as *nucleons.* This positively charged core of every atom contains almost the entire mass of the atom but only a small part of its volume. It has been calculated that the nucleus is only 1/100,000 the size of the entire atom, but it is so dense that a child's marble of the same density would weigh approximately 36,400,000 tons. The nucleus is very stable and is impervious to chemical or physical changes; however, radiation can cause changes within it.

The proton. The proton (p) possesses a known mass, which remains constant. It has a positive charge associated with it that cannot be separated from it. The charge is equal in magnitude to the negative charge of the electron. It is because of the presence of these protons within the nucleus that the nucleus possesses a positive charge. In fact, in the hydrogen atom, the proton *is* the positive nucleus. In all other atoms the proton is one of the constituents. The mass of the proton is much greater than that of the electron. It has a mass 1,836 times that of the electron (see Table 1-1). The number of protons within the nucleus determines the type of atom; for example, all carbon atoms have 6 protons and all atoms containing 6 protons are carbon atoms.

The neutron. The neutron (n) also possesses a known mass that remains constant. This mass is just slightly greater than the mass of a proton (1840). This particle, as the name implies, has no electrical charge. Because of the neutral charge it cannot attract or repel charged particles. In fact it is this very property that makes the neutron important. With a lack of charge, the neutron cannot be affected by the charged particles in the atom and can penetrate right into the

Table 1-1. Mass and charge of particles of the nucleus

Particle	Charge	Mass
Electron	Negative	1*
Proton	Positive	1,836
Neutron	Neutral	1,840
Neutrino	Neutral	~ 0

*Reference Mass

heart of the atom. Under proper conditions, the neutron can actually be incorporated into the nucleus or disrupt it. The former is referred to as neutron activation; the latter is referred to as fission. Both of these phenomena will be discussed later.

The mystery of the nucleus. The nucleus can be considered to be an aggregate of positive charges because of its proton constituents. According to Coulomb's law, the protons should repel one another and the repulsive effects of the positive charges should cause the nucleus to fragment. However, this does not seem to be the case. An explanation is that the protons—and, therefore, the nucleus—are contained through binding energy. The nucleus expends some of its energy to keep the nucleons bound to one another.

The neutrino. The neutrino cannot be considered a normal constituent of the nucleus, but it results from interactions within the nucleus. This particle plays a more or less important role in nuclear medicine, since it is emitted during several methods of atomic decay. At the present time, only a description of the particle is warranted. The neutrino (v) is, as the name would indicate, a particle possessing a neutral charge. The mass of the neutrino approaches zero mass.

The mass and charge of all these particles are summarized in Table 1-1.

Energy shells

The atom has been defined as the smallest unit of matter that exhibits the chemical properties of an element. It is composed of a nucleus containing protons and neutrons of varying numbers and is surrounded by one or more negatively charged electrons circling in rather well defined orbits or *energy shells.* The number of electrons in each energy shell varies according to the chemical element. Each shell can contain only a certain number of electrons. That number is based on the *$2n^2$ formula,* in which n is the number of the energy shell. The energy shells are numbered beginning with that shell closest to the nucleus and proceeding outward numerically. According to the $2n^2$ formula, the first energy shell can contain no more than 2 electrons. The second energy shell can contain no more than 8 electrons, the third energy shell can contain no more than 18 electrons, the fourth energy shell can contain no more than 32 electrons, and so on. Rather than being designated by numbers, the shells are labeled alphabetically beginning with K and proceeding outward. Therefore, the K shell can have no more than 2, the L shell no more than 8, and the M shell no more than 18 electrons.

PERIODIC CHART OF THE ATOMS

At the present time, 103 elements have been identified. All of these elements can be arranged into a table in which they are grouped according to increasing weight and chemical similarities. This arrangement is known as the periodic chart of the atoms (Fig. 1-2).

The periodic chart is an outgrowth of observations recorded by early investigators who saw that the periodicity or rhythm of atomic behavior could be shown graphically. The chart is a natural repository of our knowledge of the atoms, a compilation of some thirty physical and chemical facts about each element. Many scientists and scientific workers have aided in perfecting the new theory of the

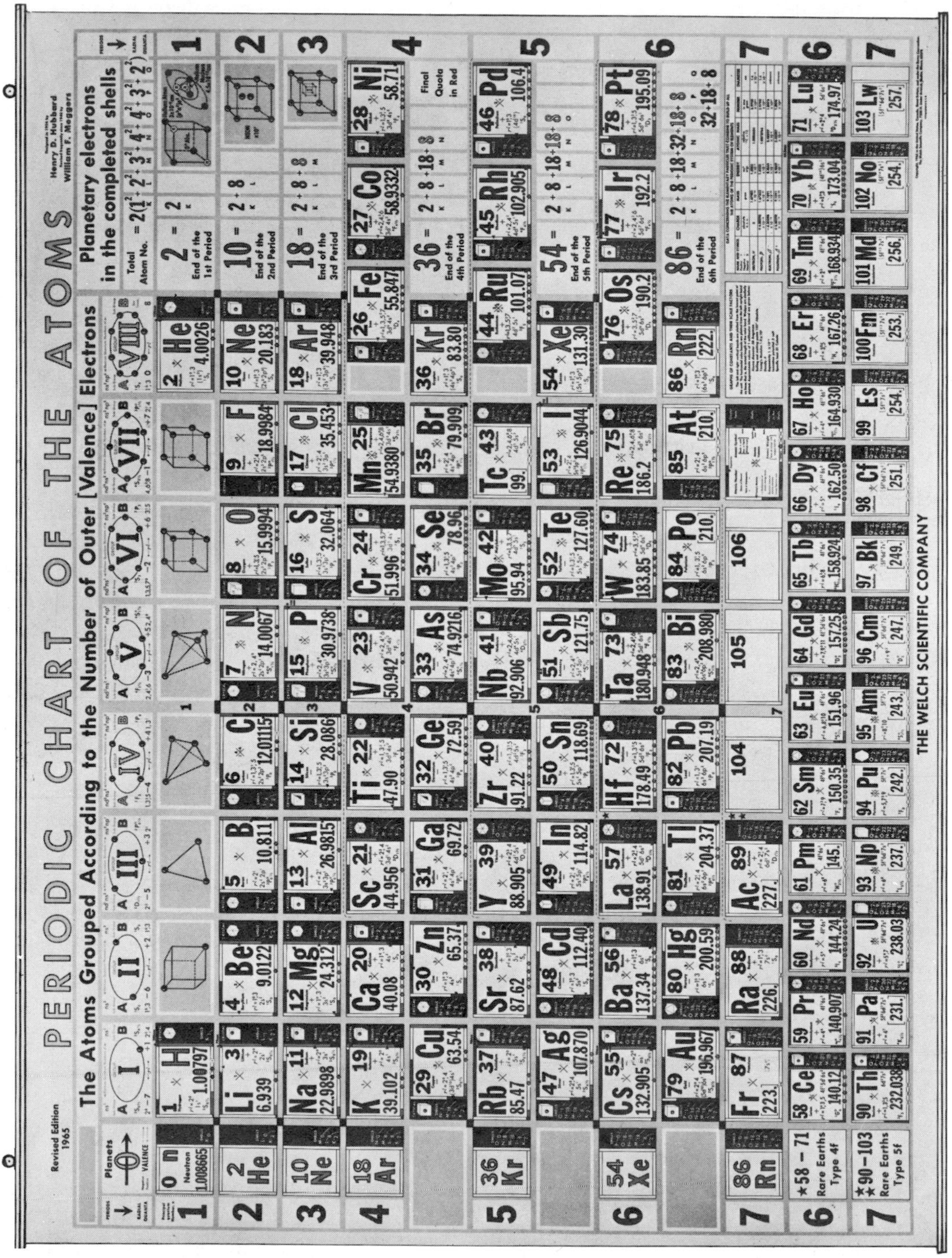
PERIODIC CHART OF THE ATOMS
The Atoms Grouped According to the Number of Outer [Valence] Electrons
Planetary electrons in the completed shells
Revised Edition 1965
Henry D. Hubbard
William F. Meggers
THE WELCH SCIENTIFIC COMPANY

Fig. 1-2

atom, and their work finds expression in the periodic chart of the atoms. The chart enables modern scientists to predict the existence and properties of undiscovered elements.

The chart of the atoms is a serial list of atoms. The atoms are arranged in numerical order and are catalogued according to column number and row number. The column number appears as a Roman numeral along the horizontal axis at the top of the chart. The row number appears as an Arabic number along the vertical axis on the left side of the chart. Each of these systems carries its own significance.

Group number. Each column of the chart contains atoms which have electrons in the outermost shell consistent with the number of the group itself. All atoms under group I have 1 electron in their outermost shell, all atoms in group II have 2 electrons in their outermost shell, and so on. In general, the number of electrons in the outermost shell determines the chemical properties of the atom. Since all atoms in the column have the same number of electrons in the outermost shell, they have similar chemical properties. The atoms comprising such a column can be called a family of atoms. Those atoms that comprise group VII (such as fluorine, chlorine, bromine, and iodine) are often referred to as the halogen family. Those atoms belonging to group VIII are usually referred to as the inert gas family (helium, neon, argon, krypton, and so on).

Row number. Each row following the Arabic number contains atoms having the same number of orbital rings consistent with the row number itself; for example, all atoms in row 1 have 1 orbital shell in their atomic structure and all atoms in row 2 have 2 orbital shells in their atomic structure. Each successive row adds one new set of electron shells. The successive addition of electrons, one at a time, needed to complete a new shell of 8 outer electrons is called a *period*. Group I begins the first period and with each new group an electron is added and the properties of the atom change. Because of an irregularity in row 1, it might be well to use row 2 as the example. Group I of row 2 begins with lithium (Li). From its placement on the chart it is known that lithium has 2 energy shells and 1 electron in the outermost shell. The next atom in sequence is beryllium (Be). Beryllium has 2 energy shells and 2 electrons in the outermost shell. Each new row repeats its sequence of behavior change from atom to atom across the chart. The rhythmic recurrence of typical behavior gives the name "periodic" to the chart.

A typical rectangle. Approximately thirty different physical and chemical properties are given in the rectangle an atom occupies. In a treatment of the periodic chart, such as this, only a few of these will be discussed. Those facets of each atom which have immediate importance to the nuclear medicine technologist are the atomic name and symbol, the atomic number, the atomic weight, and the electron shell groups.

Atomic name and symbol. The name and symbol for each atom can be observed on the chart. The symbol of each atom is that adopted by the International Atomic Weights Committee. The vertical alignment of symbols is designated to place similar atoms in the same vertical line. The atomic name appears in small letters in the upper portion of each block and the atomic symbol is the large letter(s) occupying the large portion of the rectangle.

Atomic number. The atomic number (chemical number) is the large Arabic numeral found in the upper corner of each rectangle. The atomic number is the most fundamental fact about an atom. The number represents the net number of positively charged units (protons) within the nucleus of that atom, and these protons govern the structure and behavior of the atom. The atomic number also reflects the number of orbital electron sets in a neutrally charged atom, since the number of protons and electrons are equal.

Atomic weight. The atomic weight is the fractional number found at the base of the rectangle. Since the atomic weight is considered fundamental for the chemist, it appears on the periodic chart. The atomic weight is an average of the weight of all stable nuclides of the element with respect to their percent of abundance in nature (see pp. 18 to 19). These atomic weights are redetermined periodically.

Electron shell groups. The number of electrons in each shell can be found by close inspection of the edge of each rectangle. All atoms that contain 8 electrons (group VIII) in their outermost shell constitute an inert gas and cannot undergo a chemical reaction with another atom in any way. Therefore, neon, argon, krypton, xenon, and radon are all inert gases. An irregularity exists within that group. Helium contains only 2 electrons in its outermost shell. Nevertheless, helium falls into the inert gas group, rather than in group II, because its 2 electrons constitute the full complement of electrons in the K shell. Any time an atom has its full complement of electrons in the outermost shell, that atom is chemically inert.

Since a periodic chart of the atoms organizes each atom according to atomic structure and similarities in chemical and physical properties, it becomes a wonderful tool to learn about the atom. Because the atom, its constituents and its properties are necessary knowledge for the chemist, physicist, technician, and student, the chart is an indispensable compilation of facts.

NUCLEAR SHORTHAND

In every phase of business and professional life, there is a need to express oneself in concise, definitive terminology. Nuclear physics is no different. For this reason, a shorthand system has been devised to specify every atom and every form of that atom. This identification process is carried out with the aid of the *chemical symbol,* the *atomic number,* and the *mass number* in accordance with the following format:

$$_{Z}^{A}X$$

X represents the chemical symbol
A represents the mass number
Z represents the atomic number

The *mass number* (A), has the superscript position immediately preceding the chemical symbol and indicates the number of protons and neutrons in the nucleus. (In the past, this number held the superscript position immediately following the chemical symbol.) The *atomic number* (Z), has the subscript position immediately preceding the chemical symbol and indicates the number of protons in the nucleus just as it does on the periodic chart of the atoms. Since the proton number of any element is synonymous with the element itself, this shorthand method has been shortened even further by indicating only the element and the mass number. These two terms are sufficient to identify the atom. The *neutron number* (N), can be found by subtracting the atomic number from the mass number:

$$N = A - Z$$

THREE SIMPLEST ATOMS

In a detailed study of the three simplest atoms—hydrogen, helium, and lithium—some basic principles can be learned of the nature of the more complex atoms which occur in nature (Fig. 1-3). These principles will be delineated following the discussion of each of these atoms.

Hydrogen

The simplest of all atoms is the hydrogen atom (H). This element is a colorless, odorless gas that occurs throughout all living material. It represents 10% of the body weight of the biochemical standard man. Hydrogen, the simplest atom in the periodic chart of the atoms (see Fig. 1-2) possesses the atomic number 1, indicating 1 proton and, therefore, 1 electron. The number of neutrons in the nucleus of any atom can be learned by rounding off the atomic weight, found at the bottom of the rectangle in the periodic chart, and subtracting the atomic number. The rounding off of the atomic weight of hydrogen, 1.0079, would result in the number 1. Since the atomic number is 1, there are no neutrons in the most abundant form of the hydrogen atom. The symbol for this form is $_1^1$H.

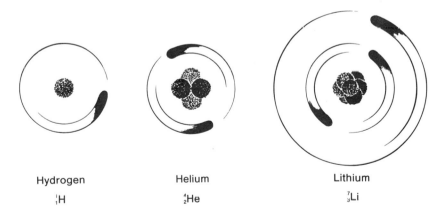

Hydrogen   Helium   Lithium

$_1^1$H $_2^4$He $_3^7$Li

Fig. 1-3. The nuclear components and the electron configurations of the three simplest atoms—hydrogen, helium, and lithium. It should be noted, however, that these atoms have not been drawn proportionally. If the constituents of the hydrogen atom, for example, were depicted correctly, it would be impossible to display the atom on the page. It has been calculated that if the nucleus of the hydrogen atom were the size of a baseball, the electron would be circling in an orbit wide enough to encompass New York City. It should also be remembered that atoms are three-dimensional. The electrons do not circle the nucleus in a flat field relationship as depicted here, but can circle the nucleus from an infinite number of angles.

11

Helium

Helium (He), occupying the next position on the periodic chart, is also a colorless and odorless gas. It has an atomic number of 2 and an atomic weight of 4.0026. The helium nucleus consists of 2 protons and 2 neutrons, accounting for the symbol $_2^4$He.

In order that the helium atom be electrically neutral, 2 orbiting electrons are required because there are 2 protons in the nucleus. This same pattern is followed throughout the entire periodic chart of the atoms.

Lithium

Lithium (Li) is a metal considered not essential for biologic materials. Lithium occupies the next position in the order of complexity, having an atomic number of 3 and an atomic weight, when rounded off, of 7. This would indicate that the lithium atom has 3 protons, 4 neutrons, and in an electrically neutral atom, 3 orbiting electrons, indicated in the symbol $_3^7$Li.

Principles. In studying these three simplest atoms, four important principles are demonstrated:

1. To maintain electrical neutrality, the number of orbiting electrons must equal the number of protons within the nucleus. Hydrogen has 1 proton and, therefore, 1 electron. Helium has 2 protons and, therefore, 2 electrons. Lithium has 3 protons and, therefore, 3 electrons.

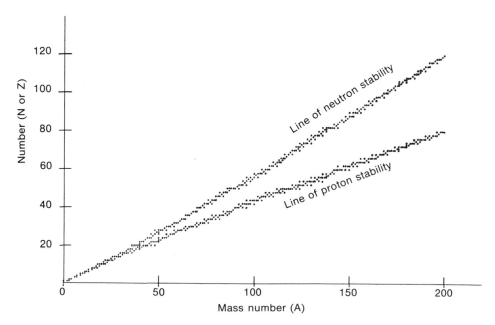

Fig. 1-4. Graph showing the number of neutrons to the number of protons for all known stable forms of an element and plotted against their mass number. The graph displays neutron and proton lines of stability. The graph also illustrates the fact that as atoms become more complex, more neutrons are required to maintain stability.

2. The mass of the electron lends very little to the total mass of the atom under study. In the hydrogen atom, the nucleus consists of 1 proton. Since the proton is 1,836 times greater than the electron in mass, the nucleus is of the same order of magnitude. In the helium atom, the nucleus is 7,350 times greater in weight than that of the electron. The mass of any atom is very closely equal to the sum of the masses of the protons and the neutrons comprising its nucleus. The mass of the orbital electrons can in general be disregarded.

3. The electron configuration of each atom has a certain order. In hydrogen, the electron is added to the K shell. In helium the second electron is added to the K shell, thereby completing that shell's full complement of electrons according to the $2n^2$ formula. In the lithium atom, the third electron must be added to the L shell, since the K shell has received its full complement of electrons. A somewhat similar orderly progression continues throughout the entire chart of the atoms, although many irregularities exist, especially beyond potassium (K).

4. The number of neutrons within the nucleus varies with respect to the number of protons that exist within the nucleus. In the case of hydrogen, there are no neutrons. Helium contains an equal number of protons and neutrons. Lithium has a larger number of neutrons than protons. In fact, proceeding from lithium in complexity, the number of neutrons must increase at a faster rate than the number of protons in order to maintain nuclear stability; that is, in order to maintain a nonradioactive status (Fig. 1-4). This relationship begins to express itself as early as the third atom in the order of complexity. It continues until an atom such as polonium 210 is reached, which contains 84 protons and 126 neutrons. Even with this obvious abundance of neutrons, the nucleus cannot maintain stability and the atom is subject to radioactive decay.

EXTRANUCLEAR STRUCTURE AND BONDING

Generally speaking, an atom is chemically stable when its outermost energy shell is completely filled. Should this shell not be filled, it will tend to react with any element which will give to the shell its full complement of electrons, either by giving up all the electrons in the outermost shell or by adding electrons to the shell to alleviate the deficit in electrons. An atom such as carbon can react chemically in many ways since it has only 4 electrons in the outermost shell. This element can either give up 4 electrons or it can accumulate 4 more electrons in order to achieve chemical stability. Since carbon falls midway in the number of necessary electrons, it has the capability to go either way and does so. These reactions with which atoms react with other atoms are called bonding; the type of bond indicates the method by which atoms are held together to form molecules. There are three basic types of chemical bonds: covalent, ionic, and hydrogen bonds.

Covalent bonding. Oxygen has 6 electrons in its outermost shell, 2 electrons short of a completed shell; therefore, oxygen falls into group VI of the periodic table. Its tendency is to gain 2 electrons rather than to lose 6. Carbon dioxide (CO_2) is well known as a product of human metabolism and it serves as an example of covalent bonding. The covalent bond of CO_2 is illustrated in Fig. 1-5.

Two oxygen atoms with 2 electrons in their outermost shell combine with 1

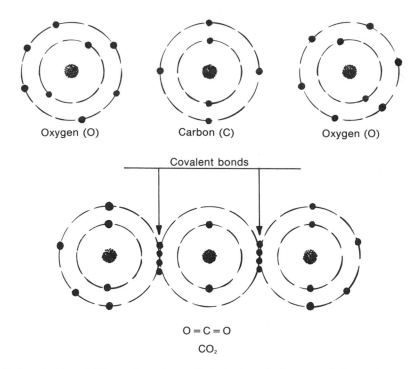

Oxygen (O)   Carbon (C)   Oxygen (O)

$$O = C = O$$
$$CO_2$$

Fig. 1-5. Covalent bond. The carbon atom with 4 electrons in its outer shell and 2 oxygen atoms with 6 electrons in their outer shells combine and share electrons in order that the full complement of electrons for those shells is realized.

carbon atom, which has 4 electrons in its outermost shell. In combining, all three atoms are actually *sharing* electrons to the extent that all 3 atoms have completed the electron shells to their maximum number of 8. In order to do so, each oxygen shares 2 electrons with the carbon atom, thereby giving the carbon atom a maximum of 8 electrons. The carbon atom reciprocates by sharing 2 of its electrons with each of the oxygen atoms, thereby completing the outer orbital rings of oxygen to a total of 8 electrons. In this way carbon dioxide becomes a very stable compound. Another example of this type of bond is water (H_2O).

Ionic bonding. A glance at the group VII atoms (halogen family) of the periodic chart of the atoms would suggest that these atoms are highly reactive because they have 7 electrons in the outermost shell and would be actively competing to acquire the eighth electron. This would apparently be true also of atoms in group I. However, atoms in group I, since they have only 1 electron in the outer shell, constantly search for situations where they can give up the 1 electron, thereby eliminating the outer shell. This would leave the atom with its full complement of electrons in the next inner shell. Such is the situation in the second form of bonding, the ionic bond.

The ionic bond is a type of bonding in which 2 atoms are held together by their attraction of unlike charges. These atoms are no longer atoms, but are actually ions having an electric charge; one ion is positively charged and the other ion is negatively charged. A typical example of the ionic bond is salt, sodium chloride

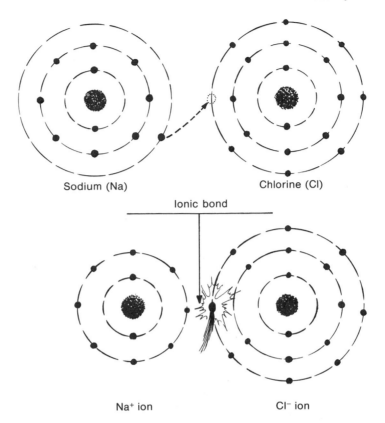

Fig. 1-6. Ionic bond. The sodium atom with 1 electron in its outer shell is given up to the chlorine atom, which has a vacancy in its outer shell. Through this reaction, the sodium and chlorine atoms become positive and negative ions, respectively, and are bound by electrostatic attraction.

(see Fig. 1-6). In this case, the sodium atom is a member of group I of the periodic chart. A perfect companion of sodium would be one of the members of the halogen group (group VII of the periodic chart). Chlorine has 7 electrons in the outermost shell and it is actively searching for another electron in order to receive its stable complement of 8 electrons. This electron is provided by the sodium atom. The sodium atom actually gives to the chlorine atom the single electron in its outermost shell. In this way, the atom abolishes its own outer shell and completes the stable complement of electrons in the chlorine atom (8 electrons). In so doing, the sodium atom has 1 *less* negative charge in its shells, so it becomes a sodium ion with a *positive* charge of 1. The chlorine ion now has 1 *more* negative charge in its shells, so it becomes an ion of chlorine with a *negative* charge of 1. An attraction exists, therefore, between the positively charged sodium ion and the negatively charged chlorine ion, which holds these 2 ions together. This is known as the ionic bond. It differs from the covalent bond in that there is no sharing of electrons.

Hydrogen bonding. The third type of bond, the hydrogen bond, is unlike the covalent bond and the ionic bond in that there is neither sharing of electrons, nor giving of electrons to the sister atom. The hydrogen bond does have a similarity with the ionic bond in that the attraction of unlike charges plays a role. This

15

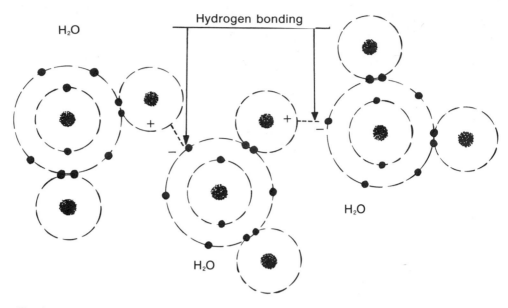

Fig. 1-7. Hydrogen bond. This form of chemical bonding is exemplified by water molecules; the water molecules themselves are examples of covalent bonds. The two water molecules are bound together by the slight electrostatic attraction between the two molecules.

attraction, however, is not between 2 ions of unlike charges but between 2 molecules of unlike charges. An example of this type of bonding can be seen between 2 molecules of water (Fig. 1-7). Between each *atom* comprising a molecule of water, the classic example of covalent bonding prevails. Between two *molecules* of water, the bond is a hydrogen bond. Such a bond, although weak, exists because of a slight differential in electrical charge between the oxygen atom of one molecule and the hydrogen atom of the other. In all covalent bonds the electrons are free to travel in either the oxygen circuit or the hydrogen circuit. Since it requires a longer period of time to travel around the oxygen than the hydrogen, the electron spends more time in the oxygen portion of the molecule than in the hydrogen portion. Therefore, the oxygen portion of the molecule has a slightly negative charge and the hydrogen portion a slightly positive charge.

In 2 molecules of water in close proximity to one another, a slight electrical attraction of unlike charges would exist. This attraction is based on the slightly negative charge of the oxygen of one molecule and the slightly positive charge of the hydrogen of the other molecule. Since this phenomenon occurs between all molecules of water and, indeed, between any molecule having hydrogen as a covalent component, it is easy to imagine that all of these molecules are bonded together through the hydrogen bond to form one large molecule. Since almost all organic compounds have hydrogen as one of their normal constituents, many molecules are all held together by these hydrogen bonds.

Chapter 2

Nuclides and radionuclides

In recent years, the terms *isotope* and *radioisotope* have fallen into disfavor. These two terms had been used for many years to describe all forms of all elements. Since this is not entirely correct usage of the two terms, they have been replaced by the terms *nuclide* and *radionuclide,* respectively. The term nuclide was proposed as a more precise term than isotope since the meaning of nuclide is any nucleus plus its orbital electrons. The term isotope refers to two or more forms of the same element. It would be incorrect to say iodine 127 is the only stable isotope of iodine, since there is only one stable form, not two or more. It would be more meaningful to describe iodine 127 as the only stable nuclide of iodine. Further, it would be improper to refer to ^{197}Hg and ^{131}I as radioactive isotopes (radioisotopes). They are actually radioactive nuclides (radionuclides) because they are two different elements. A correct usage of the term radioisotopes would be that ^{197}Hg and ^{203}Hg are radioisotopes, because they are two forms of the same element.

ISOTOPES

An isotope may be defined as one of two or more forms of the same element having the same atomic number (Z), differing mass numbers (A), and the same chemical properties. These different forms of an element may be stable or unstable (radioactive). However, since they are forms of the same element, they possess identical chemcial properties. These chemical properties remain the same even though, if unstable, their radioactive properties differ. Another way of defining isotopes is that they are forms of the same element, but each form has a different weight because of the varying number of neutrons in the nucleus (Fig. 2-1).

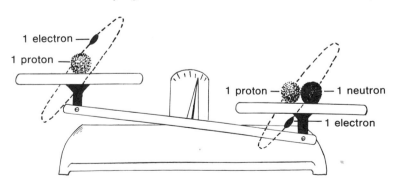

Fig. 2-1. Diagram illustrating that the difference between two isotopes can be expressed as a weight differential, caused by an increased or decreased number of neutrons in their nuclear configurations.

There are over 270 known nuclidic forms of stable elements; 40 of these exist in nature and are termed *naturally occurring* nuclides. In addition to these, more than 900 radionuclides have been produced artificially.

Three isotopes of hydrogen. The periodic chart lists atomic numbers (chemical numbers) as whole numbers and atomic weights as decimal fractions. It would seem that if the nucleus consists of protons and neutrons and each nucleon represented one unit of atomic weight (the electrons not adding significantly to the weight of the atom), then all atoms should have an atomic weight which would be a multiple of one. However, this is not the case. For example, hydrogen has an atomic weight of 1.008. This must have, at some point in time, caused great concern to early investigators, since the earliest known form of hydrogen had only 1 proton and should have had an atomic weight of 1.000. This not being the case, early investigators found it necessary to hypothesize the existence of some other form of the element which reacted identically to hydrogen, but was heavier. This would cause the resultant weight to be something greater than 1.000. The existence of isotopes was postulated as one of the possible factors in this obvious discrepancy. Hydrogen was found to occur in nature in two different forms, ordinary hydrogen and deuterium.

Hydrogen. Ordinary hydrogen, $^1_1$H (sometimes called protium), is the most abundant form of the element hydrogen. Its nucleus has only 1 proton (Z = 1) and no neutrons (A = 1) (Fig. 2-2). It is naturally occurring and stable.

Deuterium. Another isotope of hydrogen is deuterium. Deuterium, $^2_1$H, consists of 1 proton (Z = 1) and 1 neutron (A = 2), and is the least abundant form. It occurs in a ratio of 8 parts to every 1,000 parts of ordinary hydrogen. Deuterium is naturally occurring and stable. It has also been called "heavy hydrogen." Since ordinary hydrogen has 1 proton, and deuterium has 1 proton plus 1 neutron, deuterium is twice the weight of the most abundant form.

It is interesting to note that deuterium occurs at a ratio of 8:1,000 parts of all hydrogen atoms in nature. This ratio of abundance would justify the atomic weight differential of the hydrogen atom as 1.008. The atomic (chemical) weight of an element is derived from all the *stable* forms of the element, considering the atomic weight of each form of the element and its percent abundance in nature. For

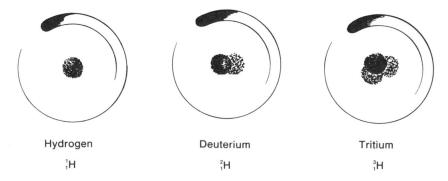

| Hydrogen | Deuterium | Tritium |
| $^1_1$H | $^2_1$H | $^3_1$H |

Fig. 2-2. Three isotopes of hydrogen—ordinary hydrogen, deuterium, and tritium. The number of protons and electrons remains the same for all three forms, but the neutron number increases.

example, if both forms occurred in nature at a rate of 50:50, and since ^2H is twice the weight of ^1H, the atomic weight would be 1.500.

Tritium. There is a third isotope of hydrogen, but it does not occur naturally. It is the artificially produced tritium, ^3H. Tritium is sometimes symbolized as ^3T. This isotope contains 1 proton (Z = 1) and 2 neutrons (A = 3), and is, therefore, three times the mass of the most abundant form. It is sometimes referred to as "extra-heavy hydrogen." Since hydrogen is an intimate part of body chemistry, the use of tritium plays an important role in medical and agricultural research. It is also used as one of the nuclides measured in the Atomic Energy Commission's stratospheric sampling program. It is formed by neutron bombardment of nitrogen 14 after the detonation of an atomic device, yielding carbon 12 and tritium.

All three forms have only 1 proton in their nuclei and only 1 electron in their orbits (Fig. 2-2). Since the electrons determine the chemical characteristics, and their number is the same on all three forms, these isotopes, whether stable or unstable, react identically in a chemical situation. The difference in mass is due solely to the number of neutrons within the nucleus.

Neutron to proton ratio. From studying these isotopes of hydrogen, the principle of neutron to proton ratio and nuclear stability can be observed. In the cases of ordinary hydrogen and deuterium, the presence or absence of 1 neutron does not alter the stability of the nucleus. In both cases, the nucleus is nonradioactive. However, the incorporation of 1 more neutron into the nucleus, as in the case of tritium, exceeds the bounds of nuclear stability. Why the nucleus becomes unstable at that point is not clearly understood, but tritium becomes an unstable or radioactive nuclide of hydrogen because there are too many neutrons.

This principle is also true with all other nuclides. Each element has its own unique ratio or combination of neutrons and protons. Any deviation from this, either too few neutrons and too many protons or too many neutrons and too few protons, results in nuclear instability.

The method by which a nuclide decays (changes into another nuclide) is that method which will result in the nucleus becoming stable or closer to stability. If the decay process contains only one step, then the resultant new nuclide is stable. If the decay process contains many steps, then the nuclide formed following the first step will be unstable and more than one step is necessary before a stable form of an element is reached.

OTHER "ISOS"
Isobar

By definition, isobars are 2 atoms that have the same mass number but different atomic numbers and, therefore, different chemical properties. To state it another way, the nucleus of each of these atoms contains the same sum of protons and neutrons, but the division between protons and neutrons is different. An example of isobars would be lithium 7 (^7_3Li) and beryllium 7 (^7_4Be). Both nuclides have a total of 7 nucleons. Lithium has 3 protons and 4 neutrons, and beryllium has 4 protons and 3 neutrons. Isobars in nuclear medicine are of no particular importance per se.

19

Table 2-1. Summary of the differences between isotopes, isobars, and isotones

	Atomic number (Z)	Mass number (A)	Neutron number (N)	Chemical properties
Isotopes	Same	Different	Different	Same
Isobars	Different	Same	Different	Different
Isotones	Different	Different	Same	Different

Isotone

Isotones are nuclides having the same number of neutrons. In no other way are 2 isotones similar. They differ in atomic number, mass number, and chemical properties. They are mentioned primarily because the trilinear chart of the nuclides has been formulated on the basis of isotopes, isobars, and isotones. An example of isotones would be $^{131}_{53}I$ and $^{132}_{54}Xe$. In each case $N = 78$.

Table 2-1 summarizes the differences between isotopes, isobars, and isotones.

Isomer

An isomer is one of two or more nuclides that has the same mass number and atomic number as the others, but exists for measurable times in the excited state. When a nucleus is in an excited state and decays by gamma emission, the transition from the higher to the lower energy usually takes less than 10^{-13} second. Nuclei that take longer than 10^{-9} second are called isomers. Two examples of isomers are technetium 99m and strontium 87m.

ATOMIC ENERGY LEVELS

Both x-rays and gamma rays represent energy releases as a result of changes in energy levels either within the nucleus or in the extranuclear structure. X-rays are releases of energy as a result of changes within the orbital pattern of the electrons. Gamma rays are releases of energy as a result of changes occurring within the nucleus itself. To understand these energy releases an explanation of both the orbital energy levels and the nuclear energy levels is warranted.

ORBITAL ENERGY LEVELS

Although it has been said that an electron is more or less assigned to a definite orbit, the analogy of an atom to a miniature solar system is to some degree an oversimplification. Unlike the planets circling the sun, the electron can actually exist anywhere, although it is most often found in its regularly assigned orbit. Unlike the usual illustrations of the atom, it has been suggested that the electron does not follow a circular path around the nucleus but more nearly an elliptical path. In fact, some scientists subscribe to the theory that the K shell electron(s) has such an elliptical pattern that the orbit of the K shell electron actually passes through the nucleus. Furthermore, since like charges repel one another, the electrons repel each other in their respective orbits so that these electrons are actually arranged in space symmetry. There are two types of energies involved in the

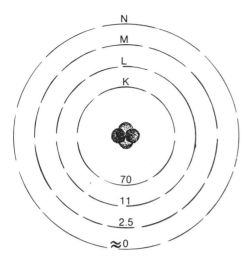

Fig. 2-3. Representative electron binding energies of a hypothetical atom. The binding energy is larger for those electrons circling closer to the nucleus. To remove an electron from its orbit, the removing force must possess an energy equal to or greater than the binding energy.

course of an electron and each plays a definite role in the action and subsequent reaction of electron disturbance. These energies are the binding energy and the energy state of the electron itself.

Binding energy. The binding energy of the electron is the energy required to remove the particle from its orbit. If the binding energy of a K shell electron of a particular atom was 70,000 electron volts (70 kev), as in Fig. 2-3, that electron must be supplied with an energy equal to or greater than 70 kev to remove it from its energy shell. This energy could be supplied to that electron by a high energy particle or photon radiation, at which time the energy of the interacting particle or ray would be decreased in energy by an amount equal to the binding energy. The same principle is true for an L shell electron except that less energy is required to remove it, since the binding energy becomes less as the electron is positioned farther away from the nucleus. In a typical atom, in which the K shell electron would have a binding energy of 70 kev, the binding energy of the L shell electron may be reduced to as little as 11 kev, the M shell electron to 2.5 kev, and the N shell electron ≈0, the latter being the case with all outer shell electrons. In each of these cases, energy equal to or greater than that of the binding energy of the electron must be supplied in order to remove that electron from its orbit.

Energy state of the electron. The energy state of an orbital electron can, perhaps, best be described by comparing it, through a crude analogy, to a race track (Fig. 2-4). In order for each car to stay abreast with the others it must possess a different speed (energy). According to the illustration, the car on the outside track (the M track) must travel at 75 mph to keep abreast with the car on the inner track (the K track) traveling at 65 mph. Therefore, the 75 mph car has a greater energy state than does the car on the inner track. Should the car on the inside track drop from the race, either the car in the middle track or the car on the outside track would have the ability to take its place. To do so, each car must decrease its speed, that is, decrease its energy state in order to maintain its position in the race.

21

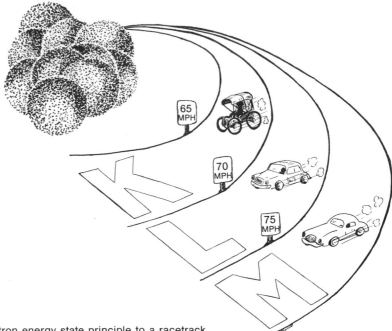

Fig. 2-4. Comparison of the electron energy state principle to a racetrack.

Such is also the case of the orbiting electrons. Should the K shell electron be removed from its orbit for some reason, the L or the M shell electron would take its place. To do so, there would necessarily have to be a decrease in the energy state of that orbiting electron. At the same time, there would be an increase in the binding energy, since the electron is assuming the role of the K shell electron which possesses more binding energy. Should a K shell electron be removed, the probability that that space would be filled by the L electron and the L space filled by the M electron would be greater than of the M falling down into the K shell electron. In any case, just as nature abhors a vacuum, an electron shell abhors a vacancy. By depicting the energy states of the electrons as analogous to a race track, the intention is to simplify the phenomena of *optical radiation* and *characteristic radiation*.

Optical radiation. The ability of atoms under certain conditions to emit radiations which fall into the visible spectrum allowed scientists a means of identifying the atom by identifying the color of the light. This type of radiation is termed optical radiation. It results from the fact that when an atom is given a certain amount of energy (termed *excited state*), the electron will move to a certain corresponding path (suborbit) farther from the nucleus. This move would not be enough to move it into another orbit. (In the case of the racing car, the car would not move into the 80 mph race track, but would move into a suborbit which might correspond to the outer portion of the 75 mph track, thereby necessitating the car to go 77 mph in order to keep aligned.) In order to go to this suborbit, the electron would have to assume additional energy, just as would the racing car. As soon as the source of energy is removed, the electron jumps back to the original path and emits a photon of an energy corresponding to the energy loss by the electron. The photon would be of a frequency and wavelength equal to some form of the visible light spectrum, thereby serving as a means of color identification.

This same principle applies to *excitation* of an atom by a passing particle (α or β) or electromagnetic radiation (γ- or x-radiation). An orbital electron is raised in energy state with the subsequent release of that energy, and the electron falls back into its regular orbit.

Characteristic radiation. The same principle holds true for electrons falling into an orbit closer to the nucleus. In the event that a K shell electron would be removed from its orbit, the vacancy would be filled by either the L shell electron or the M shell electron. Since the L shell electron would have to decrease in energy state by assuming the role of a K shell electron, the energy differential must be released in the form of x-radiation. This is known as characteristic radiation. It is important to note that these emissions are not known as gamma radiations. The only difference between gamma and x-radiation is their *source* or origin. X-rays originate from the orbital structure of the atom and gamma rays always originate from the nucleus. At no time could these characteristic radiations be referred to as gamma rays. The term "characteristic radiation" has been applied because the energy of the resultant x-ray is characteristic of the energy loss by an electron falling from an orbit distant from the nucleus to an orbit closer to the nucleus. All electrons falling into the K shell, regardless of their origin, would emit x-rays, called characteristic K-radiation; all electrons falling into the L shell would emit characteristic L-radiation, and so on.

Nuclear energy levels

The concept of energy states as discussed regarding the orbital structure is also applicable to the nucleus, except that the release of energies resulting from changes within the nucleus are of much greater magnitude than those of the electrons. There are two possible results should an elevation in energy state (excited state) be experienced by the nucleus. There may be particle emission caused by conditions involving binding energy, or photon (gamma) emission caused by conditions involving the energy state of the nucleus.

Binding energy. Just as there is a binding energy involved with the orbiting electrons, so also is there a binding energy involved with the nucleus. The binding energy in the nucleus is the energy required to remove a single proton, neutron, or alpha particle from the nucleus. The existence of binding energy can be demonstrated by comparing the mass relationship of an intact helium 4 nucleus (2 protons, 2 neutrons) to the weight of 2 protons and 2 neutrons weighed separately (Fig. 2-5). The intact helium 4 atom actually weighs less than the sum of its constituent parts, because some of the actual mass of the helium 4 nucleus has been converted to energy (binding energy). The nuclear binding energy is the equivalent energy difference between the sum of the masses of the protons and neutrons as they would exist separately and the equivalent energy of the mass of the nucleus itself. This difference is also called *mass defect* (see Chapter 3).

It is believed that the protons and neutrons are in a constant state of motion.

23

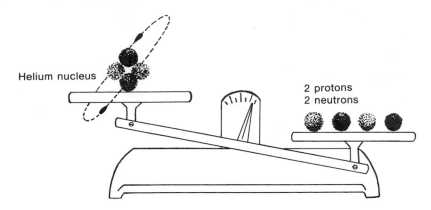

Fig. 2-5. Proof of nuclear binding energy. The weight of the intact helium 4 nucleus weighs less than the individual components weighed separately. This suggests that some of the nuclear mass has been converted to binding energy.

When energy is supplied to an atom, the degree of motion increases. This condition can be caused by the absorption of a photon, collisions with other particles or systems, or the natural radioactivity of the nucleus.

Since the nucleons are in motion, there are many chances for collisions between nuclear particles. When energy is added to the nucleus, the number of collisions increases. When a collision occurs, some or all of the energy of the colliding particle is transferred to the particle into which it collides. By this transfer of energy, the particle receives and retains an inordinate amount of energy until such time as it would lose that energy by a subsequent collision. If the energy that the particle receives exceeds the binding energy of that particle in the nucleus, the particle will be subject to ejection from the nucleus if no subsequent collision occurs. This would, then, constitute *particle emission.*

This phenomenon could be compared to a pool table. A dormant cue ball can be supplied with energy through the action of striking it with a cue stick. As the cue ball is propelled over some distance of the pool table, it collides with other balls on the table. Through this collision the cue ball transfers some, or possibly all, of its energy to other balls on the table. Should the energy transferred to another ball on the table be sufficient, the ball could possibly exceed the limits of the rebound cushions and be ejected from the pool table. This would be analogous to particle emission. Energies transferred to the nucleons which exceed their binding energy result in the loss of a particle from the nucleus, just as energy transferred to the pool balls, sufficient to overcome the containing effect of the table cushions, results in the loss of a pool ball from the table. This analogy typifies one mode of decay exactly. The analogy must be altered somewhat for other modes of decay, which result in the production of particles other than protons and neutrons. These "foreign" particles, then, receive high energies with their subsequent emission from the nucleus.

Energy state of the nucleons. The concept of energy state of the electron is also applicable to that of the nucleus. When energy is added to the nucleus, but not enough to cause particle emission, the nucleus may merely be raised to another

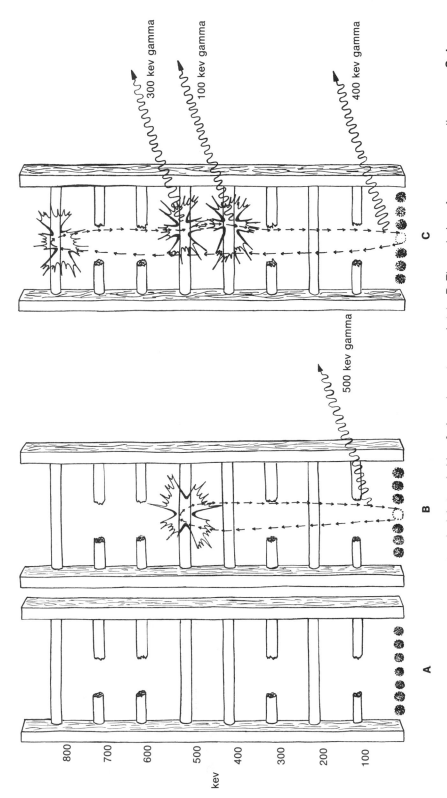

Fig. 2-6. Comparison of the nuclear energy state principle to a ladder. **A,** A nucleus at ground state. **B,** The emission of a monoenergetic gamma. **C,** A more complex decay scheme.

energy state. The most frequent cause for this is particle emission. The particle does not require all of the energy given to the nucleus to bring about its ejection. Therefore, energy remains in the nucleus, raising it to an excited state. Actually, both the protons and the neutrons have their own set of discrete energy levels to which either nucleon can be raised if sufficient energy is supplied to the nucleus. A nucleus is in its *ground state* when all of its lower energy levels are filled. This can be compared to step ladders with several missing rungs (Fig. 2-6). Only the intact rungs in the ladder would be representative of energy levels to which the nucleons could be raised. If each rung of the ladder represented 100 kev, the nucleons could be raised only to an energy level of 200 kev, 400 kev, 500 kev, or 800 kev. In Fig. 2-6, *A,* the nucleus is in its ground state, because all the nucleons occupy the lowest rungs (or energy levels). In part *B* of the diagram, an excited state of the nucleus is represented in which a nucleon has been raised to an excited level of 500 kev. When this occurs the nucleus instantaneously returns to ground state and releases energy corresponding to the energy differential. This energy release is known as gamma radiation. The return to ground state could occur as a one-step, one-gamma affair (monoenergetic), as in Fig. 2-6, *B,* or as a series of jumps with more than one gamma being released as in Fig. 2-6, *C.* It is not un-likely that in exciting the nucleus, the nucleus would not receive sufficient energy to raise the excitation state of the neutron to 500 kev, but may only raise it to 400 kev. The reverse could also be true; the nucleus may have received a greater amount of energy, thereby raising the nucleus to 800 kev. It is impossible to predict which particular atom in a given sample of atoms would receive more energy or less energy so that these variations in neutron and proton excitation levels would be known. It is possible, however, to predict the percentages of nuclei receiving these varying energies.

The concept of atomic energy levels is extremely difficult. The analogies of race tracks, pool tables, and ladders would, without hesitation, be considered over-simplifications. There is no such thing as a perfect analogy, and these are certainly no exceptions. They are included to assist the student of nuclear medicine in the understanding of extremely difficult principles. Any one of them could be subject to criticism, should the analogy be extended beyond its intended purpose.

Electron volt

In all exposures to the fundamentals of physics and electricity, terms that have become commonplace are words such as volt, ampere, and erg. In nuclear medicine, the unit of definition seems to center upon the term the electron volt (ev). As the name implies, an electron volt has a relationship to an electron and to the volt. In physics, the fundamental unit of work is the erg. A more useful energy unit for nuclear medicine purposes is the electron volt, with its multiples, thousand electron volts (kev) and million electron volts (mev). The electron volt is defined as the amount of kinetic energy acquired when an electron falls through a potential difference of 1 volt. In some instances, kev is similar to kv (used on x-ray equip-ment). If 1 electron falls through a potential difference of 1 volt, it is equivalent to 1 ev; therefore, if 1 electron falls through a potential difference of 1,000 volts, it is equivalent to 1,000 ev (1 kev). Both kv and, in this instance, kev relate to 1,000 volts potential difference. In other instances, kev is totally different from kv; if 1,000 electrons fall through a potential difference of 1 volt, it is also equivalent to 1,000 ev (1 kev). In this example, the potential difference is 1 volt and quite unlike kv.

The amount of work performed by 1 electron volt, expressed in ergs, is found to be the product of the charge of the electron and the potential difference through which that electron falls. The charge of 1 electron is known to be 4.80×10^{-10} electrostatic unit (esu). The potential difference of 1 volt is known to be $\frac{1}{300}$ of 1 electrostatic unit:

$$1 \ \text{ev} = \tfrac{1}{300} \times 4.80 \times 10^{-10} \ \text{ergs} = 1.60 \times 10^{-12} \ \text{ergs} \qquad (2\text{-}1)$$

Therefore, 1 electron volt has the capacity to do the work of 1.60×10^{-12} ergs. Through the use of this formula, the electron volt has been converted to ergs, the fundamental unit of work. This conversion figure will be used in the following chapters.

Nature of radiation

Every human being is exposed daily to a variety of radiations whether he recognizes it or not. The popular concept of radiation, however, is somehow synonymous only with radiations emanating from an x-ray tube, from radioactive materials, or from fallout. In addition to these, there are several other types of radiations, all of which manifest themselves in different ways. Some of these radiations can be felt, such as the radiant energy whereby heat is transferred. Other radiations are audible, or at least the devices which receive these radiations, such as the radio, translate them to audible sound. Other radiations can be seen, such as light, which when focused through a prism, can be further subdivided into all the colors of the spectrum.

There are other radiations that can neither be heard, seen, felt, nor otherwise perceived by the human senses. Examples of these are x-rays and gamma rays. All of these radiations are among the members of the electromagnetic spectrum, and are spoken of in terms of waves of energy.

ENERGY WAVES AND THEIR CHARACTERISTICS

A wave in the electromagnetic spectrum is not unlike a wave resulting from a disturbance within a body of water. Throwing a rock into a large body of water would result in the familiar ripples, beginning at the point where the rock touched the water and progressing outward in a circular fashion. Close inspection of these waves would reveal that each wave is an entity in itself, each having a definite length. Those waves occurring near the point of impact occur more frequently than those at a distance from the point of impact, and they travel away from the point of impact. The *wavelength* is defined as the distance from a point on one wave to the same point on the subsequent wave. It could be said that the wavelength of those waves at the point of impact is shorter than those at a distance. The *frequency* is defined as the number of wave formations per unit time. It could be said that the frequency of waves would be greater near the point of impact than distant to the point of impact. The *velocity* is defined as the speed at which these waves travel.

All electromagnetic waves possess these same three characteristics of wavelength, frequency, and velocity. The velocity (c) of an electromagnetic wave is a constant. All waves travel at the same velocity regardless of their position on the electromagnetic spectrum. The speed of light waves is 186,000 miles per second (3.0×10^{10} cm/sec), and all members of the electromagnetic spectrum travel at this velocity. Wavelength (λ) and frequency (n) are variables, and are *inversely proportional* to

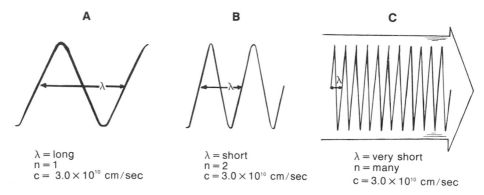

A

B

C

λ = long
n = 1
c = 3.0×10^{10} cm/sec

λ = short
n = 2
c = 3.0×10^{10} cm/sec

λ = very short
n = many
c = 3.0×10^{10} cm/sec

Fig. 3-1. Characteristics of electromagnetic waves. **A,** The wavelength, frequency, and velocity of a wave. **B,** As the wavelength decreases, the frequency increases and velocity remains unchanged. **C,** The quantum nature of radiation; the wave behaves like a bundle of energy, having direction and traveling at the speed of light.

one another. This is readily apparent in Fig. 3-1. If the wavelength is decreased, the frequency with which that wave would occur per unit time would necessarily increase (Fig. 3-1, *B*).

For electromagnetic waves there is a very important relationship between wavelength, frequency, and velocity according to the following formula:

$$c = n \times \lambda$$

c = velocity in cm/sec
n = frequency in waves (vibrations) per second
λ = wavelength in cm

Since c = 3×10^{10} cm/sec, that value can be substituted immediately. If the frequency is known, the wavelength can be calculated, or, conversely, if the wavelength is known, the frequency can be calculated. Since the wavelength of radiations of interest to nuclear medicine personnel is extremely small, the angstrom unit (Å) has been devised as an expression of length, rather than the centimeter. The angstrom unit has a value of 10^{-8} cm.

ELECTROMAGNETIC SPECTRUM

The electromagnetic spectrum is usually displayed on the basis of wavelength in angstrom units. It could also be displayed in terms of frequency or energy. Fig. 3-2 attempts to incorporate all three variables in its display of the electromagnetic spectrum.

The spectrum may best be discussed by imagining ourselves to be in a room containing a variety of electrical and electronic instrumentation, seated before an instrument that has a capacity of dialing in wavelengths ranging from 10^{17} Å to 10^{-5} Å. By setting the dial of the instrument at 10^{17} Å, the operator would feel heat since heat waves occur at this wavelength. If the dial were turned slightly, to decrease the wavelength, the radio would begin to play. A further turn of the dial would allow reception by the television set. When the dial is turned even farther to allow reception of even shorter wavelengths, the radar monitoring scope would begin to indicate reception of information. With another turn of the dial an intense

29

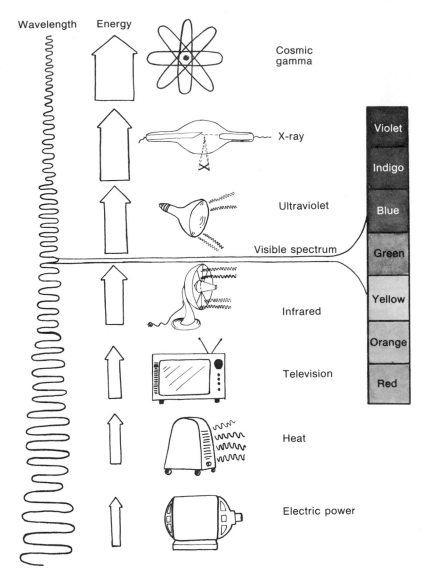

Fig. 3-2. The electromagnetic spectrum.

and deeply penetrating heat in the form of infrared radiation from a heat lamp would be experienced. As the dial is turned further, the room would become illuminated by a deep red light. Subsequent turns of the dial would change the color of the light from red to orange, orange to yellow, yellow to green, green to blue, blue to indigo, and indigo to violet. Eventually the sunlamp will glow, allowing exposure to ultraviolet radiation. Up to this point, changes in wavelengths have demonstrated phenomena, which, with appropriate aids, could be felt, seen, or heard. Further changes in wavelength, indicating reception of even shorter waves, cannot be perceived by the human senses. The first of these that would be encountered would be that of x-rays, next would be gamma rays, and finally, at the shortest wavelength setting possible, would be cosmic radiation. In this hypothetical situation, a variety of waves of energy would be experienced, all of which differ from one another in wavelength, frequency, and energy.

It is important to note that although emissions from radioactive materials are spoken of in terms of alpha particles, beta particles, and gamma rays, alpha and beta particles do not appear on the electromagnetic spectrum. Only gamma rays exist as electromagnetic waves. Alpha particles and beta particles are particulate matter, and, therefore, possess mass. They are not waves of energy, and for this reason, are not seen on the spectrum, even though these particles sometimes behave as waves of energy, and waves of energy sometimes behave as particles.

Relationship of wavelength to frequency

Since the electromagnetic spectrum is based on wavelength, it is apparent that the wavelengths of the various entities must be known. Red light, which has the longest wavelength of the visible light spectrum, has a value of 0.00007 cm or 7,000 Å. Green light is known to have a wavelength of 5,000 Å, and blue light has a wavelength of 4,000 Å. If the wavelength of the radiation is greater than 7,000 Å or shorter than 4,000 Å, the radiations are no longer visible to the human eye and fall into the infrared and ultraviolet ranges, respectively. According to formula 3-1, the frequency of radiation from blue light (4,000 Å) can be calculated as follows:

$$n \times \lambda = c \tag{3-1}$$
$$n = \frac{c}{\lambda} = \frac{3.0 \times 10^{10}}{0.00004} = 7.5 \times 10^{14} \text{ waves/sec}$$

Proceeding further up the electromagnetic spectrum, the wavelength begins to become very short and the corresponding frequency begins to become very great. At this point, the quantum nature of radiation must be considered.

Quantum nature of radiation. Sometimes electromagnetic waves produce results that cannot be explained by the action of waves of energy. A question arises as to whether these waves can actually be regarded as waves at all, or whether they should be regarded as mass. This is especially true with such waves as x-rays, gamma rays, and cosmic rays, which have very short wavelengths. These waves can assume properties, not of waves, but of particles, as is seen in Fig. 3-1, *C*. They can be likened to bullets possessing great energy and traveling in a given direction. This bundle of energy is called a *quantum* or a *photon,* and the amount of energy carried by the photon depends upon the frequency of the radiation. The frequency, in turn, is an inverse function of wavelength. The *energy of the photon is directly proportional to frequency* as indicated by the following formula:

$$E = h \times n \tag{3-2}$$
$E =$ energy in ergs
$h =$ Planck's constant in ergs/sec
$\quad (6.61 \times 10^{-27} \text{ ergs/sec})$
$n =$ frequency in seconds

Since the energy of the photon is directly proportional to frequency, and frequency is inversely proportional to wavelength, then, *energy is inversely proportional to wavelength* also. As the wavelength decreases, the energy of the photon increases, and vice versa.

Relationship of wavelength to energy

It has already been demonstrated in formula 2-1 that 1 electron volt is equal to 1.6×10^{-12} ergs. Using this value and formulas 3-1 and 3-2 it is possible to calculate the energy of any photon of radiation, given the wavelength. To express a photon with a wavelength of 1.0 Å in terms of energy, three steps are required:

1. Convert wavelength to frequency (formula 3-1)*

$$c = n \times \lambda$$
$$n = \frac{c}{\lambda} = \frac{3 \times 10^{10}}{10^{-8}} = 3 \times 10^{18} \text{ waves/sec (equivalent to 1 Å)}$$

2. Convert frequency to energy in ergs (formula 3-2)*

$$E = h \times n$$
$$E = 6.61 \times 10^{-27} \times 3 \times 10^{18}$$
$$E = 19.83 \times 10^{-9} \text{ ergs (equivalent to 1 Å)}$$

3. Convert ergs to electron volts by comparing it to the value of 1 ev., that value being 1.6×10^{-12} ergs.

$$1 \text{ Å} \approx \frac{19.83 \times 10^{-9}}{1.6 \times 10^{-12}} = 12.4 \times 10^3 \text{ ev (or 12.4 kev)}$$

With these formulas, given the wavelength of any type of radiation, it is possible to convert wavelength to energy in electron volts or conversely, energy in electron volts to wavelength. Since energies of the various radionuclides are known, it is possible to place them in their proper positions on the electromagnetic spectrum.

If 1.0 Å is equal to 12.4 kev as determined above, then .01 Å is equal to 1,240 kev or 1.24 mev, and this relationship holds true for any wavelength. Since this is the case, another relationship can be formulated whereby wavelength can immediately be converted to energy in electron volts without going through the three steps just discussed.

$$E = \frac{12,400}{\lambda}$$

E = energy in electron volts   (3-3)
λ = wavelength in angstrom units

MASS-ENERGY EQUIVALENCE

For centuries it was believed by all that mass was mass and energy was energy; no thought was given to the possibility that the two were interconvertible. It was not until the present century that the possibility was advanced and proved. Einstein's contribution to nuclear science was an extremely important one and helped to explain some of the phenomena of nuclear disintegration. He explained that

---

*Since formula 1 is $n \times \frac{c}{\lambda}$ and formula 2 is $E = hn$, formula 1 can be substituted into formula 2 to read:

$$E = \frac{hc}{\lambda}$$

mass is really a form of energy, and that mass and energy could be converted from one to the other by the following relationship:

$$E = mc^2 \qquad (3\text{-}4)$$

E = energy in ergs
m = mass weight in grams
c = velocity of light in cm/sec

By this equation it is possible to calculate the amount of energy released if 1.0 gm of matter were completely destroyed and converted to energy:

$$E = 1.0 \text{ gram} \times (3 \times 10^{10})^2$$
$$= 1.0 \times 9 \times 10^{20}$$
$$= 9.0 \times 10^{20} \text{ ergs}$$

The conversion of ergs to the more useful electron volt would yield an immense number, not of particular importance at this time.

More important, just as one can convert 1 gm of mass to energy, so also one can calculate the energy released should an atom become annihilated, or even more appropriate, should a subatomic particle (a proton, neutron, or electron) be converted to energy. This is accomplished by the use of the *atomic mass unit* (amu). The atomic mass unit is defined as $\frac{1}{12}$ of the arbitrary mass assigned to carbon 12 ($^{12}_{6}$C). It is known that 1 amu is equal to 1.49×10^{-3} ergs. According to formula 2-1, 1 ev is equal to 1.6×10^{-12} ergs and 1 mev is equal to 1.6×10^{-6} ergs; therefore:

$$1 \text{ amu} = \frac{1.49 \times 10^{-3}}{1.6 \times 10^{-6}} = .9312 \times 10^3 \text{ mev or } 931.2 \text{ mev} \qquad (3\text{-}5)$$

This figure (931.2) becomes of value as a conversion factor to convert mass to an equivalent amount of energy whenever a loss of mass has been observed following any nuclear reaction or interaction. Examples of its use in a nuclear reaction will be shown in the following chapter. An example other than a nuclear reaction is that of a helium atom. It has previously been discussed that the intact helium atom actually weighs less than the sum of its constituent parts weighed separately, because some of the mass has been converted to binding energy. The actual energy realized by such a loss of mass can be calculated by the use of this relationship between atomic mass units and energy. Helium 4 is composed of 2 protons, 2 neutrons, and 2 electrons. It has an amu value of 4.003874. The sum of its component particles however, is indicated in the following:

amu of protons = $1.007597 \times 2 = 2.015194$
amu of neutrons = $1.008986 \times 2 = 2.017972$
amu of electrons = $0.000548 \times 2 = 0.001096$
sum of components = 4.034262

Based on the above values, the component particles of helium 4 weighed separately are heavier than the intact helium 4 atom by 0.030388 amu (4.034262 − 4.003874 = 0.030388 amu). Since 1 amu has been determined to be equal to 931.2 mev (formula 3-5), the binding energy within the atom of helium 4 is equal to 28.2973 mev according to the following calculation:

$$E = 0.030388 \times 931.2 \text{ mev} = 28.2973 \text{ mev}$$

What has actually occurred is that the atom, in order to keep itself intact, must convert 0.03 units of atomic mass into 28.3 mev of energy. The atom uses a small fraction of this energy as binding energy to keep the electrons in their energy shells. The major part of this energy is used by the nucleus to keep its nucleons (primarily the protons carrying the positive charges) from repelling one another to the point of disrupting it.

The fact that the nucleus possesses the ability to convert units of mass to pure energy tends to place the entire phenomenon into the realm of sheer fantasy. The possibility of having a piece of matter in one instance and have it converted to invisible energy in another instance is a fact that sometimes seems difficult to understand. However, this same type of phenomenon occurs almost every time a reaction or interaction occurs in a nucleus.

A better example of the conversion of mass to energy is that of the reaction between a positron and an electron. It is known that when these 2 units of mass collide, they completely annihilate one another and all of their mass is converted to energy according to the following calculations:

$$\begin{aligned} \text{amu of electron} &= 0.000548 \\ \text{amu of positron} &= \underline{0.000548} \\ &\;0.001096 \\ 0.001096 \times 931.2 &= 1.02 \text{ mev} \end{aligned}$$

The resultant energy of the annihilation reaction between a positron and an electron is 1.02 mev. Actually the energy is not represented as 1 photon of 1.02 mev but as 2 photons of 0.51 mev emitted at exactly opposite directions from one another. (See sections on positrons and on pair production, pp. 49 and 53.)

GENERAL CLASSIFICATIONS OF RADIOACTIVITY

In general, there are two classifications of radioactivity and of radioisotopes: natural and artificial. Naturally occurring radionuclides are those nuclides that emit radiation spontaneously. No additional energy is necessary to place them in an unstable state. Artificial radioactivity is that radioactivity resulting from man-made unstable nuclides. Such nuclides are made unstable by bombarding stable nuclides with high energy particles. Both types of radioactivity play an important role in nuclear medicine.

Natural radioactivity

It has been suggested that particles within the atom are in a constant state of motion. This motion within the nucleus results in collisions between nucleons whereby energy is transferred to other nucleons. This transfer of energy sometimes results in a nucleon achieving energy greater than the binding energy, in which case the particle is allowed to escape the nucleus. This particle escape is termed a *disintegration.* The process of *decay* and the act of particle escape allow the nucleus to reduce the number of protons and/or neutrons to a point where the binding energy can contain the remainder of the nucleons. In this way, stability is eventually achieved.

All nuclides with the atomic number (Z) greater than 82 are radioactive because they possess an unstable number of protons or neutrons. Many of these are naturally occurring. There are also instances of naturally occurring radionuclides of lesser atomic number, such as potassium 40 and carbon 14.

These naturally occurring radionuclides occur in all parts of the world; therefore, all the peoples of the world are subjected to their radiation effects. The amount of radiation caused by these nuclides would vary from place to place based on local geographic conditions. Some of the genetic mutations are attributable in part to such exposures to naturally occurring radioactivity. These radiations could also have contributed to some of the phases of the evolutionary process. The source of these radiations is both extraterrestrial and terrestrial. Cosmic rays arising from outside the earth's atmosphere constitute the radiations of extraterrestrial origins. Those of terrestrial origin are found in the earth's crust, and radioactive materials having gaseous form are found in the air.

Generally, in the process of decay, only a few steps are necessary before a stable ratio of neutrons to protons is reached. Occasionally, however, the process of achieving stability will require as many as 18 different steps. Such a sequence of events is called a *radioactive series*. There are currently 4 such series in existence: the thorium series, decaying to stable lead 208; the actinium series, decaying to stable lead 207; the uranium series, decaying to lead 206; and the neptunium series, decaying to bismuth 209. It has been suggested by some scientists that there may have been more radioactive series that existed at some point in time, but they have all since attained stability.

Artificial radioactivity

Artificial radioactivity is the same as natural radioactivity, except that the radionuclides are man-made. It is possible to subject stable nuclides to high energy particles to produce instability. This instability can be effected by subjecting a stable nuclide to such devices as a cyclotron or a nuclear reactor (pile), wherein the stable nuclides are bombarded with neutrons, protons, deuterons, or alpha particles. In such bombardment, some of these bombarding particles will be absorbed by the nucleus of the target material. In each case, an alteration has occurred in the proton to neutron relationship. By such changes in the nucleus, the number of particles within the nucleus is altered to a point where the binding energy can no longer contain them. Accordingly, a particle is ejected from a nucleus, and a new nuclide is formed, which may be either radioactive or stable. If it is a stable nuclide the reaction ends. The manner in which these artificial radionuclides are produced will be discussed in Chapter 5.

Chapter 4 Methods of radioactive decay

IDENTIFICATION OF EMISSIONS

There are basically three emissions from radionuclides—alpha, beta, and gamma rays. A means of identifying these radiations had to be devised, and this problem became the doctoral thesis of Mme. Marie Curie at about the turn of the twentieth century. To carry out the experiment of identification, Mme. Curie devised a very simple technique. She took a large block of lead with a hole in its center into which she placed a source of radium. In this manner, since the radiations emanate at an infinite number of angles from the source, those that did not radiate upwards through the hole would be absorbed by the surrounding lead. A piece of photographic film was placed above the lead block. In this way, radiations emanating from the radium source and going through the hole in the lead block would be detected by an area of darkening on the film. In an effort to learn if these radiations had electrical charges, Mme. Curie included a magnetic field in a direction perpendicular to the direction of the emissions (Fig. 4-1). She reasoned that, if charged, the positively charged emissions would be deflected to the right according to the rules of physics for positive charges in a magnetic field, and the negatively charged emissions would be deviated to the left. Those with no charge would remain unaffected by the magnetic field. Further, in the presence of the magnetic field, if all 3 types of emissions were present, 3 areas of darkening would be seen on the photographic plate. Since Mme. Curie did detect 3 areas of darkening, she arbitrarily labeled the emissions after the first three letters of the Greek alphabet. Those that were deflected to the right and had a positive charge were called *alpha* emissions; those that were deflected to the left and negatively charged were called *beta* emissions; and those that remained undeflected and having no charge were called *gamma* emissions.

CHARACTERISTICS OF EMISSIONS

Many experiments have been performed to learn more about radioactivity. In addition to the conclusions of Mme. Curie's experiment, many other characteristics are now known.

It is an accepted fact a radioactive nuclide will emit one, two, or all three of these basic radiations. There are comparatively few radionuclides that possess the ability to decay by both alpha and beta emission with the subsequent release of a gamma ray. Most radionuclides decay by either alpha emission or beta emission. In either case, gamma emission could be a subsequent reaction. Those radio-

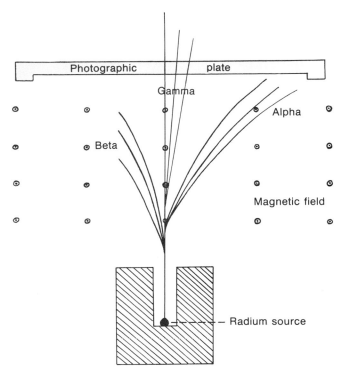

Fig. 4-1. Electrical properties of radioactive emissions. An illustration of Mme. Curie's experiment to prove that alpha emissions are positively charged, beta emissions are negatively charged, and gamma emissions are neutrally charged.

nuclides that decay by alpha emission only or beta emission only are termed *pure alpha emitters* and *pure beta emitters,* respectively.

It is also known that the process of decay creates other nuclides which may be either radioactive or stable. (Note the word *nuclides,* not isotopes.) ^{203}Hg, for instance, does not eventually decay to ^{197}Hg (an isotope); it decays by beta-gamma emission to ^{203}Tl (another nuclide). This is called *transmutation,* the conversion of one element into another.

Another indisputable fact is that the process of decay is a series of random events. It is impossible to predict exactly which atom is going to undergo disintegration at any given time. However, it is possible to predict, on the average, how many atoms will disintegrate during any interval of time. Because of this predictability, the rate of disintegration can be used as a method of quantitative analysis. These disintegrations can be detected; those detected can be counted and the results can be expressed as counts per unit time.

It has also been demonstrated that temperature, pressure, or chemical combination have absolutely no effect on the rate of decay. Radioactive materials can be placed in a freezer without any demonstrable change in the half-life. The same is true should a source of radioactivity be subjected to heat and pressure, as in an autoclave for sterilization purposes.

The fact that chemical combination does not alter the radioactive characteris-

37

tics is the rationale responsible for labeling or "tagging" chemicals, by replacing stable atoms of a compound with radioactive atoms. ^{197}Hg-labeled chlormerodrin, a mercurial diuretic, is an example. In labeling this compound, the stable form of mercury is replaced by the unstable form. In this way, neither the mercurial diuretic nor the ^{197}Hg is altered in any way and the body reacts to either form similarly.

METHODS OF DECAY

The original radionuclide in any method of decay is called a *parent;* the nuclide to which it decays is called a *daughter,* which may be stable or unstable. If a daughter nuclide is stable, the decay process is terminated. If the daughter is unstable, a new decay process begins which may differ entirely from its predecessor.

Alpha emission

Definition and origin. The alpha particle (α, $^4_2\alpha$, or $^4_2$He) is a helium nucleus consisting of 2 protons and 2 neutrons. This particle is the same as the helium atom with the exception that there are no orbital electrons. Because there are no negative charges to neutralize the positively charged nucleus, the alpha particle possesses an electrical charge of $+2$ upon emission. Since the particle is without electrons, it will not be satisfied until it acquires 2 electrons, making it an electrically neutral helium atom.

Alpha particles originate in the nuclei of heavier atoms. For the most part, these atoms occupy the upper one-third of the chart of the nuclides. It is obvious that if alpha emissions occurred as a result of nuclear changes in the lighter nuclides, the nuclide would be discarding a major portion of its nucleus. Alpha decay is a fast and efficient means of bringing the neutron to proton ratio closer to a stable ratio. Since an alpha particle removes 2 protons and 2 neutrons from the parent nuclide, the new nuclide contains 2 fewer protons and 2 fewer neutrons. In effect, the atomic number (Z) would be decreased by 2, the neutron number (N) would be decreased by 2, and the mass number (A) would be decreased by 4.

Ionization and penetration. Since an alpha particle has an electrical charge of $+2$, its immediate purpose is to acquire 2 electrons in order to become electrically neutral. As the alpha particle passes through matter, it attracts electrons from near-by atoms (Fig. 4-2). Because of the strong electrical attraction of the alpha particle and the almost nonexistent binding energy of outer shell electrons, the alpha particle can actually overcome the binding forces of the electron's parent atom, causing the electron to be released in space. As a result the electron is free to ionize other atoms in the surrounding media (provided it has enough energy to do so), to combine with positive ions in the vicinity, or to become one of the free electrons which occur in all matter. This process of removal of an electron from an atom is called *ionization.* The results of this ionization process is the creation of an *ion pair* consisting of a negative ion (the electron) and a positive ion (the atom from which the electron was removed). *Primary ionization* is that produced by the originally charged particle; *secondary ionization* is that subsequently produced by the ions that resulted from the primary event (electrons, primarily).

This process of attracting the electron by the alpha particle causes a slowing

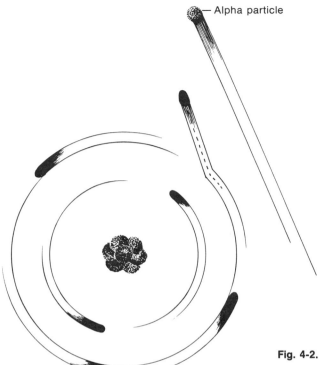
— Alpha particle

Fig. 4-2. Ionization of matter by a passing alpha particle.

down and loss of kinetic energy of the particle itself, because the alpha particle uses some of its energy to remove the electron. This process of ionization will continue many, many times with subsequent atoms in the path of the alpha particle. The particle will create more ion pairs until it loses all of its kinetic energy and comes to *rest mass*. The particle picks up the 2 electrons necessary for electrical neutrality, and comes to rest as a helium atom, a chemically inert gas. At this point, it ceases to be of radiobiologic significance.

An alpha particle loses an average of 34 ev per ionization event in air. If energy loss by the alpha particle were the only consideration, this would mean that an alpha particle with 3,400,000 ev of energy (3.4 mev) would undergo 100,000 ionization events (100,000 ion pairs) before expending all of its energy and coming to rest mass. It would require less than 2 cm of air to expend all the energy of such an alpha particle. As matter increases in density, less distance is required to expend the energy of the alpha particle; therefore, penetration decreases.

The *range* of an alpha particle, that is, the distance the charged particle travels from its point of origin to the place where it no longer acts as a destructive radiation particle, is about 4 cm in air. This value changes considerably in tissue, in which the range is reduced to a few thousandths of a centimeter. For this reason, an alpha particle is unable to penetrate the epidermis of the skin. It is not to be assumed, however, that an alpha particle is without injurious radiation effects because it cannot penetrate the skin. The most common methods of alpha contamination are inhalation or ingestion of alpha-laden materials. This is not of

39

particular importance in the usual nuclear medicine laboratory, since alpha emitters are not used in routine nuclear medicine procedures.

Ionization is often spoken of in terms of *specific ionization,* that is, the number of ion pairs formed per unit of path traveled by a moving charged particle through matter. For particles of the same energy the specific ionization increases with mass and charge. For this reason, alpha particles have a higher specific ionization than other particles because they have more mass and 2 positive charges. Further, specific ionization is inversely proportional to velocity, since the slower moving particle spends more time in the vicinity of the atom, and therefore, has a greater chance to ionize it. The specific ionization in air for a 1 mev alpha particle is about 60,000 ion pairs per centimeter of path traveled.

An alpha particle is also capable of *excitation* of an atom as it approaches or passes through it. To excite an atom is to increase the energy state of an orbital electron by the transfer of some of the energy of the alpha particle to the electron. By increasing the energy state, the electron assumes a new suborbit distant to the nucleus. The electron cannot stay in this excited state, so it immediately releases the excess energy and returns to its original orbit.

Example

Since an alpha particle consists of 2 protons and 2 neutrons, there would necessarily be 2 fewer protons and 2 fewer neutrons in the parent atom. A typical alpha emitter is $^{226}_{88}$Ra. The reaction of alpha emission is seen below:

$$^{226}_{88}\text{Ra} \rightarrow {}^{222}_{86}\text{Rn} + {}^{4}_{2}\text{He}$$
$$(\text{radium}) \rightarrow (\text{radon}) + (\text{alpha})$$

Accordingly, the new nuclide, radon 222, has a mass number reduced by 4 and an atomic number reduced by 2.

Beta emission

A beta particle (β) is a high velocity electron ejected from a disintegrating nucleus. The particle may be either a negatively charged electron, termed a *negatron* (β^-) or a positively charged electron, termed a *positron* (β^+). Both types of beta particles have the same mass, regardless of their charge. Although the precise definition of "beta emission" refers to both β^- and β^+ particles, the common usage of the term refers only to the β^- particle, as distinguished from positron emission which refers to the β^+ particle. The remainder of this text will treat β^- and β^+ particles as betas and positrons, respectively.

Beta decay

Definition and origin. The beta particle (β^-) is a high velocity, negatively charged electron emitted from a nucleus of an atom undergoing disintegration. The beta particle is identical to the orbital electron in mass and electrical charge. Both possess a charge of -1 and a mass $\frac{1}{1,836}$ that of a proton and equivalent to 0.000548 amu.

Since a β^- particle is defined as being ejected from the nucleus, the question arises of how an electron can be emitted from the nucleus when there is no electron in the nucleus. What actually happens is that a neutron is converted into a proton, an electron (β^-), and a neutrino as shown below:

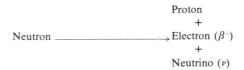

The immediate result of the neutron breakdown is that the electron (β^-) and the neutrino are ejected from the nucleus, while the proton remains. The parent atom is increased in atomic number by 1, with no change in mass number. (Mass number is protons plus neutrons and one has been converted to the other, so there is no change in the total number.)

Examples

An example of a beta emitter is phosphorus 32. It decays to sulfur 32 with the emission of a beta particle and a neutrino according to the following:

$$^{32}_{15}P \rightarrow {}^{32}_{16}S + \beta^- + \nu$$

In the above reaction, no gamma is released; therefore, ^{32}P is a pure beta emitter. Others are carbon 14 ($^{14}_{6}C$), cesium 137 ($^{137}_{55}Cs$) and strontium 90 ($^{90}_{38}Sr$).

An example of a beta-gamma emitter is iodine 131. ^{131}I decays by beta emission to xenon 131 according to the following:

$$^{131}_{53}I \rightarrow {}^{131}_{54}Xe + \beta^- + \nu + \gamma$$

Other beta-gamma emitters are mercury 203 ($^{203}_{80}Hg$), gold 198 ($^{198}_{79}Au$), iron 59 ($^{59}_{26}Fe$), molybdenum 99 ($^{99}_{42}Mo$), and sodium 24 ($^{24}_{11}Na$).

Debit mass and credit energy. It is important to realize that whenever the disintegration of a nucleus occurs, regardless of the method of decay, there is a release of energy. The source of this excess energy is the nucleus itself because of a disparity in the mass of the new nuclide. This unaccounted mass is expressed in atomic mass units (amu) in the calculations of the ^{32}P reaction that follow: (amu values are taken from Appendix C, p. 359).

amu $^{32}_{15}P$	31.984030
less amu 15 electrons $= 0.000548 \times 15 =$	0.008120
amu of $^{32}_{15}P$ nucleus	31.975910 (A)
amu $^{32}_{16}S$	31.982200
less amu 16 electrons $= 0.000548 \times 16 =$	0.008668
amu of $^{32}_{16}S$ nucleus	31.973532 (B)
amu of $^{32}_{15}P$ nucleus	31.975910 (A)
less amu of $^{32}_{16}S$ nucleus	31.973532 (B)
mass difference	0.002378
less β^- mass	0.000548
less neutrino mass	0.000000
unaccounted mass	0.001830

It was not until Einstein that this question of what happened to the rest of the mass could be answered. He said that mass or energy could not be destroyed but that each could be converted into the other. In these reactions, some mass is always lost, but an equivalent amount of energy is always gained. It has already been shown (formula 3-5) that 931.2 is the conversion factor to convert mass (amu) to energy expressed as mev. Therefore, the energy released from decay of ^{32}P to ^{32}S is as follows:

$$\text{Energy released in mev} = 0.00183 \times 931.2 = 1.70 \text{ mev}$$

The energy resulting from this neutron breakdown is expended in three different ways: (1) Some of the energy goes to the electron in order that it may be ejected from the nucleus. (2) Some of the energy goes to the neutrino in order that it may be ejected from the nucleus. (3) In any radionuclide other than a pure beta emitter, some of the energy is retained by the nucleus. The latter elevates a nucleon to a new energy level. The consequence of this elevated energy level or excited state is that, with the exception of isomeric transition (see p. 51), the excess energy is instantaneously released in the form of gamma radiation. The energy levels to which the excited nucleus is elevated are discrete energy levels and are well known. Therefore, the energy released in the form of gamma radiation is also well known. This is not the case with the β^- particle and the neutrino. The amount of energy that is expended on the beta particle or the neutrino is quite unpredictable from one atom to another, but the energy distribution is known based on percentages.

Energy distribution of a pure beta emitter. In the pure beta emitter, all the energy resulting from a neutron breakdown is expended on the beta particle and neutrino to eject it from the nucleus. There is no elevated energy state of the nucleus, and therefore, no subsequent gamma emission. Fig. 4-3 shows the distribution of energy to the ^{32}P beta particle as a function of energy plotted on the abscissa (horizontal axis) versus frequency of occurrence on the ordinate (vertical axis). As indicated, the maximum energy (E_{max}) of any beta particle from this radionuclide is that of 1.7 mev. The number of atoms in a given sample producing a beta particle of 1.7 mev is very, very low. Conversely, the number of atoms in the given sample producing a beta particle of 0.6 mev is much higher. E_{max} indicates that the maximum energy resulting from the neutron breakdown is 1.7 mev. Since all of the energy in a pure beta emitter is expended on either the beta particle or the neutrino, whatever portion of that energy that the beta particle does not receive, the neutrino receives. Therefore, an atom that supplies the beta particle with all of the energy resulting from the neutron breakdown would have a neutrino that has just enough energy to be ejected from the nucleus. However, one of its sister atoms in the same sample which gives only 0.6 mev of energy to the beta particle, would have a neutrino possessing the energy difference of 1.1 mev. According to Fig. 4-3, the situation in which a beta particle receives 0.6 mev and the neutrino receives 1.1 mev of energy occurs much more frequently than that in which the beta particle receives the total energy and the neutrino very little or vice versa. This whole concept of energy distribution can be crudely summed up as whatever energy the beta particle does not use, the neutrino receives. If this were actually the case, the beta particle must be considered as most charitable. However, most

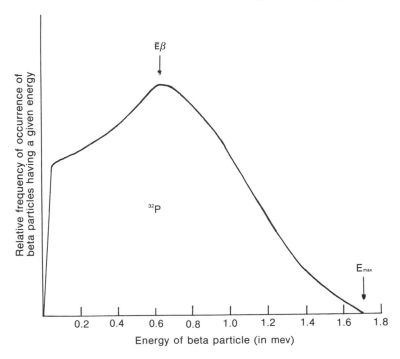

Fig. 4-3. Distribution of resultant energy to ^{32}P beta particles following the conversion of a neutron to a proton with the expulsion of an electron and a neutrino from the nucleus.

of the beta particles need only approximately one-third of the available energy, leaving the other two-thirds for the neutrino. This energy value is generally considered to be its average energy represented by the symbol $\bar{E}_\beta$ (E bar beta). Since it is approximately equivalent to one-third of all the available energy, $\bar{E}_\beta \approx \frac{1}{3}E_{max}$. In any nuclide that is not a pure beta emitter the nucleus would contribute some of its energy to the nucleus itself. Energy distribution between the beta particle and the neutrino would remain similar.

Purpose. When a nucleus undergoes beta disintegration, the daughter nuclide possesses a nucleus with an atomic number increased by 1 and the mass number remains the same. A neutron has been changed into a proton; therefore, the proton number is increased by 1. However, the mass number has not been changed because what has been lost in neutrons has been gained in protons. This type of decay would occur in any nuclide having too many neutrons and/or too few protons. Beta decay is the only method available to such an unstable nucleus. The neutron number is decreased and the proton number is increased in order to attempt to achieve stability. It may be, however, that the new nuclide may also be unstable for the same reason, and it may subsequently disintegrate by the same method. This process will continue until a stable proportion of neutrons and protons exists. (Disintegration of a nucleus means only that it changes in composition, not that it no longer exists.)

The above situation exemplifies the conditions that exist in every atom of tin 127 ($^{127}_{50}$Sn) (Fig. 4-4). ^{127}Sn contains 77 neutrons and 50 protons. For some reason not

43

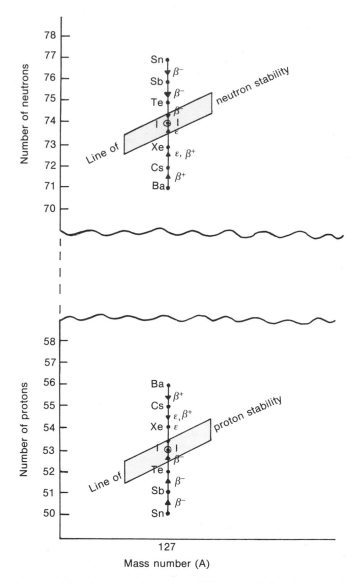

Fig. 4-4. Magnification of Fig. 1-4 at the level of A = 127 demonstrating that unstable atoms decay to stability by whatever method is required to achieve a stable ratio of neutrons to protons.

completely understood, this neutron to proton ratio is unstable because there are too many neutrons and too few protons. Its only course of action is beta decay. In decaying by beta emission, ^{127}Sn becomes antimony 127 ($^{127}_{51}$Sb); this nucleus with 76 neutrons and 51 protons is still unstable. Consequently, it decays by beta emission to tellurium 127 ($^{127}_{52}$Te) and this nucleus with 75 neutrons and 52 protons is unstable also. Finally, it decays by beta emission to iodine 127 ($^{127}_{53}$I) which has a stable ratio of 74 neutrons to 53 protons, and the decay series ends. ^{127}I happens to be the only stable isotope of iodine, and is that form of the element which is found in iodized salt, fish, and so on.

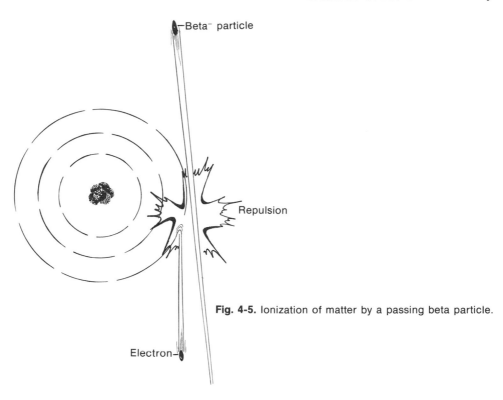

Fig. 4-5. Ionization of matter by a passing beta particle.

Since the unstable parent atom decays by beta emission to a daughter atom that has the same mass number but a different atomic number, and therefore different chemical properties, it can be said that beta decay gives rise to an isobar. The process is termed *isobaric formation.*

Ionization and penetration. Beta particles also possess the ability to excite and/or ionize atoms. The method of ionization, however, is somewhat different from the ionization of alpha particles. An alpha particle attracts an orbital electron and thus creates an ion pair. The beta particle repels the orbital electron from its energy shell to create an ion pair (Fig. 4-5). Each ion pair produced by the β^- particle represents a loss of energy by the beta particle. These processes of excitation and ionization continue until the beta particle loses all of its kinetic energy. At this point, the beta particle is said to have attained rest mass. It can now combine with some positively charged ion to make it a neutral atom once again. This process is termed *deionization.* It can also become a free electron, in which capacity it does not combine with anything. The specific ionization of a 1 mev beta particle in air is about 45 ion pairs per centimeter of path traveled. Compared to an alpha particle, the specific ionization of a beta particle is greatly reduced. This is largely because the charge of an alpha particle is twice that of a beta particle. Further, an alpha particle has a lower velocity than a beta particle and is in the area of any one atom for a longer period of time, which increases its probability of attracting an orbital electron to it.

As with alpha particles, beta particles lose an average energy of 34 ev per

45

ionization event. Similarly, considering only the loss of particle energy, a 3.4 mev beta particle would undergo 100,000 ionization events before losing its radio-biologic significance. It differs from the alpha particle, however, in its penetration. As the specific ionization values indicate, a beta particle incurs fewer ionization events per unit of path traveled, so it travels farther than an alpha particle of equal energy. The penetrating power of beta particles is approximately 100 times as great as that of alpha particles. However, the penetration power of beta particles is only a small fraction of that of gamma rays. Alpha particles are completely absorbed by a thin sheet of paper, whereas, an inch of wood or $\frac{1}{25}$ inch of aluminum is required to stop a beta particle. In tissue a 1 mev beta particle has a range of 0.42 cm. However, this particle is not harmless from a radiobiologic standpoint. It is well to remember that phosphorus 32, a pure beta emitter, is used as a therapeutic agent for such clinical states as leukemia, polycythemia, and ascites. In each case the epidermis is bypassed either by intravenous or intracavitary administration.

Bremsstrahlung. Bremsstrahlung is the German word for "braking radiation." Bremsstrahlung is the production of electromagnetic radiation by the acceleration that a fast, charged particle undergoes when it is deflected by another charged particle. The charged particles in the case of Bremsstrahlung are the beta particle and the nucleus of an atom near which the beta particle passes. When a beta particle passes near an atomic nucleus, its path of travel will be changed somewhat in the direction of the nucleus because of the attraction of unlike charges. This change in direction is spoken of as acceleration, but it is a negative acceleration.

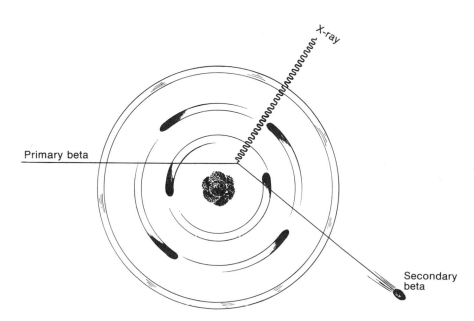

Fig. 4-6. Bremsstrahlung. A beta particle passes near the nucleus of an atom and is attracted to it. This results in a loss of energy and change in direction. That loss of energy is expressed as x-ray, or Bremsstrahlung.

The beta particle slows down and loses energy. In these instances, the energy lost is released in the form of x-rays (Fig. 4-6). These x-rays are equal in energy to that energy lost by the beta particle. This is one of the phenomena that occur in x-ray tubes and their subsequent x-ray production. In the case of x-ray machines, however, electrons are used rather than beta particles.

Positron decay

Definition and origin. The positron (β^+) is a high velocity, positively charged electron emitted from the nucleus of an atom undergoing disintegration. The positron differs from the electron and the beta particle only in that it has an opposite electrical charge. It has the mass of an electron, but the electrical charge of a proton. The nuclear origin of the positron is the proton. A proton, under the influence of all the nucleons in its nucleus, is converted into a neutron, an electron with a positive charge (positron), and a neutrino, as shown below:

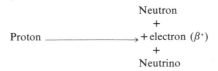

The immediate result of the proton breakdown is that the positive electron (β^+) and the neutrino are ejected from the nucleus while a neutron remains. The parent atom is reduced in atomic number by 1, with no change in mass number. (Similar to beta decay, one of the units comprising the mass number is converted to the other so there is no change. In positron decay, however, it is the opposite of beta decay; a proton becomes a neutron.)

Examples

An example of a positron emitter is nitrogen 12. It decays to carbon 12 with the emission of a β^+ particle, and a neutrino according to the following:

$$^{12}_{7}\text{N} \rightarrow ^{12}_{6}\text{C} + \beta^+ + \nu$$

In the above reaction, no gamma is released; therefore, ^{12}N is a pure positron emitter. ^{18}F is another.

A further example of a positron emitter and one more pertinent to nuclear medicine is gallium 68. It decays to zinc 68 with the emission of a positron, a neutrino and energy (γ) according to the following:

$$^{68}_{31}\text{Ga} \rightarrow ^{68}_{30}\text{Zn} + \beta^+ + \nu + \gamma$$

The reader is also referred to the decay scheme (p. 61) for this reaction. Another important positron emitter is sodium 22 ($^{22}_{11}$Na).

Debits and credits. Just as with beta decay, the disintegration of a nucleus, with the subsequent emission of a positron, yields energy as a result of loss through conversion of mass. The mass-energy equivalence can be calculated since amu values are known. A calculation of the ^{12}N reaction follows:

amu $^{12}_{7}$N	12.022780
less amu 7 electrons $= 0.000548 \times 7$	0.003836
amu of $^{12}_{7}$N nucleus	12.018944 (A)

amu $^{12}_{6}$C	12.003803
less amu 6 electrons $= 0.000548 \times 6$	0.003288
amu of $^{12}_{6}$C nucleus	12.000515 (B)

amu of $^{12}_{7}$N nucleus	12.018944 (A)
amu of $^{12}_{6}$C nucleus	12.000515 (B)
mass difference	0.018429
less β^+ mass	0.000548
less ν mass	0.000000
unaccounted mass	0.017881

Having determined the mass difference, the mass-energy equivalence can be determined as follows:

$$\text{Energy released (mev)} = 0.017881 \times 931.2 = 16.65 \text{ mev}$$

Purpose. By undergoing positron decay, the proton number is decreased by 1 and the neutron number is increased by 1. This would result in a daughter product having 1 less atomic number and the same mass number, another example of isobaric formation. This type of decay is exactly opposite to beta decay. This type might occur in an unstable nucleus in which there are too many protons and/or too few neutrons to bring the number of neutrons and protons to a stable ratio. In many instances, positron emission is in competition with electron capture (see p. 49), since both methods of decay have identical results.

It may be, however, that positron emission will only bring the neutron to proton ratio closer to stability. This is the case with barium 127 ($^{127}_{56}$Ba), (Fig. 4-4). ^{127}Ba contains 71 neutrons and 56 protons. This ratio of neutrons to protons is not stable so it decays by β^+ emission to cesium 127 ($^{127}_{72}$Cs). ^{127}Cs is still unstable, so it decays by β^+ emission or electron capture (primarily the latter) to xenon 127 ($^{127}_{73}$Xe). ^{127}Xe still contains an unstable ratio of neutrons and protons and it decays entirely by electron capture to iodine 127 ($^{127}_{74}$I). The series has finally reached stability at this point because iodine 127 has 74 neutrons and 53 protons, and these are the numbers necessary for stability.

It is of particular importance to learn what happens to the positron once it is ejected from the nucleus. Three reactions are of importance: ionization, Bremsstrahlung, and the annihilation reaction.

Ionization and penetration. The degree of ionization and Bremsstrahlung is similar to that which occurs with the beta particle for as long as the positron survives. The methods, however, are different because of an opposite electrical charge. Ionization occurs when the positron attracts the negatively charged orbital electron from its orbit; the beta particle repels it from its orbital path.

Bremsstrahlung. Bremsstrahlung differs also since the nucleus has a preponderance of positive charges and the positron is also positive. The negative acceleration seen in the Bremsstrahlung phenomenon would be that of a repulsion away from the nucleus rather than an attraction toward it. This negative acceleration is, as in

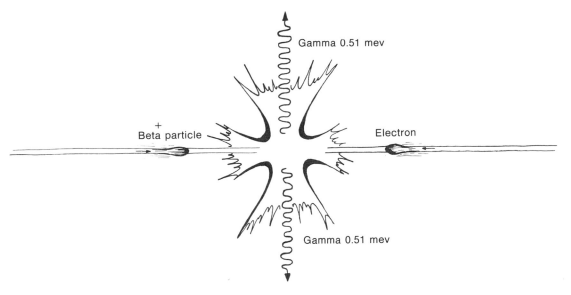

Fig. 4-7. Annihilation reaction. A positron is attracted to an electron, whereupon both particles are annihilated and converted to energy (2 gamma photons each with an energy of 0.511 mev).

the beta particle, a loss of energy to that positron and this energy is released in the form of x-ray. The x-ray is equal in energy to the energy lost by the positron particle.

Annihilation reaction. The most important reaction of the positron following ejection is the annihilation reaction. It is for this reason that the positron is short-lived; the average life is approximately 10^{-9} seconds. The annihilation reaction is the result of a collision between the positively charged positron which has lost all of its kinetic energy and an always present negatively charged electron. The masses of both particles are completely annihilated. Accordingly, energy must be released equivalent to the masses of 1 electron and 1 positron. That mass energy equivalence is 1.02 mev of energy as indicated below:

$$
\begin{aligned}
\text{amu of electron} &= 0.000548 \\
\text{amu of positron} &= \underline{0.000548} \\
&\quad\ \ 0.001096
\end{aligned}
$$
$$0.001096 \times 931.2 \text{ mev} = 1.02 \text{ mev}$$

The energy that results is not 1 photon with an energy of 1.02 mev but 2 photons of 0.511 mev radiating in exactly opposite directions of one another. The available energy is equally divided between the 2 photons. This reaction is seen in Fig. 4-7.

Electron capture

Another mode of radioactive decay used by unstable nuclei having too few neutrons and too many protons is that of electron capture (ε). Electron capture is similar to positron decay in that the end results are similar, but the methods used to achieve these ends differ. As stated previously, it is believed by some scientists that energy shells are not perfectly circular around the nucleus but are elliptical

49

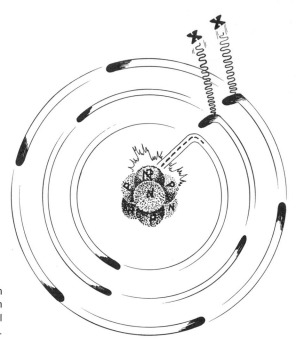

Fig. 4-8. Electron capture. The nucleus attracts an orbital electron, which combines with a proton to form a neutron. The secondary process of filling the orbital vacancy results in emission of characteristic x-radiation.

in shape. It is even thought that possibly the K-shell electron passes through the nucleus during one of its orbits and is captured by the nucleus. Whatever the case, it is known that 1 of the orbiting K-shell electrons is captured by the nucleus. When this electron is captured, the nucleus transforms a proton into a neutron and a neutrino is ejected (Fig. 4-8). It is usually the K-shell electron that is captured by the nucleus (K-capture). This method of decay is known to exist with electrons from the L energy shells as well. In these cases, the phenomenon is known as L-capture. Capture of unbound (free) electrons by nuclei has not been observed to date. Whatever electron is captured, a vacancy will exist in that shell that must be filled. Electrons fall down into the vacancy and characteristic x-radiation results, as described in Chapter 2.

By the decay process of electron capture the parent nucleus produces a daughter nucleus with a neutron number increased by 1 and a proton number decreased by 1. In so doing, the daughter product becomes an isobar of the parent. This is the third method of isobaric formation. Chromium 51 ($^{51}_{24}$Cr) is an example of electron capture and its decay scheme is shown at the end of this chapter (p. 00). Other pertinent radionuclides that decay by electron capture are iodine 125 ($^{125}_{53}$I), mercury 197 ($^{197}_{80}$Hg), cobalt 57 ($^{57}_{27}$Co), strontium 85 ($^{85}_{38}$Sr), selenium ($^{75}_{34}$Se), and germanium 68 ($^{68}_{32}$Ge).

Gamma emission

Radioactive decay by alpha emission, beta emission, positron emission, or electron capture usually leaves some of the energy resulting from these changes in the nucleus. As a result, the nucleus is raised to an excited level. None of these excited nuclei (with the exception of isomeric transition) can remain in this high energy state. They must instantaneously release this energy so the nucleus can return to ground state or its lowest possible energy state. This energy is released in the form of gamma radiation, and the gamma has an energy equal to the change in energy state of the nucleon. These photons are members of the electromagnetic spectrum and have a wavelength corresponding to very short x-rays. As stated previously, a gamma ray differs from an x-ray only in its origin; gamma rays originate in the nucleus, x-rays originate in the orbital electron structure. Although of different origin, gamma rays and x-rays have precisely the same characteristics. Their powers of excitation, ionization, and penetration are exactly the same. For this reason they are used interchangeably in medical diagnosis and treatment.

Gamma rays carry no electrical charge; therefore, they are not subject to forces of attraction or repulsion as are alpha, beta, and positron particles. Unlike these particles, gamma rays are the only emissions from an unstable nucleus that fall into the electromagnetic spectrum. Since they are not particles, the postemission product differs from the preemission form of the element only in a decreased energy state. There is no change in atomic number, neutron number, or mass number. Further, some nuclear reaction or interaction must have preceded the gamma emission in order for the nucleus to be in an excited state. Reactions include neutron bombardment and charged particle bombardment. Interactions include alpha decay, beta decay, and positron decay.

Ionization and penetration. Gamma rays are also capable of producing ionization. It is referred to as *indirect* ionization, however. Gamma photons are capable of striking orbital electrons, thereby ejecting them from their orbits at very high velocities. These rapidly moving secondary electrons ionize the atoms in the surrounding media. The same is true of x-rays.

The degree of penetration by a gamma ray is much greater than that of the other nuclear emissions. Penetration is such that, theoretically, enough shielding could never be provided to entirely stop all gamma rays. Even with a mile of lead there would be some gamma rays not totally absorbed but passing its full length. The degree of absorption or degree of attenuation can be predicted (see pp. 101 and 102).

Isomeric transition. An isomer, in nuclear terms, is one of 2 nuclides having the same mass number and the same atomic number but which can exist for measurable times in the excited state. This differs from the chemical meaning of the term. It has been stated before that, in most cases, this state of excitation must be instantaneously relieved by the emission of a gamma ray. In some radionuclides, however, this does not occur instantaneously. Isomeric transition is the radioactive transition from one nuclear isomer to another of lower energy. It is part of the decay process of certain radionuclides. An example of this would be molybdenum 99 ($^{99}_{42}$Mo). Molybdenum 99 decays by beta-gamma emission to technetium 99 ($^{99}_{43}$Tc). In the process of decay a point is reached at which the nucleus is able to retain its excited level (142 kev) for a half-life period of 6 hours. Since the molybdenum nucleus has ejected the beta particle and the neutrino, it has already lost 1 neutron and gained 1 proton. It is no longer molybdenum 99, but technetium 99. Further, it can only be technetium 99 when the nucleus is at ground state, which it is not. It acts as though it were another radionuclide, a semistable technetium 99 atom. For this reason, the atom that can exist in this increased energy state of the nucleus is referred to as being in a *metastable* state. This state is signified by *m* after the mass number (technetium 99m). Not until the nucleus loses that energy is it known as a true technetium 99 atom. Isomeric transition is regarded as a form of decay because of the emission of the gamma ray. It only represents a change in energy state, not a change in nuclear compositon. Other pertinent radionuclides that decay by isomeric transition include strontium 87m (^{87m}Sr) and barium 137m (^{137m}Ba).

Interactions with matter. There are three ways that gamma photons can interact with matter. These are the Compton effect, the photoelectric effect, and pair production. All three methods result in the loss of energy by the gamma ray and its eventual absorption.

Compton effect. The Compton effect (Fig. 4-9) occurs when an incident gamma ray (primarily of medium energy) interacts with a free or loosely bound (outer shell) electron. In this interaction with matter, a portion of the energy of the incident gamma ray is transferred to the electron. The energy expended depends on the angle at which the incident gamma ray hits the electron. If the electron is hit head-on, then a major portion of the energy is given to the electron. If the hit is one of a glancing nature, very little of the energy is transferred to the electron. As a result, the electron (Compton electron) is ejected from the orbital structure and a gamma ray of reduced energy (*secondary, Compton,* or *scatter*) emerges from the atom with a change in direction. The incident gamma ray has been reduced in energy by two factors. First, it has had to use some of its energy to overcome the binding energy of the electron which was removed. Secondly, it has transferred

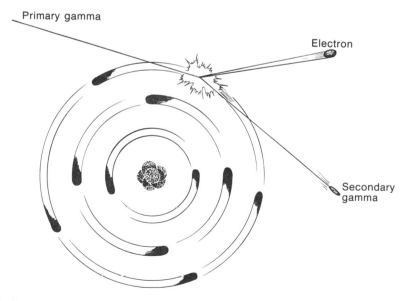

Fig. 4-9. Compton effect. A gamma photon of medium energy strikes an outer orbital electron and releases it from its orbit. This results in the production of a secondary gamma of reduced energy.

some of its energy to that electron. Therefore, the energy of the secondary gamma ray is equal to the energy of the incident gamma ray, less the binding energy of the electron which was released, less the energy given to that electron. Inasmuch as this secondary gamma is changed in direction and is of reduced energy, it becomes of extreme importance to nuclear medicine. (Without knowledge of instrumentation [namely, spectrometry] and Compton scatter, results from scanning techniques and function studies could be misinterpreted. This will be discussed in greater detail under Spectrometry, Chapter 8.)

Photoelectric effect. The photoelectric effect (Fig. 4-10) occurs when an incident gamma ray (primarily of low energy) interacts with an inner-orbital electron. When this reaction occurs, the entire energy of the gamma ray is transferred to the electron and the gamma is totally absorbed. The electron, called a *photoelectron* is released from its energy shell and the atom. Since the electron had a binding energy to contain it within its orbit, energy had to be used by the incident gamma ray to overcome that binding energy. Therefore, the electron would have the energy of the gamma ray less the amount of energy required to overcome the binding energy. Since a vacancy exists within that inner orbit, other orbital electrons will fall into that vacancy with a subsequent emission of characteristic x-rays.

In the process of absorption of gamma rays, the gamma ray usually goes through a series of Compton collisions, progressively reducing it in energy until it can finally be totally absorbed by the photoelectric process.

Pair production. Pair production is the third way in which gamma rays interact

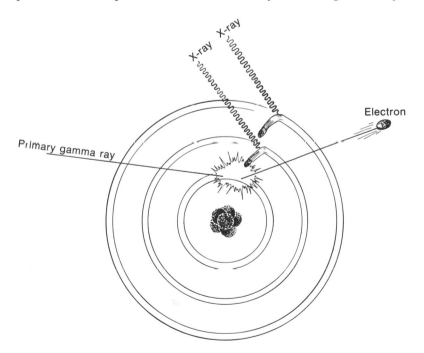

Fig. 4-10. Photoelectric effect. A low energy gamma photon strikes an inner orbital electron and releases it from its orbit, which effects total absorption of the gamma photon. Characteristic x-radiation results from the filling phenomenon.

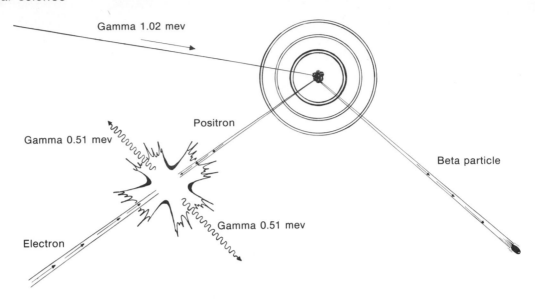

Fig. 4-11. Pair production. A high energy gamma ray interacts near the nucleus producing two particles, a beta particle (negatron) and a positron. The positron annihilates almost immediately.

with matter. This phenomenon occurs when high energy gamma rays interact in the vicinity of the nucleus. In pair production the energy of the gamma ray is completely absorbed in the vicinity of the strong electrical field of the nucleus with a subsequent production of a negatron and a positron (Fig. 4-11). In order for this to occur, the incident gamma ray must have a minimum energy of 1.02 mev. If these conditions are met, the positron and the negatron are ejected from the atom. The beta particle acts as other beta particles in that it passes through matter creating ion pairs along its path until such time as it is incorporated into an atom or becomes a free electron. The positron, however, almost instantaneously collides with an electron. This results in the subsequent annihilation of both particles and the emission of 2 gamma rays of 0.511 mev. Since the conversion of the mass of 2 beta particles is equal to 1.02 mev, and since that amount of energy is equally divided between the 2 annihilation gamma photons regardless of the energy of the incident gamma ray (provided it is greater than 1.02 mev), the energy of the annihilation gamma rays would always be equal to the 0.511 mev. If the incident gamma ray is greater in energy than 1.02 mev, the excess energy is given to the β^+ and β^- as kinetic energy which must be lost before the β^+ can undergo annihilation. Regardless of the energy of the incident gamma ray (provided it is 1.02 mev or greater), the energy of the annihilation gamma ray is always 0.511 mev. This gamma interaction represents an energy-to-mass-to-energy relationship. The reaction was begun with energy (gamma), it was converted to mass ($\beta^- + \beta^+$), which in turn was converted to energy (2 gammas of 0.511 mev).

Internal conversion. Following almost all nuclear interactions, the nucleus is left in an excited state. This elevated energy state is usually decreased to ground state immediately by the emission of a gamma ray equal to the change in energy

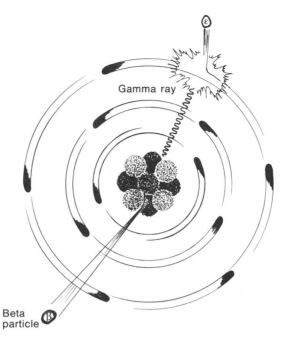

Fig. 4-12. Internal conversion. A gamma photon, being released from the nucleus following beta decay, strikes and ejects one of the orbital electrons from the parent atom.

level. In some cases, however, when this gamma ray emerges from the nucleus, the gamma ray can be naively regarded as transferring all of its energy to one of its own orbital electrons, usually the K-shell electron (Fig. 4-12). The electron is then ejected from the atom and possesses an energy equal to that of the gamma ray less the binding energy. The gamma ray has internally converted its own atom, hence the name internal conversion. The electron that is ejected from the atom is called the *conversion electron.*

The neutron. Since the neutron has no charge and is a comparatively large particle, it is unaffected by other particles containing electrical charges. The neutron can penetrate through the orbital structure directly into the nucleus where it is either absorbed, as in the case of neutron capture and transmutation (see Chapter 5), or it can possibly disrupt the nucleus, as in the case of fission. Another special consideration of neutrons is that they are produced in enormous quantities in the fission process, either controlled as in the case of a nuclear reactor, or uncontrolled as in the detonation of a nuclear bomb. Neutrons can have energies from as low as 0.025 ev (thermal neutrons) to higher than 1 million ev (fast neutrons)

The ionizing effects of neutrons are greater than those of gamma or x-rays. They also have one special feature regarding their ability to ionize hydrogen, which is a major constituent of all biologic materials. Ordinary hydrogen has a nucleus composed of only 1 proton, which is less in mass than the neutron. Upon subjecting biologic materials to neutron bombardment, the neutron possesses the unique quality of ionizing its hydrogen atoms by removing the nucleus, rather than the usual orbital electron.

55

DECAY SCHEMES
Principles

A decay scheme provides a ready reference for a variety of data. Quick identification is possible of such information as mode of decay, energy states of the nuclei and their subsequent gamma emissions, and the nuclide to which the radionuclide decays. These decay schemes have a wide variation in complexity. Those which decay directly to the daughter product without emitting electromagnetic radiation are the simplest forms. These would include the pure alpha emitters and pure beta emitters. Those decay schemes with resultant electromagnetic radiation vary greatly in complexity. Some, such as cobalt 60, have a very simple decay scheme. Others, such as iodine 131 and molybdenum 99, have extremely complex decay schemes.

Decay schemes are patterned by placing the parent nucleus at the top of the decay scheme. Diagonal lines extending from the right or the left of the parent indicate the mode of decay. Those diagonal lines which angle to the right represent the mode of decay whereby the daughter nuclide is of higher atomic number than the parent. Those diagonal lines that angle to the left represent the modes of decay whereby the daughter nuclide is of lower atomic number than the parent. Alpha decay, positron decay and electron capture all result in the daughter nuclide being of lower atomic number than the parent. Beta decay is the only method resulting in a daughter nuclide of higher atomic number than the parent.

A pure beta emitter is an example of the simplest form of decay. ^{32}P is representative of such a scheme. The parent radionuclide, phosphorus 32, has a 14.28-day half-life and decays by β^- directly to sulfur 32, which is stable. One hundred percent of all ^{32}P nuclei decay by this method; the maximum energy is 1.7 mev. All of the energy is distributed to the beta particle and the neutrino. The nucleus does not receive any energy from this reaction; therefore, the nucleus is neither raised to an excited level, nor is there a subsequent gamma emission. Note that in this mode of decay the diagonal line is angled to the right indicating an increase in atomic number by the daughter. The atomic number of phosphorus 32 is 15 decaying to sulfur 32 with an atomic number of 16. Simple decay schemes can also be represented by pure alpha emitters, pure positron emitters, or in nuclides that undergo 100% electron capture. In these cases, all diagonal lines would be angled to the left because in all cases the daughter has a lower atomic number than the parent.

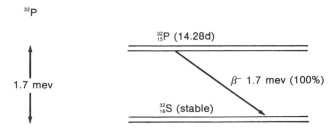

In general, the scintillation crystals used in routine diagnostic nuclear medicine procedures detect only gamma emissions. For the nuclide to be of importance to diagnostic nuclear medicine, gamma emission must be a part of its decay scheme. There are exceptions to this, such as beta emitters used with liquid scintillation detectors and positron emitters. In order that gamma rays be emitted, the radionuclide must decay in such a way that only part of the energy involved in the transition from parent to daughter is distributed in the ejection particles. When this occurs, the nucleus is raised to an excited energy state and in returning to ground state this energy is emitted in the form of gamma rays. These increases in energy state are represented by horizontal lines drawn between the parent and daughter nuclide and are representative of the various energy levels to which the nucleus can be raised. These horizontal lines would be analogous to the rungs on the step ladder used previously to describe the nuclear energy levels. A relatively simple example of such a decay scheme involving gamma emission would be that of cobalt 60. Cobalt 60 is an unstable nucleus with a half-life of 5.26 years and it decays by beta decay to the stable nickel 60. In this transition, however, only a portion of the energy resulting from the change within the nucleus is distributed to the beta particle and the neutrino. The remainder of the energy is retained by the nucleus and the nucleus is raised to an excited state. The energy state to which the nucleus of cobalt 60 is raised following the emission of the beta particle is 2.5 mev. Rather than decaying from this elevated energy state with one release of energy to achieve ground state it releases 2 gamma quanta in order to achieve ground state. In jumping from 2.5 mev to 1.33 mev energy state, there is a release of a gamma photon (γ_1) of 1.17 mev in energy, the energy difference between the two energy states. There is a subsequent release of another gamma photon of 1.33 mev (γ_2) representative of the change in energy state from the 1.33 mev level to ground state. The total energy involved in the transition of cobalt 60 to nickel 60 is 2.81 mev; the beta particle has a maximum energy of 0.31 mev, 1 gamma has an energy of 1.17 mev, and 1 gamma has an energy of 1.33 mev.

^{60}Co

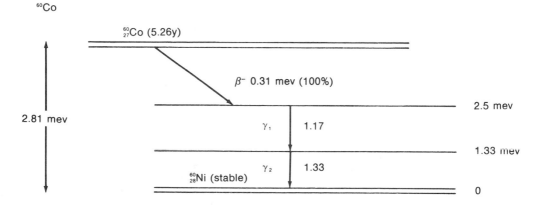

Decay schemes are simplified methods to describe the mode of decay and subsequent energy release in the form of gamma radiation due to changes in an unstable nucleus. The direction of the arrows that represent the modes of decay, although not intended, assume a similarity to the Madame Curie experiment discussed at the beginning of this chapter. The negatively charged particle, representing the beta decay, is angled in one direction; the positively charged particles, representing alpha decay and positron decay (also electron capture), are angled in the opposite direction; the gamma ray with no charge is drawn perpendicular to the parent nucleus.

Alpha decay

Alpha decay can be represented by the decay of radon 222 as follows. Almost 100% of the atoms of radon 222 (Z=86) decay by an alpha particle of 6.28 mev to polonium 218 (Z=84). Since an alpha particle is a helium nucleus, the parent atom loses 2 protons and 2 neutrons (an atomic number of 2 and a mass number of 4) to become polonium 218. Less than 1% of all atoms of radon 222 decay by an alpha particle which leaves the nucleus in an excited state with a new energy level of 0.51 mev. It instantaneously emits a gamma ray of 0.51 mev to become polonium 218. The daughter product has a decreased atomic number, so the angle of the charged particle is to the left. Polonium 218 itself is an unstable nucleus and is referred to as radium A. Being unstable, polonium will continue to decay and does so by alpha emission. This is a portion of the series which will eventually decay to stable lead 214. This chain of decay can be easily followed by referring to Brucer's trilinear chart of the nuclides. Radon 222 is a very simple alpha decay scheme. There are others much more complex in nature.

Alpha decay

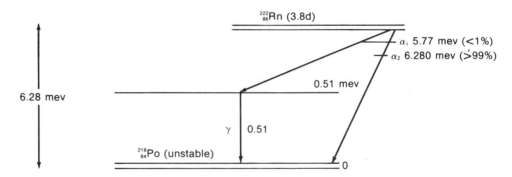

Beta decay

The decay scheme of a pure beta emitter, phosphorus 32, has already been discussed in the introduction of this section. This is a simple decay scheme in which no electromagnetic radiation is emitted. As energies to the beta particles vary and as energy states of the nucleus vary, the decay scheme becomes more and more complex.

Gold 198. A more complex decay scheme involving 3 beta particles of different energies and 3 gamma photons of different energies is that of gold 198. Gold 198 (Z=79) decays by beta decay to stable mercury 198 (Z=80). The percentage of all gold 198 atoms which decay with a beta particle having a maximum energy of 0.96 mev (β_2) is 98.6%. This leaves the nucleus in an excited energy state of 0.412

Beta decay

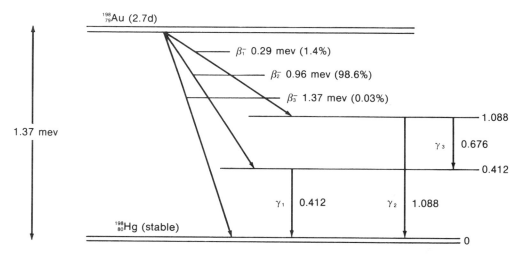

mev. This state of excitation is instantaneously relieved by the emission of a gamma ray of 0.412 mev (γ_1). This path of decay represents an energy differential between parent and daughter nuclei of 1.37 mev; the beta particle has a maximum energy of 0.96 mev and the gamma has an energy of 0.412 mev.

The percentage of all gold 198 atoms which emit a beta particle with a maximum energy of 0.29 mev (β_1) is 1.4%. The energy state of the nucleus is raised to 1.088 mev. There are two ways to relieve this excited state. The nuclei may reach ground state immediately by the emission of a gamma ray of 1.088 mev (γ_2); or they may do it in a two-step fashion by the emission of a gamma ray of 0.676 mev (γ_3) plus a gamma ray of 0.412 mev (γ_1). Both paths represent an energy differential between parent and daughter of 1.37 mev just as the β_2-γ_1 route does.

There is also a possibility that 0.03% of all gold 198 atoms would distribute all of their energy to the beta particle and the neutrino, in which case the atom decays directly by beta decay (β_1) to stable mercury 198 with no emission of electromagnetic radiation. The maximum energy of such a beta particle would be 1.37 mev, the energy differential between parent and daughter.

The largest number of beta particles (98.6%) decay in such a manner as to elevate the nucleus to an energy state of 0.412 mev. This being the case, the energy used in detecting gold 198 with radiation detection devices is 0.412 mev. In addition to the 98.6%, contributions are received from β_1 since one of its paths in relieving its excited state is by the 0.412 mev route, which further increases the percentage of atoms decaying by that energy emission. In looking at a gamma spectrum of gold 198, if the detection device was sensitive enough, three gamma peaks would be displayed: a very large peak at 0.412 mev and two much smaller peaks at 0.676 mev and 1.088 mev. The peak of choice to use in any study using gold 198 would be the peak of 0.412 mev.

Iodine 131. An even more complex beta-gamma spectrum is that of iodine 131. Iodine 131 decays by beta to stable xenon 131, by way of a metastable state of xenon 131. The nuclei of iodine 131 can decay by four different methods repre-

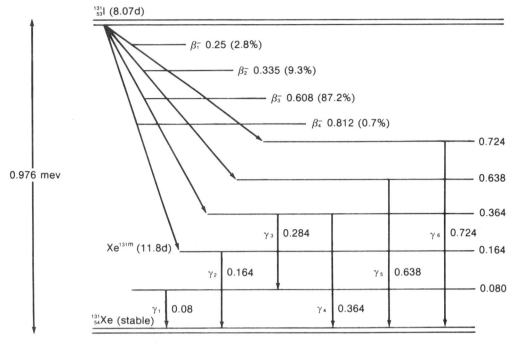

sented by four different beta particles all varying in energy. The differential between parent and daughter is 0.976 mev regardless of which beta-gamma pathway is calculated. Since 87.2% of all nuclei of iodine 131 decay by the β_3^--γ_4 pathway and γ_4 has an energy of 0.364 mev, the energy used to detect iodine 131 is 0.364 mev. With iodine 131 there are no contributors from other beta pathways to increase the percentage of 0.364 mev gammas, as was the case of gold 198. In fact, the opposite is true. The β_3^- pathway results in three different gammas (γ_1, γ_3, and γ_4) each having varying energies. In effect, this would actually reduce the percentage of nuclei giving the 0.364 gamma. This is realized by the study of gamma percentages. Of the 84.2% of iodine 131 atoms that decay by the β_3^- route only 80% continue the decay process by the γ_4 route (0.364 mev); the remaining 7.2% of all iodine 131 atoms decay by the γ_3-γ_1 route.

Electron capture

Germanium 68. A simple decay scheme representing the electron capture phenomenon is that of germanium 68 (Z=32). Germanium 68 decays by electron capture directly to gallium 68 emitting no electromagnetic radiation. Gallium is, itself, unstable and will decay further. The daughter, gallium, has an atomic number which is less than the parent, so the diagonal line is angled to the left. The germanium-gallium decay scheme is part of the basis of a generator system (see Chapter 5) for positron emitters (gallium 68). The entire decay scheme is discussed on p. 61.

Chromium 51. Another radionuclide used in nuclear medicine procedures and which involves electron capture is chromium 51. Chromium 51 decays to vanadium 51 by two methods of electron capture. Ninety percent of all atoms of chromium

Electron capture

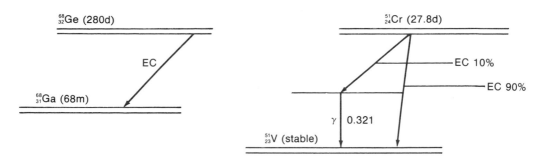

51 decay by electron capture to the ground state of vanadium 51, while 10% leave the nuclei in an excited energy state. The 10% which decay via the excited nucleus do so by raising its nuclear energy state to 0.321 mev. That energy state is instantaneously relieved by the release of a gamma photon equivalent to the change in energy state (0.321 mev). Vanadium 51 is a stable form of the element vanadium. As with the decay of germanium 68 to gallium 68, chromium 51 produces a daughter nuclide which is reduced in atomic number and, therefore, the diagonal of the decay scheme is angled to the left. It is interesting to note that this gamma peak of 321 kev represents only 10% of all the available atoms of chromium in any sample. The other 90% go undetected by standard detection methods.

Positron decay

Gallium 68 is an example of a positron emitter. Gallium 68 (Z = 31) is a daughter of germanium 68 via electron capture and decays to zinc 68 (Z = 30), which is stable. The nuclei of gallium 68 can decay by two different methods represented by two different positron particles, β_1^+ and β_2^+.

Only 3% of all atoms decaying by positron emission from gallium 68 are β_1^+ atoms. In these 3%, the nucleus is left in an increased energy state equivalent to

Positron decay

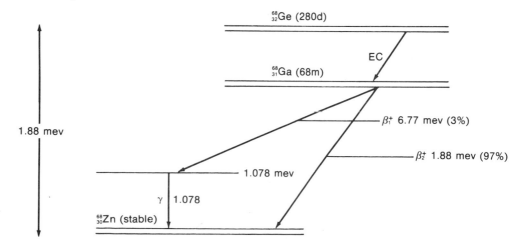

1.078 mev. The alternative positron emitted from gallium 68 (β_2^+) represents 97% of all positrons emitted from that radionuclide. These atoms decay directly to their ground state, zinc 68. Three percent of all gallium 68 atoms are responsible for the gamma energy peak of 1.078 mev. The energy differential between the daughter and parent is 1.88 mev. The daughter product has a decrease in atomic number so the diagonals are angled to the left.

Isomeric transition

Cesium 137. A simple example of a decay scheme representing isomeric transition is cesium 137. Cesium 137 (Z=55) decays by 2 beta particles of 0.514 mev and 1.18 mev. The beta particle having a maximum energy of 0.514 mev (β_1^-) represents 92% of all cesium 137 atoms; the 1.18 mev beta particle (β_2^-) represents only 8% of all the atoms of cesium 137. β_2^- decays directly to ground state barium 137 (Z=56) which is stable. β_1^- decays to an excited state of the nucleus. Unlike other forms of decay in which there is an excited state of the nucleus, this excitation state can be held for a half-life of 2.55 minutes. This isomeric state is known to be barium 137m (Z=56). The isomer decays to ground state, barium 137, releasing a gamma photon of 0.662 mev. The transition from parent to daughter represents an energy differential of 1.18 mev. The daughter product has an increased atomic number, so the diagonals are angled to the right.

Isomeric transition

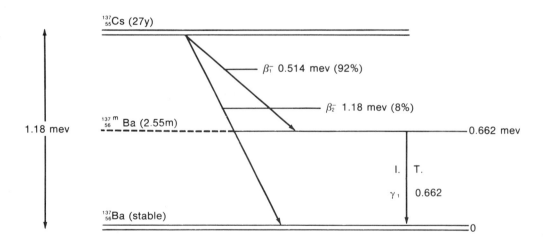

Molybdenum 99. A more complex decay scheme representing isomeric transition and pertinent to nuclear medicine is molybdenum 99. All atoms of molybdenum 99 (Z=42), have a 67-hour half-life and decay by 1 of 3 beta particles to technetium 99 (Z=43), through the isomeric state of technetium 99m. This isomeric state has a half-life of 6 hours and is the form of the radionuclide which is of interest in nuclear medicine procedures. Molybdenum 99 decays primarily by a beta particle, having an energy of 1.23 mev, to the metastable form of technetium with an increased energy state of 0.142 mev. It relieves that energy state by two pathways.

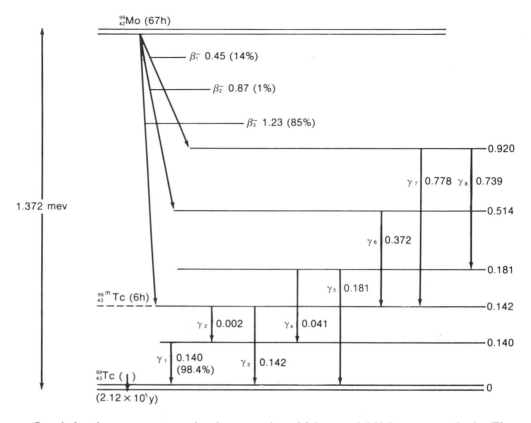

One is by the γ_2-γ_1 route, releasing energies of 2 kev and 140 kev, respectively. The other is by the γ_3 route, releasing a gamma photon of 142 kev, the latter being the lesser route. It is interesting that even though β_3^- represents 85% of all the beta particles emitted, γ_1, with an energy of 140 kev, represents 98.4% of all gammas emitted. The obvious conclusion is that β_1^- and β_2^- also contribute to this 140 kev gamma. β_1^- contributes by the γ_7-γ_2 route and the γ_8-γ_4 route, while β_2^- contributes by the γ_6-γ_2 route. The transition from molybdenum 99 to technetium 99 represents an energy change of 1.372 mev regardless of which pathway the nucleus decays. Technetium 99 is itself unstable having a half-life of 2.12×10^5 years and decays by beta with no electromagnetic radiation to ruthenium 99, a stable form of that element.

Origin of nuclides

The following is a discussion of five methods whereby nuclides are produced, not all of which are currently used to obtain the nuclides used in a nuclear medicine department.

FISSION

Fission, stated simply, is the production of small nuclei from a large nucleus. It may be strictly defined as an exergonic (energy-liberating) process of splitting certain heavy nuclei into 2 more or less equal fragments. These fragments are known as fission products. Fission may occur spontaneously or may be induced by the capture of bombarding particles, primarily neutrons. In addition to fission fragments, neutrons and energy in the form of gamma rays are usually by-products. The fission products from such reactions are usually from atomic numbers 42 (molybdenum) to 56 (barium), but may range from atomic numbers 30 through 64. Approximately 200 different radioactive nuclides are formed as fission products in the detonation of a nuclear device (atomic bomb). Uranium and plutonium are usually used in a nuclear reactor to produce some of the radioactive materials used in nuclear medicine. There are 40 or more different ways in which the nuclei of uranium and plutonium can split when fission occurs so that 80 or more different fission products can be produced.

Fission is a process which can either be controlled (the energy released does not reach explosive quantities) or it can be made uncontrolled as in an atomic device. The latter results in a nuclear explosion. The controlling of a fission reaction is based primarily on the slowing down of the highly energetic neutrons released from the reaction. A typical example of a fission reaction is described below:

$$^{103}_{42}\text{Mo} \xrightarrow{\beta^-} {}^{103}_{43}\text{Tc} \xrightarrow{\beta^-} {}^{103}_{44}\text{Ru} \xrightarrow{\beta^-} {}^{103}_{45}\text{Rh} \text{ (stable)}$$

$$^{235}_{92}\text{U} + {}^{1}_{0}\text{n} \longrightarrow {}^{236}_{92}\text{U} \qquad + 2{}^{1}_{0}\text{n} + \text{energy}$$

$$^{131}_{50}\text{Sn} \xrightarrow{\beta^-} {}^{131}_{51}\text{Sb} \xrightarrow{\beta^-} {}^{131}_{52}\text{Te} \xrightarrow{\beta^-} {}^{131}_{53}\text{I} \xrightarrow{\beta^-} {}^{131}_{54}\text{Xe} \text{ (stable)}$$

Uranium 235 absorbs a neutron to become uranium 236, liberating 2 neutrons, plus energy in the form of gamma photons. Uranium 236 splits into approximately 2 equal parts to begin two fission chains. One of these chains begins with molybdenum 103 and continues to stable rhenium 103; the other begins with tin 131 and continues to the stable xenon 131. Involved in these two fission chains are several radionuclides, other forms of which are used in nuclear medicine procedures (radioisotopes of molybdenum, tin, iodine, and xenon). Obviously, this could be one method of producing radionuclides for use in nuclear medicine.

According to the above reaction, each fission process liberates 2 neutrons. Assuming that each neutron generates another fission process, 4 neutrons would be released in the second generation. If each of these neutrons generated a fission process, the third generation would release 8 neutrons; the fourth, 16 neutrons; the fifth, 32 neutrons, and so on. Should this fission process go uncontrolled, the amount of energy and continued production of neutrons would reach the point of explosion. Such is the case of the atomic bomb. It has been calculated that in fewer than 90 generations the neutron yield would be sufficient to cause the fission of every nucleus in 110 pounds of uranium. This would result in the liberation of the same amount of energy as in the explosion of 1 million tons of TNT. If uncontrolled, this nintieth generation will be attained in less than one-millionth of a second.

Fortunately, with the use of nuclear reactors, fission can be controlled through the use of absorbing media resulting in a self-sustaining reaction. In this way, by-products of fission can be continuously produced and used for peaceful purposes.

FUSION

Fusion can be defined simply as the joining of light nuclei to form a heavier nucleus. When this occurs, neutrons and energy are released. This is also an exergonic process. A typical example of fusion is illustrated below:

$$_1^2H + {_1^2}H \rightarrow {_2^3}He + {_0^1}n + 3.22 \text{ mev}$$

Two deuterium molecules are brought together against extremely large forces of electrostatic repulsion until they actually fuse to produce a new nucleus. This fusion can only be accomplished by the acceleration of these deuterium particles to extremely high velocities. These velocities represent temperatures of millions of degrees. Only at this point will the particles collide with sufficient energy to fuse.

Although this is not a way in which radioactive materials are produced for nuclear medicine uses, it does represent a very interesting and hopefully useful source of energy. Its importance lies in the fact that water could be used as a source of energy since deuterium (^2H) occurs in 8 parts per 1,000 of ordinary hydrogen (^1H). The present problem is that, unlike the fission reaction, the fusion reaction is not self-sustaining. It requires the constant application of extremely high temperatures to sustain the reaction. In order that it be self-sustaining, the energy released from fusion must be fed back into the reaction. To date, no such method is available, although many researchers are working on the problem. When and if such a method is devised, it has been estimated that a cubic mile of water will provide enough energy for all man's needs forever.

A nonpeaceful use of the fusion reaction is the thermonuclear weapon. The term thermonuclear weapon is used because the weapon relates directly to the fusion reaction and can be brought about only in the presence of very high temperatures. This thermonuclear weapon is commonly referred to as the hydrogen bomb as opposed to the fission atomic bomb. The million degree temperature necessary to bring about a nuclear fusion reaction is provided by the initiation of the reaction with a nuclear fission reaction. A quantity of deuterium is combined with a fission weapon and upon detonation a combined fission-fusion reaction takes place with

65

the release of enormous energy. Weight for weight, the fusion of deuterium nuclei provides over three times as much energy as the fission of uranium or plutonium. It has been calculated that 1 lb of uranium produces as much energy as 8,000 tons of TNT, while 1 lb of deuterium produces energy equivalent to 26,000 tons of TNT.

NEUTRON ACTIVATION (NEUTRON CAPTURE)

One of the most common production methods of radioactive materials used in the nuclear medicine departments is neutron activation (neutron capture). Neutron activation involves the capture of a neutron into a stable nucleus with the subsequent emission of a gamma ray. This process is usually referred to as an (n, γ) process. Production of gold 198 from gold 197 by neutron activation is written as follows:

$$^{197}Au + {}_{0}^{1}n \rightarrow {}^{198}Au + \gamma$$

A shorthand method for indicating this neutron activation phenomenon is:

$$^{197}Au \ (n, \gamma) \ ^{198}Au$$

The product is always an isotope of the target element, but since it has incorporated a neutron into its nucleus, the product has a mass number increased by 1. The process usually involves neutrons of relatively low energy called *slow neutrons*. The bombardment of stable forms of an element by neutrons is usually carried out in nuclear reactors.

Since the product of such a reaction is an isotope of the target element, there is no possible way to separate these on a chemical basis. Further, it is impossible to create a situation in the reactor whereby all atoms of gold 197 incorporate a neutron to become gold 198. The material which is removed from the reactor following bombardment is necessarily a mixture of the two isotopes. For this reason, the gold 198 administered to a patient will also have a certain amount of stable gold 197. The latter is referred to as a *carrier*. To inform the user of the quantity of gold 197 in the gold 198 dose, the term *specific activity* is ordinarily used (see p. 92).

Neutron activation, in addition to being a means of obtaining radionuclides, has also become a dynamic tool in research and is developing into an exciting new field in medicine. Many areas of utilization have not even been touched yet. Some, however, are well known. Neutron activation is used not only in medicine but in the field of crime detection. Neutron activation analysis has been used to determine the presence of heavy metal poisons in tissues. This has been extremely valuable in medical-legal problems. It can also be used to quantitate very small quantities of elements in serum and other biologic samples. A human hair can be subjected to neutron activation for purposes of identification, chemical analysis, and so on. A paper chromatograph of a serum sample can be subjected to neutron activation analysis in an effort to determine the constituents of the serum. These are just a few of present-day applications of neutron activation.

TRANSMUTATION

Transmutation can be described as a process in which one element is converted into another. More specifically, it is the transformation of a nuclide of one element into a nuclide of a different element by nuclear reaction. Transmutation is often referred to as the answer to the alchemist's dream. Hundreds of years ago a group of "scientists" tried in vain to change common metals into gold. Their object was to bring about transmutation. Now, after years of investigation and accumulated knowledge of the nature of radioactive materials, the process of conversion from one element to another element by decay is well known. However, transmutation applies specifically, in the case of radionuclide production, to converting one stable element into another unstable element. An example of such a reaction is the conversion of stable sulfur 32 into radioactive phosphorus 32. This is accomplished by bombarding sulfur 32 with neutrons in such a manner as to eject a proton from its nucleus. In this manner, an element having one more neutron and one less proton is produced—phosphorus 32. This process is described as an (n, p) reaction according to the following:

$$\mathrm{^{32}_{16}S} + \mathrm{^{1}_{0}n} \rightarrow \mathrm{^{32}_{15}P} + \mathrm{^{1}_{1}p}$$

The shorthand method is written as follows:

$$\mathrm{^{32}_{16}S}\,(\mathrm{n, p})\,\mathrm{^{32}_{15}P}$$

As in neutron activation, transmutation also involves neutron bombardment (as well as bombardment with protons, deuterons, and alpha particles). In the case of transmutation, however, rather than bombarding with a slow neutron, the target element is bombarded with a fast neutron. The incorporation of a fast neutron into the nucleus is immediately followed by the emission of a proton. The advantage of the transmutation process is that the target and the product are no longer isotopes but are nuclides. Being two different elements, they are subject to separation by standard chemical techniques. Phosphorus 32 can easily be separated from the sulfur 32. In this way a pure product of phosphorus 32, referred to as *carrier-free,* is obtained. In a shipment of phosphorus 32 from a radiopharmaceutical supplier, the specific activity on the label will indicate *C.F.* for "carrier-free." Ideally, this would be the method of producing all radiopharmaceuticals, but methods are not known to produce all radiopharmaceuticals in this manner.

LINEAR ACCELERATORS AND CYCLOTRONS

Under the usual conditions that prevail in the atom, charged particles are unable to enter and/or interact with nuclei of other atoms because they have insufficient energy to penetrate the orbital electrons or the nucleus. A negatively charged particle, as it nears an atom, is repelled away from the negatively charged orbital electrons. Likewise, a positively charged particle would be repelled away from a positively charged nucleus. However, if sufficient energy is supplied to these charged particles, they can overcome these repulsion effects and penetrate the nucleus, causing an interaction. Devices that provide the energy necessary to perform this action are called particle accelerators. There are two basic types: the type which moves the particle in a straight path, called the linear accelerator, and the type which moves the particle in a circular path, such as a cyclotron, betatron, and synchrotron. Such devices can accelerate particles to the point where they possess energy from 1 million to 1 billion ev.

67

The linear accelerator is a high energy particle accelerator consisting of cylinders of increasing lengths arranged in a straight line. These linear accelerators can be as long as 2 miles in length. The particle acceleration is provided by means of a pulsing electrostatic or magnetic field.

One explanation of the function of linear accelerators is as follows. If a positively charged particle such as an alpha particle, proton, or deuteron (nucleus of deuterium atoms) were used at the beginning of the linear accelerator, and the first cylinder was charged negatively, the particle would be attracted by electrostatic attraction through the first cylinder, thereby gaining energy. As the particle nears the second cylinder, which is increased slightly in length, the charge of the cylinder through which it has just passed is reversed to a positive charge and the cylinder toward which it is approaching is charged negatively. The particle is attracted by the unlike charge in the second cylinder and repelled by the like charge in the cylinder through which it has just passed. This process of reversal of charges between cylinders continues throughout the entire length of the linear accelerator; each time it occurs the particle is accelerated further. In this way the particle can achieve tremendous energy levels. By achieving such high energies, the particles can overcome the repulsive effects of the nucleus and actually interact with it. In this way, stable nuclei are made unstable and accelerators become a source of radionuclides.

Another explanation of the internal workings of the linear accelerator is that electrons are fed into one end of the tube down which an electromagnetic wave of radiofrequency is traveling. The electrons are carried forward on this wave not unlike a surfboard being carried by an ocean wave. Linear accelerators of this type are used for radiotherapy. In this way, very high energy electrons (4 to 8 mev) may be produced through a distance of 1 to 2 meters. It is important that charged particles are used. Neutrons, gamma rays, and neutrinos are unacceptable as a bombarding material in this type of unit.

The principle of reversed electromagnetic charges is used in the cyclotron. The cyclotron was first described in 1931 by Lawrence and Livingston as a type of particle accelerator. In the cyclotron the particles are repeatedly accelerated through intermediate voltages to achieve high energy. The cyclotron consists of two hollow semicircular pieces of metal with a short gap between them. These semicircular pieces of metal are called "D's" because of their shape. The D's are mounted between the poles of the large electromagnet with the straight side of the D's abutting one another. Two D's arranged in this manner assume the shape of a circle; hence the name cyclotron. The particles are attracted into the first D which has an opposite electrical charge. The particle moves through the semicircular path of the D until it reaches the gap. At this point the electromagnetic fields are reversed. The D through which it just passed changes in charge so as to have a repulsive effect and the D into which it will now move will have an attractive effect. In this way the particle is accelerated. This process continues throughout the extent of the cyclotron until it reaches the target material. The particle now possesses extremely high energies and interacts with the target material to produce an altered nucleus, which is unstable. The source of the particles is arranged in the center of the circle formed by the two D's and the particles proceed outward in a spiral fashion until they reach the target material.

The cyclotron is generally a more versatile device compared to a reactor or a linear accelerator. It has an advantage over the linear accelerator because space does not present the problem for a cyclotron that it does for a linear accelerator. It has more advantages over a nuclear reactor because of the wider variety of nuclear particles it can employ. Another major advantage is that it is capable of producing certain useful radionuclides, primarily short-lived, which are not produced in significant quantities in nuclear reactors. A further advantage over reactors is that radioisotopes may be produced with much higher specific activity; they are often carrier-free. The disadvantage to the cyclotron over the nuclear reactor is that of operating costs. The operating cost for cyclotrons is much greater than that for nuclear reactors.

Protons are commonly used as a bombarding material in the cyclotron. Their source is a small amount of hydrogen placed in the center of the cyclotron. The hydrogen is then bombarded with electrons from tungsten filament removing the single electron in the orbit of the hydrogen atom and leaving the positive ion in the source. The nucleus of the hydrogen atom is a proton. At the present time, most of the standard nuclear medicine radionuclides are by-products of a nuclear reactor for economic reasons. Cyclotrons are employed for radioisotope production when they offer a significant advantage over reactors.

GENERATORS

Another method of radionuclide production is the generator. The generator has become a very convenient method of obtaining short-lived radionuclides at places distant to large-scale production sites. Their use has gained wide acceptance in the field of nuclear medicine because, by using such short-lived radionuclides, larger doses of radiopharmaceuticals can be injected with resultant decreased radiation dose to the patient and organs of interest, increased statistics necessary for more meaningful imaging results, and a continuous availability of a short-lived radionuclide in the nuclear medicine laboratory. Examples are molybdenum 99/technetium 99m generators and tin 113/indium 113m generators.

Physical characteristics. All generators are modifications of a basic physical arrangement. The generator consists of a small glass column containing an ion exchange material. The parent nuclide is firmly affixed (adsorbed) onto this material. The column of ion exchange material is held by a porous glass frit at the bottom of the column and a plastic ring at the top. An outer plastic housing is usually provided to guard against breakage during shipment and handling. Both ends of the system should be sealed to preserve sterility and pyrogen-free conditions within the column.

Principle of operation. The basis of operation for a radionuclide generator is that a relatively long-lived parent nuclide continually produces through radioactive decay a shorter-lived daughter nuclide. Separation of the daughter nuclide can be performed easily and repeatedly, usually on the basis of chemical separation techniques. This separation process is referred to as elution, or "milking."

69

The daughter nuclide is eluted from the parent nuclide (which remains on the ion exchange medium) and collected at the bottom of the column. Other elution processes are known, such as distillation, solvent extraction (MEK, methyl ethyl ketone) and precipitation; however, the simplicity of ion exchange media lend themselves well to the routine nuclear medicine laboratory. The daughter is eluted by introducing the recommended reagent through the top of the column and collecting the product solution from the bottom of the column. The product is then assayed for concentration of daughter nuclide.

This process of elution can be repeated as many times as is felt necessary; however, the percent yield will vary. After the daughter has been eluted, the daughter activity is low but begins to increase (regenerate) until it eventually attains the activity of the parent again. At this point, if undisturbed, the activity of the daughter nuclide appears to assume the half-life of the parent. The next elution repeats the cycle. (The parent continues to decay also but at a much slower rate than the daughter.) If the column has completely regenerated, the usual yield is approximately 70% of the parent activity. In the case of the ^{99}Mo-^{99m}Tc generator, regeneration requires from 18 to 23 hours. Any elutions which are performed before that time will result in lower yields per elution, however, a large net yield can be

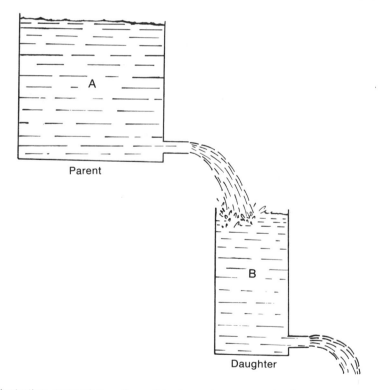

Parent

Daughter

Fig. 5-1. Illustration comparing radionuclide decay to a reservoir of water with an outlet. The number of molecules of water, the rate of flow from the outlet, and the diameter of the outlet are representative of the number of atoms in the radioactive sample, the rate of decay, and the fraction of the remaining number of atoms which decay per unit time (λ), respectively. The two reservoirs of water of varying size with outlets of the same size, in which the larger empties into the smaller, are analogous to a generator whose parent radionuclide has a longer half-life than the daughter radionuclide.

realized if several premature elutions are performed over any period of time. For example, one elution per day (at 8:00 A.M.) will yield ^{99m}Tc at approximately 70% of the activity of the ^{99}Mo, whereas two elutions per day (at 8:00 A.M. and 2:00 P.M.) will yield ^{99m}Tc at approximately 105% of the activity of ^{99}Mo. This is due to the exponential build-up of the daughter product following elution. This increased net yield carries with it a sacrifice of concentration.

The principle of generators becomes almost impossible to believe because the question always arises of how can the generator regenerate when 1 atom of molybdenum 99 with a 67-hour half-life decays to technetium 99m with a 6-hour half-life? The question is best answered, not on a one-atom-to-one-atom basis but with many atoms. An analogy may help to clarify the situation.

Radioactive decay (see Chapter 6) can be compared to a reservoir of water with an outlet at its base (Fig. 5-1). The molecules of water flowing through the outlet represent atoms undergoing the decay process, while the molecules in the tank represent radioactive atoms which have not yet decayed. The rate of flow of water molecules in both tanks is controlled only by the height of the column of water (flow rate is proportional to height of column) since the size of their outlets is the same. As the height of the column decreases by one-half, the flow rate decreases proportionally. This is also true in a sample of radioactivity; as the number of atoms in the original sample is reduced to one-half (half-life), the rate of decay is reduced proportionally. (Half-life is the time required for one-half the original number of atoms in a radioactive sample to disintegrate.)

It becomes clear from this analogy that for 2 radionuclides having two different half-lives but the same number of disintegrations per unit time, the radionuclide having the longer half-life must have a larger number of atoms in the sample. This situation is represented by the two reservoirs of water, tank A and tank B in Fig. 5-1. Since the flow rate (or disintegration rate) is exactly the same in both reservoirs, tank B will reach half height (half-life) in a shorter period of time because it has less water (fewer atoms).

The figure also demonstrates the probability of decay. It is impossible to predict which water molecules flowing from tank A to tank B will, in turn, flow from tank B. Some water molecules will flow immediately to the outlet and out of tank B, while others will flow inside tank B before being expelled. The overriding principle is that it is possible to predict the number of water molecules that will flow out of tank B per unit time. The same is true with a radioactive series of unstable parent and daughter atoms. The radioactive daughter atom may decay immediately upon being transmuted or may exist in its unstable state for a longer period of time. Although it is impossible to predict which atom will decay immediately, it is possible to predict how many atoms will decay from a given radioactive sample per unit time.

The analogy of reservoirs can also be extended to the operation of a generator. Since generators currently in use are those of relatively long-lived parents and relatively short-lived daughter products, the reservoirs of Fig. 5-1 accurately depict the situation. At the time of the initial elution, both reservoirs are full to capacity and the flow rates (decay rates, activity, disintegrations per unit time) are the same. The first elution decreases tank B to ≈30% capacity and tank A remains undisturbed. Because the height of the column of water has been reduced, the flow rate has also been reduced, analogous to decreased activity of the daughter product. As tank A continues to flow at the same rate into tank B, tank B will begin to fill up; at the same time the outflow continues at an increasingly greater rate because the column of water increases in height. The same is true in the generator. The parent nuclide continues to decay at the same rate, but because tank B following elution has fewer atoms, the rate of decay is decreased. Following elution, and since the parent nuclide continues to decay to the daughter at the same rate, the number of daughter atoms becomes increasingly greater and, therefore, the number of disintegrations per unit time (activity) becomes increasingly greater also. Eventually a point is reached at which tank B is filled to the same height as tank A and the flow rates of both reservoirs are again equal. The same point of complete regeneration is reached in the generator when the activity of the daughter nuclide is the same as the parent nuclide. Further, because the transmutation of the parent nuclide to the daughter nuclide is at the same rate as the daughter nuclide is to its successor, the half-life of the daughter appears to be the same as the parent. This is not true, of course, because the removal of the daughter from the parent allows the daughter to display its own characteristic half-life. The point at which the ratio of the two activities remains constant and both appear to decay with the half-life of the parent is called *transient equilibrium.*

Radiopharmacology. With the advent of generators, an intense interest in radiochemistry and radiopharmacology has developed. Before this time, all radiopharmaceuticals were purchased from commercial supply houses. The use of generators has allowed nuclear medicine departments to have a large quantity of radioactivity available which must be used or allowed to decay. The obvious economical answer is to use these new tools in many ways so that they might replace other radionuclides. Such has been the case with technetium 99m and indium 113m. Many radiochemical procedures have been developed that allow the nuclear medicine laboratory to utilize these short-lived radionuclides for more than one purpose. Some of these preparations are available in kit form, so a minimum of effort is necessary to produce these useful, short-lived radiodiagnostic scanning agents through "on-site" synthesis.

Technetium 99m can be used in the same form in which it is eluted (sodium pertechnetate, Na ^{99m}TcO$_4$) for both brain imaging and thyroid imaging. This is not true of indium 113m. The use of ^{113m}In in any imaging technique requires chemical manipulation. The same is true with any other form of ^{99m}Tc than that used for brain or thyroid imaging. Brain imaging has been accomplished with ^{113m}In but it must be chelated before administration. EDTA (ethylenediamine tetraacetic acid) and DTPA (diethylenetriamine pentaacetic acid) have both been used for this purpose. An advantage of indium compounds is that no radioactivity accumulates in the choroid plexus or salivary glands.

Kidney imaging is accomplished with the same chelated preparation of indium 113m. Technetium 99m can be used for kidney visualization also, but the technetium must be converted to an iron complex for this purpose.

Liver imaging can be performed with both technetium 99m and indium 113m, but both agents must be utilized as colloid preparations. ^{99m}Tc is used as a technetium sulfide colloid, stabilized by either gelatin or dextran. Reactions have been noted in patients receiving the dextran preparation. Indium 113m is used as a colloidal preparation with gelatin for the same purpose. As a colloid, the mode of action is the same as colloidal gold 198, whereby the cells of the reticulo-endothelial system selectively remove the suspended colloid particles from circulation.

Lung imaging has also been effected through the use of both indium and technetium. Just as ^{131}I-labeled macroaggregated human serum albumin (MAA) is trapped in the lung, so also is ^{99m}Tc-labeled MAA. The chemical and physical manipulations of this preparation become difficult for the routine nuclear medicine laboratory. Indium 113m has also been used for lung imaging but as an indium ferric hydroxide (^{113m}In Fe(OH)$_3$) particle. An advantage with the latter is that there is no accumulation in the thyroid as with ^{131}I and ^{99m}Tc preparations and therefore no blocking agents are necessary.

Blood pool imaging, both cardiac and placental, have been performed using both indium and technetium compounds. Technetium 99m labeled human serum albumin is the form of the technetium compound, while indium 113m stabilized with gelatin at a pH of 3.5 is the form of the indium compound, the latter is easier to prepare.

Another use of technetium has been as a spleen imaging agent. Erythrocytes from the patient are labeled with technetium which are then heat-altered. Upon reinjection into the patient the spleen sequesters these red blood cells and imaging techniques can be employed.

The future of nuclear medicine seems to rest on the greater utilization of generators and their products. As the field ages, it appears that many different types of generators will become useful and many new preparations of their products will be realized.

THE TRILINEAR CHART OF THE NUCLIDES
Marshall Brucer, M.D.

At the beginning of the twentieth century the main problem in chemistry was the periodic table of the atoms. The table was filling rapidly but some puzzling inconsistencies occurred among the naturally radioactive elements, uranium, thorium, and radium. Some substances with very different physical properties could not be separated chemically. There seemed to be more than one kind of lead; but all lead had the same chemistry.

Kasimer Fajans (a German physical chemist, now at the University of Michigan) had developed a "displacement law" to explain the pattern of radioactive decay. In 1912 he found a way to explain the puzzling inconsistencies, but it demanded more than one element in one spot on the periodic table. Soddy, in England, called these isotopes, and pointed out that if some substances had equal atomic number (chemical properties) but different atomic weight (physical properties), then there must also be some substances with equal weight but different atomic number. Eventually, the latter were called isobars.

The number of electrons in an atom was soon related to the number of positive charges (protons) in the nucleus of the atom. This was the atomic number (Z). It was postulated that the remainder of the nucleus was made up of uncharged particles much like the proton but neutral in charge (neutrons). Chadwick, in England, discovered these in 1932. The atomic number was the number of protons (iodine has 53, hence $_{53}$I). The atomic weight was the number of protons plus neutrons (one of the iodines has 53 plus 78, hence $_{53}^{131}$I). If there are isotopes with equal proton number, and isobars with equal weight, then there should also be substances with an equal number of neutrons. These were called isotones.

Discovery of radioisotopes

Atom smashing was popular about 1930 in the study of the structure of the atom. Frederick Joliot, in Paris, noticed that the target he was bombarding with radium alpha particles remained radioactive after the bombardment stopped. After careful investigation, he and his wife (the daughter of Madame Curie) found they had produced an artificial isotope of phosphorus ($_{15}^{30}$P). Thirty-six years after she and her husband had discovered the first naturally radioactive element (polonium), Madame Curie had the pleasure of hearing her daughter and son-in-law announce the discovery of the first artificial radioactive substance.

However, the neutron was thought to be a better bombardment projectile for making artificial radioisotopes. Enrico Fermi, in Italy, bombarded many elements and found about 60 new radioactive species. Physicists began to look for other new radioisotopes. Ten years earlier, Otto Hahn, a German chemist, while trying to straighten out some difficulties in the uranium chain of decay, found two substances with entirely different half-lives, but they were the same isotope, isobar, and isotone. By 1935, physicists were finding more of these unusual species. Lisa Meitner, the long-time physicist-associate of Hahn, called these isomers.

During World War II, Fermi's nuclear reactor and the newer, more powerful cyclotrons were used to create more nuclear reactions to produce even more radioactive nuclides. By 1947 there were about 800 known species; it was becoming too complex to talk about an isotope-isobar-isotone-isomer. Turner, an American physicist, in 1947, proposed the name "nuclide" to signify any specific arrangement of protons and neutrons. The term was quickly adopted and the science became nuclear, not isotope, physics; chemistry became nuclear, not isotope, chemistry. Medical societies, soon to be formed, adopted the name "nuclear medicine."

However, before World War II, the nuclear sciences had revolved around the chemical similarity of reactions of isotopes. The first chemical, and then biologic use of a nuclide had been because of its chemical isotopy. The name "isotopes" caught hold with physicians and political administrators who did not know the historical background. The newspapers picked up the catchword. By the time medical people began to use radionuclides the improper term radioisotopes was embedded in the language.

But the medical and tracer people were not using "isotopes." Once they had obtained, for example, an isotope of iodine, they measured its decay to xenon. They were using an isobar relationship. The cyclotron people were using isotone relationships.

In 1946, William H Sullivan, one of the chief chemists at Oak Ridge, Tennessee, put all the known radioactive and stable nuclides onto a chart of many hexagons.

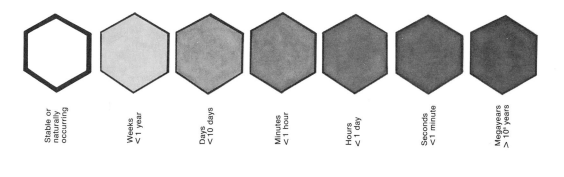

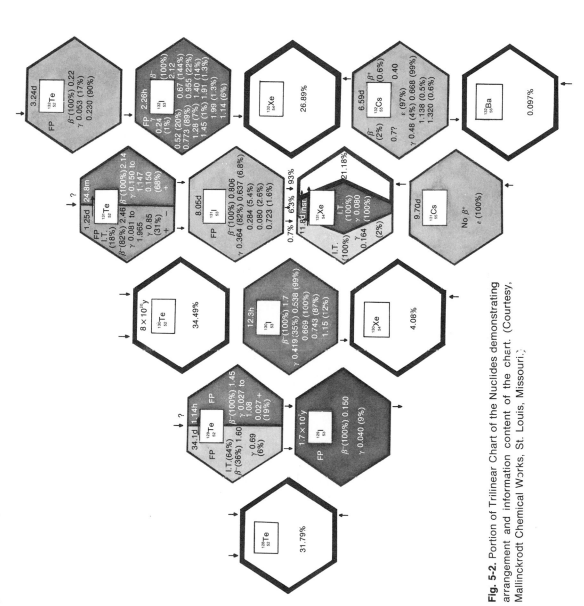

Fig. 5-2. Portion of Trilinear Chart of the Nuclides demonstrating arrangement and information content of the chart. (Courtesy, Mallinckrodt Chemical Works, St. Louis, Missouri.)

Each hexagon represented one nuclide. One axis of the hexagonal array signified isotopes; a second axis signified isobars; the third axis signified isotones. Production, chemistry, physics, or medical use didn't matter to Sullivan. He had plotted the first trilinear chart of the nuclides.

Every physicist who looked at the 1946 trilinear chart knew there were more nuclides to be discovered. By 1968, approximately 1,800 had been found and there were a few hundred (or more) yet to be discovered. If each hexagon is to be a complete designation of a nuclide, a tremendous amount of data is involved—much too much for a chart. Also, the fine details are changing with each increase in accuracy. A special journal, *Nuclear Data* and a summary "Table of Isotopes" are published periodically to keep researchers up to date.* Physicists and chemists need the complete tabular data. Clinical physicians need only a small fragment, and this much can be put in chart form. Fig. 5-2 shows 15 of the almost 1,800 nuclides.

The central box in each hexagon gives the proper name of the nuclide. All of the iodines (I) have the same number of protons ($_{53}$I). One nuclide of the iodine has 76 neutrons plus 53 protons, or 129 nucleons ($^{129}_{53}$I); one has 79 neutrons ($^{132}_{53}$I). Iodine 117 to iodine 139 have been demonstrated; and there are undoubtedly more.

Two of the 23 known iodine nuclides ($^{120}_{53}$I and $^{126}_{53}$I) have isomers. Hence, there are more than 25 different kinds of iodine. Only one kind of iodine is stable ($^{127}_{53}$I). Each hexagon shows not only a nuclide, but also an isobar, an isotone, and an isotope.

The choice of data

By the time Sullivan's chart had gone through a few editions, the data had become so complex that Sullivan had to leave something out. He wanted to make a medical chart, but with the rapid changes in medical demands, he did not know what data was important (and neither did anyone else). However, some items were obviously necessary.

Half-life. Half-life is so important in medical use that it was put immediately above the name plate. For example, iodine 132 has a half-life of 2.26 hours; iodine 129 has a half-life of 20 million years. The amount of any nuclide that can be given to a patient is probably the first consideration of a clinician. However, is the amount the physical dose of radiation or the chemical dose of the nuclide? The dose of a radionuclide is usually measured in millicuries (1 mCi is the number of atoms that will result in 37 million disintegrations per second). Because the disintegrations of iodine 129 occur over such a long time, it would take about 62 grams to produce 1 mCi. A proper large chemical dose is in the milligram range. Only picograms of iodine 132 are needed for a millicurie (a picogram is $\frac{1}{1000}$ of a nanogram, which is $\frac{1}{1000}$ of a microgram, which is $\frac{1}{1000}$ of a milligram, which is $\frac{1}{1000}$ of a gram). A true "tracer" chemical dose of the short-lived iodines (hours to weeks) can be given with an extremely large nontracer physical dose of radiation. Both concepts are implied in half-life.

*Nuclear data, Section B, New York, Academic Press, 1967 to date; Lederer, C. M., Hollander, J. M., and Perlman, I.: Table of isotopes, ed. 6, New York, 1967, John Wiley & Sons, Inc.

A 24-hour thyroid uptake could be measured with iodine 132. But even if a full millicurie were given, at 24 hours there would only be ½ of ½ of ½ of ½ . . . (10 half-lives) . . . left, and approximately three-fourths of this would have been excreted. However, in order to give the original millicurie, a day's shipping time from the pharmaceutical house would have to be allowed. A curie would be ordered to give a millicurie to measure a fraction of a microcurie—this is feasible, but not practical.

High, low, and medium radiation energy levels. Just as important as half-life is whether the energy of radiation emission is highly penetrating or below the limits of the detecting instruments. The trilinear chart gives the energy of gamma emission of iodine 132 as 773 kev plus many other energies. This is supervoltage radiation which demands tremendous shielding. On the full chart, the gamma emissions range from 520 kev to almost 2 mev. The tremendous shielding necessary might be totally impractical in a busy clinical laboratory.

A high energy gamma ray has little chance of being stopped by a piece of tissue. If it is stopped, however, it has great effect. A low energy gamma ray will not cause as much effect, but it is more likely to be stopped. The same is true in a radiation measuring instrument. Gamma rays much under 0.1 mev or much over 0.5 mev cause problems in the clinical laboratory. This is why most medical nuclides are selected from the medium range: iodine 131—0.364 mev, gold 198 = 0.412 mev, and technetium 99m = 0.140 mev.

Pattern of decay. Radium 226 with a half-life of 1,602 years decays to 3.8-day radon 222. For many medical uses the shorter-lived (and less expensive) radon is more valuable than the longer-lived radium. Early in the 1920's, Failla, a New York medical radiation physicist, devised a method to milk (elute) the radon from a large radium source.

Tellurium 132 has a 3.24-day half-life and 2.26-hour iodine 132 can be milked from a well-shielded tellurium source in the laboratory. This was the first artificial nuclide cow (generator) developed in the early 1950's. Although iodine 132 is useless for long-term medical studies, it is valuable in short-term studies. Shielding, contamination, cost, transportation, and other half-life problems can often be solved by the use of a cow system. About 118 cow systems are available and awaiting development.

Iodine 132 decays to stable xenon 132 (a white hexagon with heavy border). Xenon 132 is also naturally occurring; 26.89% of natural xenon is xenon 132.

Iodine 131 is a little more complex. Only 93% will decay to stable xenon 131 (which, incidentally, is also 21.18% of natural xenon). Xenon 131 is a triple isomer; 6.3% of iodine 131 will decay to xenon 131m. This isomer is not used in medicine because it has a half-life of only a fraction of a nanosecond. But 0.7% of iodine 131 decays to xenon 131m[1]; its 11.8-day half-life is longer than that of the original iodine 131. The 0.7% is too small to be of any concern in routine clinical work. During a long-term iodine retention study, within a few weeks there would be more xenon 131m[1] than there would be iodine 131.

The gamma emission of iodine 131 at 364 kev can easily be distinguished from the gamma emission of xenon 131m[1] at 164 kev. The older iodine 131 literature shows iodine 131 with a half-life of 8.08, 8.07, or 8.05 days. Some of the confusion was caused by whether the half-life of iodine 131 *only* was being measured, or the half-life of its decay product was included.

The 6.6-day cesium 132 nuclide shown on the sample chart decays with the emission of either a negatron (β^-) or a positron (β^+) emission. The negatron decay yields barium 132; the positron decay yields xenon 132. This double decay pattern is more common at the upper end of the periodic table where decay can be partially alpha and partially beta emission. It is not very serious in routine medical pharmacology, but it can be very serious in precise chemical work. Succeeding daughters can confuse the counting problem in routine work.

Of the 5 nuclides of tellurium shown on the sample chart, 2 are stable and 2 are double isomers, each with a double pathway of decay. Tellurium 131 forms a valuable cow system. Iodine 131 can be made more cheaply in a nuclear reactor by neutron bombardment of tellurium 130. The pharmaceutical manufacturer buys 1.25-day tellurium 131, which decays to the 8-day iodine 131 during shipping. A simple final extraction of iodine yields a very pure iodine 131.

The converse cow systems, best known in clinical medicine, are short-lived daughters from long-lived parents. The inverse system of long-lived daughters from short-lived parents is probably more important, even though the conversion occurs before the physician gets the pharmaceutical.

The most popular of the cows (technetium 99m) was an internal cow system before it was a generator in the laboratory. The first use of technetium 99m was in liver scanning, even though pertechnetate does not localize in the liver. The investigator injected 2.78-day molybdenum 99, which does localize in the liver. While in the liver, it decayed to technetium 99m, which gave off the 140 kev radiation that was used for liver scanning. Molybdenum 99 scanning is very safe and it makes the required assay of technetium generators for minute fractions of molybdenum a typical example of health physics poppycock.

Medical trilinear chart

Many details are essential to physicists and chemists. Other details are especially essential in pharmaceutical research. In ordinary clinical laboratory work, half-life, decay pattern, and proportion and energy of beta and gamma emission are about all that can be included on a simplified chart. Some health physics types would like to see the average beta energy included for dosage calculations. However, the average energy has been measured for only a few of the nuclides, and the dosage calculations are of absolutely no value. Neutron cross-sections might be of great importance in diagnostic procedures in the future. Electron spin characteristics are conceivably of future importance. However, there is no room for these data on a simplified chart.

The simplified trilinear chart of the nuclides is available to any physician or technologist using radionuclides for medical purposes. A large wall chart is available for the nuclear medicine laboratory.*

---

*Brucer, M.: Trilinear chart of the nuclides; available from Mallinckrodt/Nuclear, Box 10172, Lambert Field, St. Louis, Missouri 63145. Regular chart, no charge; wall chart, $2.00.

Chapter

6

Radiation measurement and protection

The many aspects of radiation measurement and consequent protection should become a primary consideration any time radioactive materials are used. The actual effects of radiation are not completely known, but it can generally be stated that all radioactivity is injurious; therefore, steps must be taken to prevent unnecessary exposure. A number of factors affect the radiation as to its possible injurious effect. These specific factors include type and energy of the radiation, penetration power, ionization ability, radioactive half-life, biologic half-life, and effective half-life. In addition, personnel who will use radioactive materials must be introduced to the various units of radiation measurement and must recognize the necessity for certain limitations to radiation exposure.

MEASUREMENT OF RADIATION

Basically, two parameters are used to define the various terms of radiation measurement: the ionization of matter by radiation and the energy absorbed by matter from radiation. From these two basic concepts four kinds of radiation measurement have been derived: (1) the roentgen, (2) the radiation absorbed dose (rad), (3) the roentgen equivalent, physical (rep), and (4) the roentgen equivalent, man (rem). A fifth unit describes the number of atoms that disintegrate per unit time, the curie and its submultiples. All of these are used or have been used in the past as units of radiation measurement.

The roentgen. The roentgen (r) is that quantity of x- or gamma radiation such that the associated corpuscular emission per 0.001293 gm of air produces, in air, ions carrying 1 electrostatic unit of quantity of electricity of either sign. There are two important terms to be emphasized in the definition of a roentgen. The roentgen is a measurement of radiation *quantity*, not intensity. It is a measure of the total exposure and does not involve the time over which exposure is administered. Secondly, it is a unit only of *x-rays* or *gamma rays*.

The rad (radiation absorbed dose). The rad is a measure of the amount of energy imparted to matter by ionizing radiation per unit mass of irradiated material at the place of interest. One rad is equal to 100 ergs of absorbed energy per gram of absorbing material. There are two areas which warrant emphasis in this definition. A rad includes *any* ionizing radiation, as distinguished from the roentgen, which applies only to x-rays or gamma rays. Secondly, the rad is only a measure of the energy absorbed by the material of interest and is not directly related to quantity or intensity of the radiation field.

The rep (roentgen equivalent, physical). The rep unit has become obsolete and has been replaced by the rad unit. The rep is the quantity of radiation which

79

Table 6-1. Relative biologic effectiveness of various types of radiation

Radiation	RBE
Alpha	20
Beta	1
Gamma	1
X-	1

produces per gram of tissue an ionization equivalent to the quantity of ionization of 1 roentgen of gamma radiation in air. Values have become confusing and range anywhere from 93 to 97 ergs per gram. Because of the confusion, the rad unit was adopted to take its place. The value of the rad was arbitrarily set at 100 ergs per gram by the International Commission on Radiological Units at the Seventh International Congress of Radiology, July, 1953.

The RBE (relative biologic effectiveness). RBE is a term used to indicate that different types of radiation have different effects in biologic materials or biologic systems. More specifically, it is the ratio of an absorbed dose of x-rays or gamma rays to the absorbed dose of any radiation required to produce an identical biologic effect. This definition can be written as a formula:

$$RBE = \frac{\text{dose in rads to produce effect with x-rays or gamma rays}}{\text{dose in rads to produce effect with radiation under investigation}}$$

For example, it is known that an absorbed dose of 0.05 rad of alpha radiation produces the same biologic effect as an absorbed dose of 1 rad of x- or gamma radiation. The RBE for an alpha particle would be determined by the following:

$$RBE = \frac{1.0 \text{ rad}}{0.05 \text{ rad}} = 20$$

Accordingly, the RBE value for an alpha particle is 20. Although all ionizing radiations are capable of producing similar biologic effects, the effect varies from one type of radiation to another based on the absorbed dose (rad) (Table 6-1). This relative biologic effectiveness of physically different ionizing radiations depends solely on the number of ionization events, commonly referred to as linear energy transfer (LET). Since the LET is a function of the charge and velocity of the ionizing particle, it requires less alpha radiation to produce the same biologic effect as x- or gamma radiation (see Chapter 7, p. 108).

The rem (roentgen equivalent, man). The rem is a unit of human biologic dose as a result of exposure to one or many types of ionizing radiation. It is equal to the absorbed dose in rads times the relative biologic effectiveness of the particular type of radiation being absorbed. Another way of expressing it is:

$$\text{Dose in rem} = \text{dose in rad} \times RBE$$

Should the radiation being measured be that of x-, gamma, or beta radiation, the rem value would be equal to the rad value, since the RBE value of all three types of emissions is 1.

There is a distinct difference between the three major forms of radiation measurement. The roentgen is considered the unit of exposure dose; the rad is a unit

Table 6-2. Multiples and submultiples of the curie

Units	Disintegrations/second (dps)	Disintegrations/minute (dpm)
Megacurie	3.7×10^{16}	2.2×10^{18}
Kilocurie	3.7×10^{13}	2.2×10^{15}
Curie (Ci)	3.7×10^{10}	2.2×10^{12}
Millicurie (mCi)	3.7×10^{7}	2.2×10^{9}
Microcurie (μCi)	3.7×10^{4}	2.2×10^{6}
Millimicrocurie (mμCi) also called nanocurie	3.7×10 or 37	2.2×10^{3} or 2,200
Micromicrocurie ($\mu\mu$Ci) also called a picocurie	3.7×10^{-2}	2.2

of absorbed radiation dose, and the rem is a unit of biologic dose. All three units are used in various situations in nuclear medicine. The roentgen, or more commonly, its submultiple the milliroentgen, is used as a value for most survey meter readings. The rad is used as a unit to describe the amount of exposure received by the organ of interest upon injection of a radiopharmaceutical; and the rem is the unit used to express exposure values of some personnel monitoring devices (film badges, for example).

The curie. When a radioactive nucleus changes to another nucleus, the change is called decay or disintegration. The rate of decay is spoken of in terms of disintegrations per unit of time, usually in seconds or minutes. The curie (Ci) is defined as a unit of radioactivity in which the number of disintegrations per second is 3.7×10^{10}. By multiplying this unit by 60 the definition can be expressed as disintegrations per minute (dpm), 2.2×10^{12} dpm. Multiples and submultiples of the curie unit can be expressed similarly in disintegrations per second and disintegrations per minute according to the Table 6-2.

Conversions between radiation units

Conversions can be made among all of these units, but usually only through rather complicated mathematical manipulations; roentgens can be calculated in rads, rads can be calculated in rems, and so on. The Atomic Energy Commission regulations state that roentgens, rads, and rems are almost identical and for all practical purposes x-, gamma, and beta radiations are treated as having identical values. It is felt that precise conversion methods are not within the scope of this book. There is, however, one conversion that may find practicality in the nuclear medicine laboratory. This is the conversion of units of activity (millicuries) to exposure rate (milliroentgens per hour: mr/hr). This correlation can be used to calibrate survey meters.

Having a known source of activity, one can calculate the exposure rate from any gamma point source by the following formula:

$$mr/hr = \frac{n \times I_\gamma}{s^2}$$

n = number of millicuries
I_γ = mr/hr at 1 meter/millicurie
s = distance in meters

Since this formula is for any gamma point source, a point source of cobalt 60 can be used as a calibration source. The formula and the I_γ values can be found in the *Radiological Health Handbook*.* These values are constant for each gamma source. In the case of cobalt 60, $I_\gamma = 1.23$ (Other I_γ values: $^{226}Ra = 0.84$, $^{131}I = 0.21$.)

The above formula can be used to find a survey meter reading for a 5 mCi point source of cobalt 60 at a distance of 1 meter:

$$mr/hr = \frac{5 \times 1.23}{1^2}$$
$$mr/hr = 6.15$$

A similar calculation is available for radium as the calibration source:

$$mr/hr = \frac{\text{number of milligrams of radium}}{s^2} \quad (6\text{-}2)$$
$$s = \text{distance to the source in yards}$$

The same formula using distances in terms of centimeters is as follows:

$$mr/hr = \frac{8400 \times \text{number of milligrams of radium}}{s^2} \quad (6\text{-}3)$$
$$s = \text{distance in centimeters}$$

Any of the above formulas may prove beneficial to persons working in the nuclear medicine department, because continuous calibration of survey meters is necessary. In some cases, a calibration check source is provided with the survey meter. Its value should be known and checked at each use. Should the value vary, the survey meter should be recalibrated. Too often this check source is used solely to check for functional batteries.

MAXIMUM PERMISSIBLE DOSE (MPD)

Since radiation is generally thought to be harmful to human beings, the ideal would be no radiation exposure at all. However, the use of radiation and radioactive materials, in many instances, has been proved to be beneficial to mankind. Since man is therefore going to use these radiation emitting materials, some methods must be devised to allow their use within safe limits. This establishment of a compromise became the problem of the National Committee on Radiation Protection and Measurements (NCRP). The NCRP was to establish that dose of ionizing radiation which in light of present knowledge is not expected to cause appreciable bodily injury to a person at any time during his lifetime. The acceptance of such a dose involves the acceptance of a risk as well, for there is a possibility that the radiation dose will manifest itself during the lifetime of the exposed person or in subsequent generations. The probability, however, is so low that the risk would be acceptable to the average individual. Such a dose was termed by the NCRP as a "permissible" dose, and on April 18, 1958, the Committee established the Maximum Permissible Dose (MPD). This statute allows the radiation worker to receive a maximum dose to the whole body of 5 rems per year after

---

*Published by U.S. Department of Health, Education and Welfare, Division of Radiological Health, Washington, D.C., Sept., 1960.

the age of 18 according to the following formula:

$$MPD = 5 \, (N - 18) \text{ rem}$$
$$N = \text{age in years}$$

The interpretation of this formulation is explained in Title 10 of the *Code of Federal Regulations,* Part 20.101 (10CFR20.101) by stipulating the two methods of recording and calculating the radiation exposure to occupational personnel.

The method used by most routine nuclear medicine departments is to limit the radiation exposure received by occupational personnel to doses per calendar quarter* according to the following schedule:

1. Whole body; head and trunk; active blood forming organs; lens of the eyes; or gonads—1.25 rems per quarter
2. Hands and forearms; feet and ankles—18.75 rems per quarter
3. Skin of the whole body—7.5 rems per quarter

The licensee may not permit any individual to receive a dose in excess of any of these values. Using this method the licensee is required to complete or at least be able to supply the information requested on Form AEC-5. Records are not required of the individual's accumulated occupational exposure doses prior to each quarter. A licensee may permit any employee to receive any two or all three of the specified radiation doses concurrently, provided a separate Form AEC-5 is maintained for each type of dose. All such records are preserved for 5 years.

The other method of calculating the radiation exposure to occupational personnel is to use the MPD formula in its strictest sense, a method generally considered consistent with only very hazardous uses of radioactive materials. The MPD formula is applicable to radiation exposure to the whole body, head and trunk, lens of the eye, active blood forming organs, or gonads. The formula indicates that the maximum permissible dose to these organs and sections of the body shall not exceed 5 rems multiplied by the number of years beyond age 18. The Committee also stipulates that the dose in any quarter-year (13 consecutive weeks) could be as large as 3 rems if the total occupational exposure during the lifetime of the individual does not exceed the MPD value calculated by the above formula.

The interpretation of this formula implies that one cannot work with radiation before the age of 18. Further, it places a premium on older personnel since, as one gets older, more radiation can be accumulated per year (provided the person never receives maximum exposure). According to this formula, one could build up a "bank" or reserve of permissible exposure (age-prorated maximum). One application of the use of the bank of permissible exposure is as follows. If a radiation worker had 7 rems in his bank of permissible exposure, he could receive 3 rems per quarter for the entire next year (or 12 rems for that year) before using up his bank of permissible exposure (see Table 6-3). Beyond this period of time, radiation exposures would be limited to 1.25 rems per quarter (or 5 rems per year).

*Thirteen complete, consecutive weeks; *or* the period between a date in January of any year to the same date in April, in July, and in October; *or* the quarters may be the first 14 weeks, the next 12 weeks, the next 14 weeks and the last 12 complete, consecutive calendar weeks.

Table 6-3. Exposure permissible per quarter for a person with a bank of 7 rems

Quarter	Bank at start of quarter (rem)	Suggested MPD per quarter (rem)	Total MPD (rem)	Allowable MPD per quarter (rem)	Bank at end of quarter (rem)
1	7	1.25	8.25	3	5.25
2	5.25	1.25	6.5	3	3.5
3	3.5	1.25	4.75	3	1.75
4	1.75	1.25	3	3	0

In addition to the above exposure limits to critical organs, there are several other stipulations regarding radiation exposure:

1. Accumulated dose of external exposure (radiation workers)
   a. Skin of the whole body: $MPD = 10(N - 18)$ and the dose in any 13 consecutive weeks shall not exceed 6 rems
   b. Hands and forearms; feet and ankles: $MPD = 75$ rems per year and the dose in any 13 consecutive weeks shall not exceed 25 rems
2. Emergency dose (radiation workers): An accidental or emergency dose of 25 rems to the whole body or a major portion thereof, occurring only once in a lifetime of the person need not be included in the determination of the radiation exposure status of that person.
3. Medical dose (radiation workers): Radiation exposure resulting from necessary medical and dental procedures need not be included in the determination of the radiation exposure status of the person concerned.
4. Dose to persons outside of controlled areas: The radiation or radioactive material outside a controlled area attributable to normal operation within the controlled area shall be such that it is improbable that any individual will receive a dose of more than 0.5 rems in any one year from external radiation.

In order to use this method of calculating occupational radiation exposure records, each licensee, according to 10CFR20.102, must:

1. Obtain a completed Form AEC-4, signed by the individual, showing each period of time after the individual attained the age of 18 in which the individual received an occupational dose of radiation, and
2. Calculate on Form AEC-4 . . . the previously accumulated occupational dose received by the individual, and the additional dose allowed for that individual . . . In any case where a licensee is unable to obtain reports of the individual's occupational dose for a previous complete calendar quarter, it shall be assumed that the individual has received the maximum permissible dose.*

All such records will be preserved for a period of 5 years. Regardless of the method used to calculate occupational personnel radiation exposure, any excesses are considered overexposures and must be reported to the Commission as specified in 10CFR20.403. In addition, any personnel experiencing these overexposures must be removed from all exposure to radiation for the balance of the quarter.

*The assumed MPD value should be 3.75 rems per calendar quarter before 1/1/61; 1.25 rems per calendar quarter after 1/1/61.

SPECIFIC FACTORS INVOLVED IN RADIATION PROTECTION
Type of radiation

In nuclear medicine three types of emissions are of primary concern—alpha particles, beta particles, and gamma rays. In addition, there are x-rays resulting from several phenomena of interaction with matter, but these are generally very weak in nature and of no particular concern as far as radiation protection is concerned. One fact to be considered is that of external emission versus internal emission—whether the radiation comes from outside the body and penetrates the epidermis into the body, or whether the emitters are already inside the body having been introduced via ingestion, inhalation, or intravenous injection. Gamma rays and x-rays are able to penetrate the epidermis of the skin and, therefore, present the same hazard whether they are external or internal emitters. Such is not the case with alpha and beta emitters. Alpha and beta particles cannot ordinarily penetrate the outer layers of the skin. As external emitters they do not usually constitute a serious problem with radiation protection. If they are used as internal emitters, however, the problem of alpha and beta radiation damage becomes severe.

Penetration power

As stated above, alpha particles and beta particles are not generally regarded as radiation hazards as external emitters. A 1.0 mev alpha particle has a range in tissue of 0.0006 cm and a 5 mev alpha particle has a range of 0.0037 cm. An alpha particle would require an energy of 7.5 mev in order to penetrate human skin. Under ordinary circumstances, a piece of paper will stop an alpha particle.

The penetration power of beta particles is about 100 times that of alpha particles. An inch of wood or $\frac{1}{25}$ inch of aluminum is required to stop a beta particle. The range in tissue for a 1 mev beta particle is 0.42 cm and for a 5 mev beta particle 2.2 cm. Although an external beta emitter is generally considered not to be of consequence as far as radiation protection is concerned, a beta particle can penetrate from a few millimeters to 1 cm beneath the skin. There is a rapid deceleration of the particle as a result of its interaction with tissue.

Gamma rays have extremely high penetration power and can create radiation hazards as either external or internal emitters. The gamma ray cannot be stopped by paper or small amounts of aluminum or lead. In general, protection is spoken of in terms of inches of lead and feet of concrete. In contrast to total absorption of an alpha or beta particle, only 3% of the gamma ray energy is absorbed in 1 cm of tissue. The rest is either absorbed in a much larger volume of tissue or travels through and completely out of the body.

Ionization

Ionization in tissue is thought to be the most important biologic interaction of radiation. Almost all of the damage to tissue is as a result of this phenomenon. The ability to ionize varies tremendously among alpha, beta, and gamma emissions. A term that is used to describe this phenomenon is *specific ionization,* which is defined as the number of ion pairs produced per unit of path. The specific ionization for a 1 mev alpha particle in air is 60,000 ion pairs per centimeter in air. This is greatly increased over the specific ionization for 1 mev beta particle which is 45 ion pairs per centimeter in air. The specific ionization of gamma photons is reduced even more.

There seems to be an important correlation between the ionization ability and the penetration power of the various emissions. The alpha particles are very weak in their penetration power, but the ionization ability reaches tremendous proportions. If alpha particles by-pass the epidermis, they present a tremendous problem in radiation biology. This is also true of beta emitters. Although beta emitters do not have as great an ionization ability, they have increased penetration power. However, their penetration power is not such that they can penetrate far beyond the skin. Based on their ionization ability, beta emitters can cause tremendous biologic damage provided the protective layer of the skin is by-passed. It is for this reason that phosphorus 32, a pure beta emitter, is used therapeutically in cases of leukemia and polycythemia. The rationale for its use is based solely on its ability for localized destruction of tissue function. Since most radiopharmaceuticals are beta-gamma emitters, the beta component represents the largest contribution of radiation dose as an internal emitter. In some cases, 90 to 95% of the dose is from the beta component. Although alpha and beta particles cannot penetrate the skin, there must still be protection against them. Because of their ability to ionize tissue once they have by-passed the skin, they present more of a radiation hazard than gamma photons, although the damage will be localized.

Physical half-life

The physical half-life ($T_{1/2}$ or T_p) is often called the radioactive half-life. It is defined as the length of time required for one-half of the original number of atoms in a given radioactive sample to disintegrate. This reduction of the number of atoms through disintegration of their nuclei is known as radioactive decay and is inherent to all radioactive materials. The rate of decay of a given isotope remains constant. It cannot be influenced by temperature, pressure, or chemical combination. Further, every atom in a radioactive sample has the same probability of disintegrating.

Because of decay, all radioactivity decreases with time, since fewer atoms are left as some atoms decay. Since the fraction of nuclei disintegrating per unit time is always the same, and since progressively fewer atoms are left, the fraction of remaining atoms represents fewer and fewer atoms with the passage of time. This fraction of the remaining number of atoms which decay per unit of time is called the *decay constant* (λ). The larger the fraction the faster will be the process of decay. Stated another way, the larger the decay constant, the shorter the half-life will be. Therefore, $T_{1/2}$ is inversely proportional to λ. If one were to plot on linear paper the number of atoms present in a given radioactive sample versus time, the curve shown in Fig. 6-1, *A* would be obtained. It is apparent that the same length of time is required for 100 atoms to decay to 50 atoms as is required for 50 atoms to decay to 25 atoms. The length of time during which the number of atoms diminish to one-half is referred to as the half-life. Half-lives range in value from thousandths of a second to millions of years. Notice that the curve approaches the abscissa asymptotically, which would imply that some atoms live forever in their excited state. This is not true. If an atom is excited, it must relieve that excitation with the emission of a gamma ray at some point in time. This decay curve is only applicable to large numbers of atoms. If the same curve was plotted on semilogarithmic paper with the number of atoms on the logarithmic scale and time on the linear scale, then a straight line would be obtained (Fig. 6-1, *B*). The rate of decay can, therefore, be said to have an exponential function.

Fig. 6-2 also exemplifies the concept of decay constant. It shows that one-half

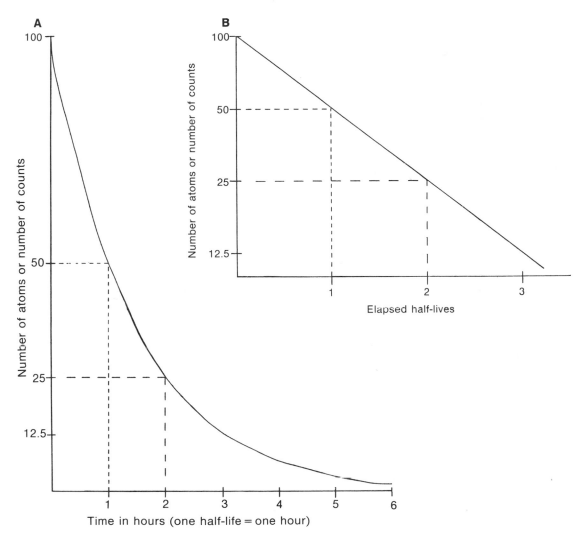

Fig. 6-1. Graph demonstrating physical decay of a radionuclide, plotting elapsed time versus the number of atoms remaining or the number of counts received. **A** expresses this relationship on linear graph paper; **B** expresses it on semilogarithmic paper. The latter can be used as a universal decay table, applying it to any radionuclide, provided the units of time are appropriately placed.

Nuclear science

of the atoms decay per unit time (in this case, the unit of time is one half-life). In the first unit of time, 100 atoms decay to 50 atoms; in the second unit of time, the 50 atoms remaining decay to 25 atoms. In each unit time, the fraction of the number of atoms remaining in the sample is constant at one-half (decay constant).

Average life expectancy (mean life). The active life of any particular radioactive atom can have any value between zero and infinity. However, the *mean life* of a large number of atoms is a definite quantity. It is related to the decay constant, being equal numerically to its reciprocal ($\frac{1}{\lambda}$). It can be described as the period of time that it would take for all the atoms of a radionuclide to decay provided that they decayed at the initial rate of decay until all the atoms were gone. Although one-half of all nuclei decay in one half-life, the fact that in the subsequent half-lives, nuclei live longer, the average life also becomes longer. The average life expectancy is always equal to 1.443 times the physical half-life (Fig. 6-2).

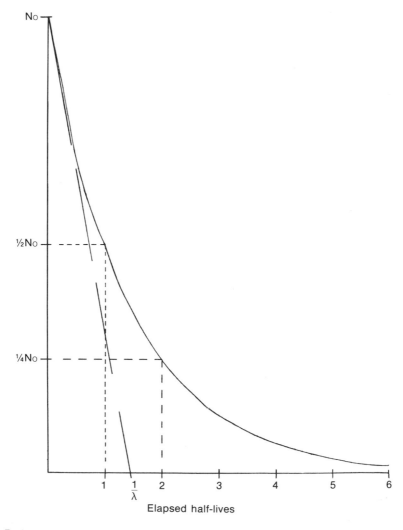

Fig. 6-2. Radioactive decay demonstrating the average life expectancy of each atom in the sample.

In Fig. 6-2, the number of nuclei originally in the sample (N_o) is plotted against time in half-lives. Accordingly, after one half-life has elapsed, only one-half of the original radioactive nuclei are still present in the sample. After two half-lives, only one-fourth of the original radioactive nuclei are present in the sample. If one were to extend the slope of the curve received at 0 half-life until it intercepted the abscissa, this extension would intercept at 1.443 half-lives. This is the life expectancy of each radioactive atom and is the reciprocal of the decay constant ($\frac{1}{\lambda}$).

The decay formula. The curve for radioactive decay can be expressed by the equation:

$$N_t = N_o e^{-\lambda t}$$

N_t = number of atoms at some point in time
N_o = number of atoms originally present
e = base of the natural logarithm, 2.718
λ = decay constant
t = time elapsed
minus sign indicates that the number of atoms are decreasing

λ can be proved mathematically to be equal to $\dfrac{0.693}{T_{1/2}}$

Substituting:

$$N_t = N_o e^{-\frac{0.693t}{T_{1/2}}}$$

The above formula can be expressed similarly in terms of activity as follows:

$$A_t = A_o e^{-\frac{0.693t}{T_{1/2}}}$$

A_t = activity after a period of elapsed time
A_o = activity in the original sample

The use of the last formula is seen in the following problem:

A sample of iodine 131 was known to have an activity of 10 mCi on January 14 at 12 noon C.S.T. What would the activity be on January 16 at 3 P.M. E.S.T.? (Note: Calculations of elapsed time must also include variations in time zones. Elapsed time in this case is exactly 50 hours.)

A_o = 10 mCi
t = 50 hours
$T_{1/2}$ = 8.1 days or 194 hours—both time units (t and $T_{1/2}$) must be the same

Solve for A_t

$$
\begin{aligned}
A_t &= A_o e^{-\frac{0.693t}{T_{1/2}}} \\
&= 10 \text{ mCi} \times e^{-\frac{0.693 \times 50 \text{ hrs}}{194 \text{ hrs}}} \\
&= 10 \times e^{-\frac{34.65}{194}} \\
&= 10 \times e^{-0.18} \\
&= 10 \times .84 \\
&= 8.4 \text{ mCi}
\end{aligned}
$$

Accordingly, the activity of the sample on January 16 at 3 p.m. E.S.T. is 8.4 mCi.

Decay tables. The factor found on any decay table for iodine 131 with an elapsed time of 2 days plus 2 hours (50 hours) is 0.84, or it may be listed at 84% remaining, the result of $e^{-\frac{0.693t}{T_{1/2}}}$ In either case, the original activity is multiplied by 0.84 to find the present activity. All decay tables for the various radio-nuclides are nothing more than the compilation of these values for various periods of elapsed time.

Since decay tables are more convenient to use, most nuclear medicine personnel prefer them to the use of the decay formula. Two practical problems involving their use should be mentioned; (1) How is the decay table used when an aliquot of the radioactive solution is needed *prior* to the calibration date, and (2) how is the decay table used when the decay factors do not cover a sufficient period of time?

The first problem could present itself when an order of radioactive material is received from a supplier prior to its calibration date. If the new source is to be used, it becomes necessary to first calculate the amount of activity on hand (this will be larger than that indicated on the label); then the volume which will represent the desired dose must be calculated. (Some tables include these factors.) The following problem will demonstrate the correct use of decay tables.

Problem

A 10 mCi source of ^{198}Au in a volume of 10 ml, calibrated for June 10 at 12 noon E.S.T. was received on June 9. What would be the activity on June 9 at 12 noon E.S.T.?

Solution (using decay table)

Decay factor for ^{198}Au after one day of elapsed time $= 0.77$. This factor may be used, but instead of multiplying the activity by the decay factor, divide by the decay factor:

$$\frac{10 \text{ mCi}}{0.77} = 13 \text{ mCi}$$

Similarly, using concentration:

$$\frac{1 \text{ mCi/ml}}{0.77} = 1.3 \text{ mCi/ml}$$

Expressing it another way:
To determine activity on hand *before* calibration date:

$$A_t = A_o - DF$$
A_t = activity on hand
A_o = activity indicated on the vial
DF = decay factor

Problem

The second problem involving decay tables presents itself when the decay factors given do not cover a sufficient period of time.

A 10 mCi source of ^{198}Au has an elapsed time of 85 hours from date of calibration and the decay table has values only to 70 hours. What is the activity on hand?

Solution

The easiest approach is to correct for one half-life, knowing that ^{198}Au has a 65-hour half-life. Then using the decay factor representative of the time differential from one half-life (65 hrs) to the remaining period of elapsed time (85 hrs), that is 20 hours (85 hrs − 65 hrs), multiply by one-half of the original activity:

1. Activity at time zero $(A_o) = 10$ mCi
2. Activity at 65 hours or 1 half-life $(A_{T_{1/2}}) = 5$ mCi
3. Elapsed time = 85 hours
4. Elapsed time − 1 $T_{1/2}$ (in this case) = 20 hours remaining time
5. Decay factor for remaining time = 0.81
6. Using $A_{T_{1/2}}$: 5 mCi × .81 = 4.05 mCi activity on hand

Accordingly, the original vial of 10 mCi ^{198}Au would contain 4.05 mCi 85 hours later.

Expressing it another way:

$$A_t = A_{T_{1/2}} \times DF \text{ (for remaining time)}$$
$$A_t = \text{activity on hand}$$
$$A_{T_{1/2}} = \text{activity after one half-life*}$$
$$DF = \text{decay factor for total elapsed time (one half-life*)}$$

The above would also apply to concentrations, if this was the desired method of record keeping.

Slide rule method. The same decay calculation may be made with a slide rule. The slide rule must have both the log scale (usually labeled LLO) and log-log scales (usually labeled LLOO). The method is as follows:

Set the hairline on 0.500 on the log-log scale (LLOO). Locate the half-life on the left half of the B scale and set this point under the hairline. To determine the decay factor, slide the hairline to the left along the B scale so that it coincides with the elapsed time in question. The decay factor may then be read from the log-log scale. If the reading runs off the left end of the scale, move the hairline to the right of the half-life and locate the elapsed time on the right half of the B scale. The decay factor should then be read from the log scale (LLO).

Specific weight. It is often the problem of the researcher to determine the specific weight of the material introduced into the human body. Knowing the specific weight becomes valuable from the standpoint of toxicity, in that the researcher does not want to approach the toxic dose of any material in order to successfully perform the study. Also, the "load" introduced into the human body must not upset the normal physiologic balance of the material. For example, if, in any thyroid diagnostic procedure, the amount of iodine exceeds the normal daily intake, the normal physiology of the thyroid is altered.

Problem

A dose of 50 μCi is used as an uptake and scanning dose. How much ^{131}I is introduced into the iodine pool? (^{131}I is used as the example, because it is carrier-free).

Solution

The determination of specific weight involves two mathematical procedures: (1) determination of the number of atoms in the sample, and (2) determination of the specific weight. These are calculated as shown on the following page.

---

*This could also be the value after 2 or more half-lives depending on the circumstances.

1. Determine the number of atoms by the formula:

$$\lambda N = A$$

A = activity in disintegrations per minute
$(1\mu Ci = 2.22 \times 10^6$ dpm; so 50 $\mu Ci = 1.11 \times 10^8$ dpm)

$\lambda = \dfrac{0.693}{T_{1/2}}$ (since A is in minute units, so must $T_{1/2}$ be in minute units)

N = number of atoms

Solving for N:

$$\frac{0.693}{8.1 \text{ days} \times 24 \frac{hr}{day} \times 60 \frac{min}{hr}} \times N = 1.11 \times 10^8 \text{ dpm}$$

$$\frac{0.693}{11664} N = 1.11 \times 10^8$$

$$5.94 \times 10^{-5} \ N = 1.11 \times 10^8$$

$$N = 1.87 \times 10^{12}$$

2. Determine specific weight of the sample by the formula:

$$W = \frac{A \times N}{K}$$

W = weight of sample
A = atomic weight of radionuclide
N = number of atoms
K = Avogadro's number $= 6 \times 10^{23}$

Solving for W:

$$W = \frac{131 \times 1.87 \times 10^{12}}{6 \times 10^{23}}$$

$$= \frac{244.97 \times 10^{12}}{6 \times 10^{23}}$$

$$= 40.83 \times 10^{-11} \text{ gm or } 4 \times 10^{-7} \text{ mg or } 4 \times 10^{-4} \ \mu g$$

It has been determined that a 50 μCi dose introduces 0.0004 μg of iodine 131 into the iodine pool. Since the daily adult intake of iodine is approximately 150 μg, the iodine pool remains physiologically unaltered. Further, approximately 20 mCi could be administered without altering the iodine pool.

Specific activity. Another parameter of interest in nuclear medicine and one which relates activity to weight is that of specific activity. Specific activity is strictly defined as the ratio of activity to the specific weight of the radionuclide. It is usually expressed as millicuries per milligram or curies per gram. Using the information just determined on specific weight and the strict definition of specific activity, the preparation in the above problem would have a specific activity of:

$$\frac{50 \ \mu Ci}{40 \times 10^{-8} \text{ mg}} = \frac{50 \times 10^{-3} \text{ mCi}}{40 \times 10^{-8} \text{ mg}} = 1.25 \times 10^5 \text{ mCi/mg}$$

The strict definition of specific activity is rarely used with commercial preparations of radionuclides, however. The specific weight used in their formula is sometimes the weight of the stable nuclide or, more commonly, the weight of the chemical compound to which the radionuclide is labeled; for example, in the case of ^{197}Hg-labeled chlormerodrin, the specific activity refers to the microcuries of mercury 197 per milligram of the chlormerodrin molecule (μCi ^{197}Hg/mg chlormerodrin).

This information regarding specific activity is found on all radiopharmaceutical labels. Even though neutron activation is the most common method of obtaining radionuclides, the inability to separate the stable form of the element (carrier) from the unstable increases the problems of chemical toxicity levels. To obtain a desired level of radioactive material in a patient, it may be necessary to introduce an undesirable level of the element or an undersirable level of the labeled compound. (A compound is said to be labeled when it consists in part of radioactive atoms, such as ^{131}I-labeled hippuran.)

The value of specific activity may be illustrated by a hypothetical example. A laboratory has just received a shipment of [197]Hg-labeled chlormerodrin. The specific activity as stated on the label is 200 μCi/mg, calibrated for Monday at 8:00 A.M. The calibration date informs the user of the radiopharmaceutical that the specific activity is true as stated only at the time of calibration. (This also holds true for two other values found on the label: activity and concentration.) The value would be different before or after the date and time of calibration.

For ease of calculation, it will be assumed that [197]Hg has a half-life of 48 hours and that the standard dose for a given study was 2.0 mCi. The following schedule would then prevail:

	Specific activity	Activity injected	Chlormerodrin injected
Monday 8:00 A.M.	200 μCi/mg	2,000 μCi	10 mg
Wednesday 8:00 A.M.	100 μCi/mg	2,000 μCi	20 mg
Friday 8:00 A.M.	50 μCi/mg	2,000 μCi	40 mg

Chlormerodrin is a well-known mercurial diuretic. Assume that 20 mg of chlormerodrin is a standard diuretic dose. By Wednesday morning at 8:00 A.M. a medical problem presents itself and by Friday it worsens. In order to inject the standard dosage of radioactivity, the patient must also receive the standard diuretic dose. Perhaps, in the medical management of some patients where diuresis is a contraindication, the nuclear medicine procedure may have to be delayed or omitted. Although this is a hypothetical situation, it demonstrates the value of specific activity, and it can be related similarly to toxicity levels.

Specific activity is not to be mistaken for concentration. This information is also found on all radiopharmaceutical labels. Concentration is defined as the ratio of activity to volume. It is usually expressed in units of millicuries per milliliter or microcuries per milliliter. A vial containing 10 mCi activity in a volume of 10 ml will be expressed as having a concentration of 1.0 mCi/ml. As with specific activity, this value is only true at the date and time of calibration.

It might be well to point out a practical problem with volume, especially as it applies to the use of a multiple dose vial. In utilizing a solution of radioactive material, whose concentration permits five or more withdrawals, a lack of volume is often encountered on the last withdrawal. The vial must be disposed of because of insufficient volume even though the inventory indicates otherwise. This is usually not an error of calculation on the part of the nuclear medicine personnel or of the radiopharmaceutical supplier. In such instances, the lack of volume can be accounted for by the "hang-up" in needles, rubber stopper, and the vial itself. Commercial suppliers of "cold" (nonradioactive) materials in multiple dose form can, in many cases, compensate for this by adjusting the volume. However, because the regulations of the Food and Drug Administration are such that volume and concentration must be included on the label, such compensatory action may not be taken. Obviously, if 1.0 ml more of diluent is added to correct for this situation, the volume and the concentration would also have to change. Calculation would then be based on the increased volume and no purpose would be served.

Biologic half-life

Biologic half-life (T_b) is the time required for the body to eliminate one-half of the dose of any substance by the regular processes of elimination. This time is the same for both stable and radioactive isotopes of any given element. The principal methods of elimination are by way of the urine, feces, exhalation, and perspiration. Biologic half-life is an important consideration when attempting to predict radiation damage to the human body from internal emitters. Any radionuclide that is retained by the body for only a short period of time will have a relatively small radiobiologic effect regardless of whether it has a long physical half-life or a short physical half-life.

Examples are mercury 203- and mercury 197-labeled chlormerodrin. Both of these compounds have an identical biologic half-life. Except for that portion of the tagged mercurial diuretic which remains in the kidneys, the radiobiologic effect would be similar, even though they vary greatly in physical half-life.

Effective half-life

Because both the physical and biologic half-lives must be taken into consideration when predicting the amount of radiation that is absorbed per unit mass of tissue, a third term is used to express the difference between the two. This is called the effective half-life.

The effective half-life is defined as the time required for the radioactivity from a given amount of a radioactive element deposited in the tissues or organs to diminish by 50% as a result of the combined action of radioactive decay and loss of the material by biologic elimination. The effective half-life (T_e) is usually experimentally determined.

A relatively simple example of experimentally determining effective half-life is that of iodine 131 in the thyroid gland. Iodine 131, labeled sodium iodide, is administered to the patient and an uptake is determined at 24 hours after administration by a standard thyroid uptake counter. Uptakes are continued every subsequent 24-hour period. By plotting the count on day 1 and comparing subsequent daily counts, one may find the activity in the thyroid reaches 50% at 6 days, even though the physical half-life of iodine 131 is approximately 8 days. Obviously, biologic elimination has acted upon the iodine 131 in the thyroid gland so that the 50% rate is reached before the physical half-life. The effective half-life in this case is something less than the physical half-life. The biologic half-life always decreases the effective half-life to a value less than that of the physical half-life. The only time that this would not be the case is in the event of no biologic elimination, as with colloidal gold in the liver. In this case, the effective half-life is equal to the physical half-life. In no case is the effective half-life larger than the physical half-life. If the biologic half-life is known, the effective half-life can be mathematically calculated by the following expression:

$$T_e = \frac{T_p \times T_b}{T_p + T_b}$$

The usual case, however, is that both the effective half-life (experimentally determined) and the physical half-life are known. Using these two values the biologic half-life can be determined by the following formula:

$$T_b = \frac{T_p \times T_e}{T_p - T_e}$$

PRACTICAL METHODS OF RADIATION PROTECTION

For personnel involved in the use of radioactive materials, methods of radiation protection should be foremost in their thoughts at all times. The actual effects of radiation are not known and may not be known for many centuries to come. However, assuming that all ionizing radiations are potentially harmful, man can cope with the problem by constantly being alert to methods of protection. Practical limitations established by national committees to assist the occupational radiation worker have already been discussed. The rationale for these limits is that even peaceful uses of the atom require some exposure to their emissions. It is impossible and impractical to shield workers from them completely. There is also a constant bombardment by cosmic radiation from outside the earth's atmosphere. These cosmic rays are highly energetic and, practically speaking, no amount of protection can shield us completely from these rays. Man has learned to live with these omnipresent cosmic radiations. Complete shielding is also impractical since many beneficial uses of atomic energy would be removed from modern medical technology, such as x-ray therapy and diagnosis and nuclear medicine therapy and diagnosis. For precisely this reason, nuclear medicine personnel must be constantly aware of the practical methods of radiation protection. These methods are distance, shielding, and time. In the judicious use of all three of these methods, the amount of radiation to which the radiation worker subjects himself can be kept at a minimum and well within the limitations established by the NCRP.

Distance

Distance constitutes one of the best methods of radiation protection and is one of the routine methods used. It is not only a very effective means of radiation protection, but in many instances it is the least expensive. As one moves away from the source of radiation, one naturally expects to receive less radiation. The novice might think that as the distance is doubled from the source at a given position, the radiation to the person would be reduced by one-half; however, the radiation is reduced by one-fourth. This is known as the inverse square law, which states that the amount of radiation at a given distance from a source is inversely proportional to the square of the distance. By doubling the distance, the dose is one-fourth the original; by halving the distance, the dose is four times the original.

95

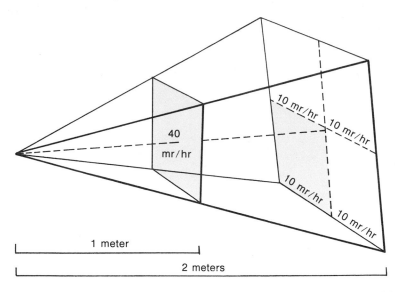

Fig. 6-3. The inverse square law. As radiations are emitted from a point source, an arbitrary area is selected at 1 meter, representative of a radiation intensity of 40 mr/hr. At 2 meters (twice the distance from the point source) that same radiation field of 40 mr/hr has expanded to an area four times the size of the original area. Consequently, the original area (gray) now receives only one-fourth of the entire radiation.

The name of the law defines the nature of the law itself. By increasing the distance by a factor of 2, the dose is decreased by the inverse square of 2 $(\frac{1}{4})$, according to the following:

Distance factor	*Inverse*	*Inverse square*
2	$\frac{1}{2}$	$(\frac{1}{2})^2 = \frac{1}{4}$

Accordingly, by reducing the distance by a factor of $\frac{1}{2}$, the dose is increased by the inverse square of $\frac{1}{2}$ (4):

Distance factor	*Inverse*	*Inverse square*
$\frac{1}{2}$	$\frac{2}{1}$	$(\frac{2}{1})^2 = \frac{4}{1} = 4$

This relationship is seen in Fig. 6-3.

The inverse square law can also be expressed as a formula. By utilization of this formula and knowing the intensity at a given distance, one can mathematically determine the intensity at another known distance or the distance at which one could receive a required intensity. The formula is seen below:

$$\frac{I}{i} = \frac{d^2}{D^2}$$

I = intensity at a distance (D) from a point source
i = intensity at a difference distance (d)

The following examples demonstrate the inverse square law:

1. 300 mr/hr is measured at 8 cm. What is the dose rate at 2 cm?

$$\frac{x}{300} = \frac{8^2}{2^2}$$

$$x = \frac{8^2}{2^2} \times 300 = \frac{64}{4} \times 300 = 4,800 \text{ mr/hr}$$

2. 600 mr/hr is measured at 10 cm. What is distance at which 150 mr/hr is received?

$$\frac{600}{150} = \frac{x^2}{10^2}$$

$$x^2 = \frac{600}{150} \times 10^2$$

$$x = \sqrt{\frac{600 \times 100}{150} \times 100} = \sqrt{400} = 20 \text{ cm}$$

Both of the above examples could have been calculated without the use of the formula. In example No. 2, the dose rate desired is one-fourth of that measured at 10 cm from the point source. According to the inverse square law, this would require twice the distance or 20 cm.

The principle of the inverse square law is easily demonstrated by any survey meter and a point source. If the point source is placed at a distance of 0.5 meter from the detector and the reading is recorded by moving the source to a distance of 1 meter, the intensity is reduced by one-fourth. The inverse square law applies most accurately with the use of gamma emitting point sources; that is, with sources in which the radioactivity is contained in a very small volume. It does not apply to extended sources or to multiple sources.

The inverse square principle explains the suggested use of long-handled tongs and remote control handling devices with application to large quantities of radiation. It also plays a role in the calculation of visiting time to a recently treated patient. It may be that a patient's family could stay only 10 minutes at the bedside, but by not allowing the visitors within 6 feet, their stay could be prolonged based on inverse square relationships.

Shielding

Shielding is also a very practical method of radiation protection. The use of shielding materials such as lead sheets and lead bricks is nothing new to even the most inexperienced radiation worker. This shield is simply a body of material used to prevent or reduce the passage of radiation. In the case of alpha and beta radiation, very little shielding is required to absorb the emissions completely. An alpha particle is stopped by a sheet of paper, a beta particle is stopped by an inch of wood, but feet of concrete or inches of lead are necessary to absorb gamma radiation (see Fig. 6-4). The general practice is to use enough shielding for complete absorption of alpha and beta particles. This is not true, however, with gamma or x-radiation. With these two types of emissions, shielding is used to reduce the amount of radiation.

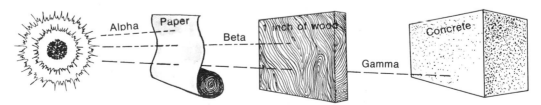

Fig. 6-4. Absorption of various types of radioactive emissions.

97

The shielding aspect of beta particles deserves special consideration. It is known that ¼ inch of plastic will stop a beta particle; therefore, a syringe will provide adequate shielding in itself. If a syringe containing ^{32}P, for example, is placed near a scintillation detector, a large number of counts will be received. The detector is actually registering the electromagnetic radiation resulting from Bremsstrahlung.

In order that radiation be completely absorbed or reduced in intensity, energy must be lost by the radiations themselves. The energy of charged particles is lost primarily by a series of ionization events or excitation of atoms within the shielding medium. Energy from electromagnetic radiation is lost by three methods: photoelectric effect, Compton effect and/or pair production, depending upon the energy of the radiation itself. For those gamma rays below 1.02 mev in energy, the process of absorbing is usually a series of Compton collisions whereby the energy gradually diminishes. Eventually the radiations are sufficiently decreased in energy that total absorption occurs through the photoelectric effect. For those gamma rays above 1.02 mev of energy, pair production occurs with the eventual formation of two gamma rays of 0.511 mev. They are eventually absorbed by the Compton and photoelectric effects.

As far as the shielding material itself is concerned, density and thickness go hand-in-hand in reducing radiation intensity. If a material 1 cm thick with a density of 10 mg/cm³ (milligrams per cubic centimeter is a standard unit of density) was placed between a source and a detector, it would have the same stopping

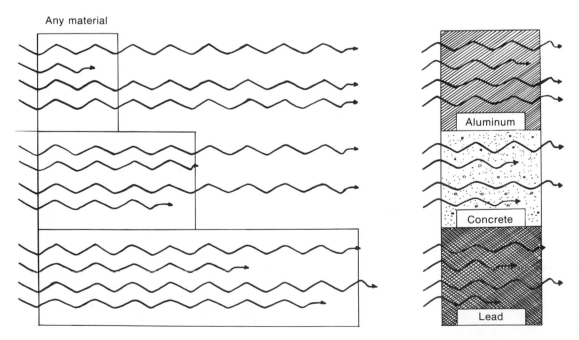

Fig. 6-5. Absorption characteristics of shielding materials. As density and/or thickness of the shielding material increases, the absorption of radioactive emissions by the material also increases.

power as a material 10 cm thick having a density of 1 mg/cm^3, placed similarly. For this reason, units of *density thickness* have become accepted in milligrams per square centimeter according to the following:

$$\frac{mg}{cm^3} \times cm = \frac{mg}{cm^3} \times \frac{1}{cm^{-1}} = mg/cm^2$$

As the shielding material increases in atomic number and, therefore, increases in density, the ability to attenuate x- or gamma radiation is increased. For this reason, aluminum would not be as good a shield as concrete for higher energy electromagnetic radiation. Similarly, concrete would not be as good a shield as lead. Aluminum may, however, serve just as effectively as lead in attenuating weak energy x- or gamma radiation, since the degree of density thickness is not important for weak radiations. It is for this reason that aluminum filtration is often used in x-ray emissions, resulting in a more uniform beam of high energy x-rays. Fig. 6-5 demonstrates the effect of thickness versus density in attenuating radiation. In addition to density and thickness, the energy of the photon or particle plays an important role. The greater the energy, the greater must be the density thickness.

Shielding formula. All of the factors influencing the effectiveness of the shielding material can be expressed mathematically as follows:

$$I = I_o e^{-\mu x}$$

I   = radiation intensity after shielding
I_o = radiation intensity before shielding
e   = base of the natural logarithm, 2.718
μ = linear absorption coefficient in cm^{-1}
x   = thickness of shield in cm
minus sign indicates that the intensity is decreasing.

The *linear absorption coefficient* is defined as the fraction of the number of photons removed from the radiation field per centimeter of absorber. This is similar to the decay constant (λ) in the physical half-life formula, for μ becomes a constant if the shield has uniform density throughout. If, for instance, the radiation intensity before shielding is 100 mr/hr and the density of the shield (absorber) is such that the fractional decrease is one-half the intensity per centimeter (50% per centimeter or 0.50 cm^{-1}), the intensity after 1 cm shielding is not 50 mr/hr as might be expected, but greater than that value because of many complicating factors, such as back-scatter and dose build-up, for which all are accounted in the formula. A μ factor of 0.50 cm^{-1} would result in a decrease in the intensity to only 61 mr/hr according to the following:

$$I = I_o e^{-\mu x}$$
$$I = 100 \times e^{-.50 \times 1}$$
$$I = 100 \times e^{-.50}$$
$$I = 100 \times .61 = 61 \text{ mr/hr @ 1 cm}$$

Calculations for 2, 3, 4, 5 and 6 cm of the same absorbing media using the above formula yield a resultant intensity of 37 mr/hr, 22 mr/hr, 13.5 mr/hr, 8 mr/hr, and 5 mr/hr, respectively. By plotting these intensity values versus thickness on linear graph paper, an exponential curve is received as in Fig. 6-6, *A*. Plotting the same parameters on semilogarithmic graph paper produces a straight line as in Fig. 6-6, *B*.

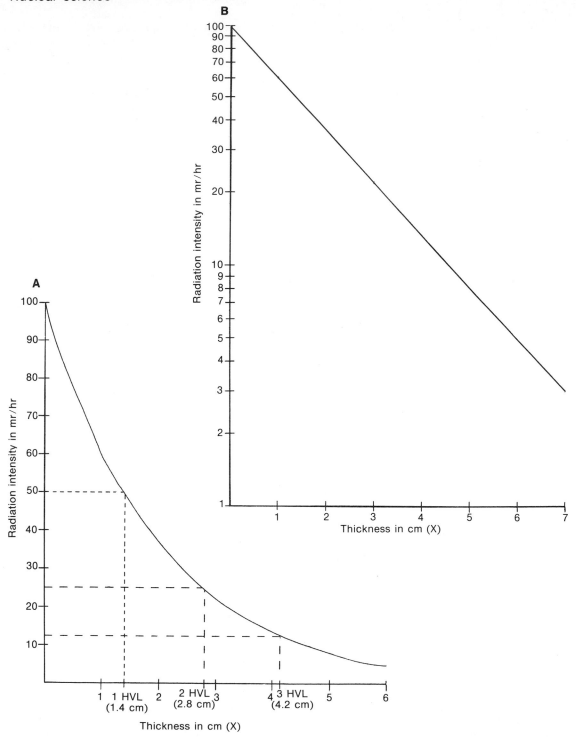

Fig. 6-6. Graph demonstrating the relationship of thickness of shielding to radiation intensity. **A** demonstrates the exponential function of the relationship. **B** reproduces the curve as a straight line plotted on semilogarithmic paper. The half-value layer (HVL) can be ascertained from either part of the graph.

The formula itself is not of major practical importance in the field of nuclear medicine. It has value in that it becomes possible to predict the attenuation of a gamma photon.

By carefully examining the shielding formula and the introductory discussion, a number of general statements may be made regarding it:

1. Three factors influence the efficacy of shielding: density, thickness, and energy.
2. As density and/or thickness of the attenuating medium increases, the after-shielding intensity decreases.
3. As the energy of the photon or particle increases, the after-shielding intensity increases.
4. Any material, regardless of the magnitude of the above 3 factors, will absorb some of the radiation and consequently decrease the after-shielding intensity.
5. The type of radiation is also an important consideration. Alpha radiation intensity can be reduced to zero (completely absorbed) by a sheet of paper. Beta radiation intensity can be reduced to zero (completely absorbed) by a quarter inch of plastic or an inch of wood. X- and gamma radiation intensity can *never* be totally reduced, although they can be attenuated in a predictable manner.
6. The shielding material must be of sufficient density and/or thickness to reduce the exposure to acceptable limits. A standard acceptable limit is 2 mr/hr at 1 meter because:

$$2 \frac{\text{mr}}{\text{hr}} \times 50 \frac{\text{hrs}}{\text{week}} \times 50 \frac{\text{weeks}}{\text{year}} = 5,000 \text{ mr/yr or 5 r/yr*}$$

This value is the MPD for occupational radiation personnel per year. For any length of time, 1 meter is a reasonable working distance from any source of radiation.

Half-value layer. Although the shielding formula per se is not of practical importance to nuclear medicine personnel, the information that can be received from its results do have practical significance. It has already been stated that x- or gamma radiation can be reduced to acceptable limits, but theoretically cannot be reduced to zero. As is evidenced by Fig. 6-6, it can be attenuated in a predictable manner. This useful information is referred to as the half-value layer (HVL). By definition HVL is the thickness of any particular material necessary to reduce the intensity of a radiation field to one-half of its original value.

Fig. 6-6 shows that by interposing 1 HVL (1.4 cm) of shielding material between the source and a detector, the radiation field is reduced to one-half of its original intensity (from 100 mr/hr to 50 mr/hr). Similarly, by interposing 2 HVLs (2.8 cm), the field is reduced by one-half again (from 50 mr/hr to 25 mr/hr). Because the exponential curve approaches the abscissa asymptotically, it can be theorized that no amount of shielding could completely stop all the photons. Continuous interpositioning of HVLs results in a continuous halving process that becomes infinite.

Half-value layers for almost all radionuclides in various media are known and can be found in any radiologic handbook. These values provide a quick calculation

---

*Actually 5 rems per year, but Title 10CFR20.4 states that, "For the purpose of the regulations . . . a dose of one rem . . . is equivalent to . . . a dose of 1 r due to x- or gamma radiation."

Table 6-4. Relationship of radiation intensity to barrier thickness

Attenuation (HVL)	Intensity (mr/hr @ 1 m)	Lead thickness (cm)
0	24	0
1	12	1.25
2	6	2.5
3	3	3.75
4	1.5	5.0

Convert to inches:

$$4.8 \text{ cm} \div 2.54 \; \frac{cm}{inch} = 1.97 \text{ inches}$$

Therefore, 2 inches of lead would be adequate to reduce radiation intensity to 2 mr/hr @ 1 meter.

of the shielding necessary to reduce the radiation intensity to acceptable limits. An example follows:

Problem

A cobalt 60 calibration source, producing a radiation field of 24 mr/hr at 1 meter requires protection. If lead is used as the standard shielding material, how much lead is required to reduce the radiation intensity to acceptable limits? (Pb HVL for ^{60}Co = 1.25 cm.)

Solution

Two inches of lead would be adequate to reduce the intensity to 2 mr/hr measured at 1 meter, the acceptable limit. Table 6-4 demonstrates this relationship.

The respect for half-value layers as a radiation protection device should become tremendously enhanced when it is realized that 1 HVL will reduce intensity to one-half, regardless of the original intensity. Accordingly, 1.25 cm of lead will reduce a cobalt 60 source with an intensity of 1,000 r/hr to 500 r/hr, just as the same 1.25 cm of lead will reduce cobalt 60 from 1 mr/hr to 0.5 mr/hr.

Time

The principle of time is also a very practical method of radiation protection. It is quite obvious that the longer an individual is exposed to a field of radiation the greater will be the total exposure. Common sense dictates that time should be used as a control of radiation exposure. In diagnostic applications of nuclear medicine, time does not become quite as important as in therapy.

There are three groups of nonoccupational personnel which deserve special time considerations. These groups are nursing personnel, visitors, and adjacent patients.

In order that time considerations become meaningful, reference must be made to the AEC regulations on the subject (10CFR20.105). These regulations stipulate that "no licensee shall possess, use or transfer licensed material in such a manner as to create in an unrestricted area*...radiation levels which, if an individual were continuously present in the area, could result in his receiving a dose in excess

---

*An "unrestricted area" is any area the access to which is not controlled by the licensee for purposes of protection of individuals from exposure to radiation and radioactive materials, and any area used for residential quarters.

of two millirems* in any one hour ... or a dose in excess of 100 millirems in any seven consecutive days."

With respect to these regulations, the three groups of nonoccupational personnel can be treated as two groups; visitors and nursing personnel in one group and the adjacent patient in another.

Visitors and nursing personnel. It is unlikely that any one of these two groups would be near the bedside of the patient any longer than 50 hours per 7 consecutive days. (This statement may be erroneous with respect to the immediate family of a seriously ill patient. In these instances, the family visitation privileges must be limited to 50 hours per week per person.) Under these conditions, this group has satisfied both phases of the AEC requirements. Their regulations regarding the exposure in any 7 consecutive days (100 mrems) concurs with that of the permissible radiation exposure in any one hour (2 millirems) because of the following relationship:

$$100 \text{ mrems} \div 50 \text{ hours} = 2 \text{ mrems/hr}$$

Since both clauses of the AEC regulations calculate to be the same, no clause takes precedence and any member of this group must be limited to 2 mrem in any one hour.

Adjacent patient. The situation of the patient adjacent to a recently treated patient presents another problem with reference to time considerations. The adjacent patient cannot be limited to 50 hours per week as can the above group of persons. It is conceivable that an adjacent patient could be subjected to this exposure every hour for 7 consecutive days (168 hours). For this group of people, the dose rate must be restricted to 0.6 mrem per hour or less according to the following relationship:

$$100 \text{ millirems} \div 168 \text{ hours} = 0.6 \text{ mrem/hr}$$

Since one clause of the A.E.C. regulations states 2 mrems in any one hour, and the other clause calculates to a permissible exposure rate of 0.6 mrem/hr, the latter takes precedence. Therefore, the exposure rate of all patients adjacent to a recently treated patient must be less than 0.6 mrem/hr.

This regulation automatically rules out placing therapy patients in multibed wards following administration of therapy. The patient requires a private room. This statement is made based on the assumption that all therapies of 30 mCi or less are treated on an out-patient basis.† If, in the opinion of the physician, a patient treated with less than 30 mCi requires hospitalization, the patient may not require a private room. This is entirely dependent on the dose and the subsequent radiation field surrounding the treated patient. These regulations do not apply to the patient receiving x-ray or cobalt teletherapy treatments, since the radiation-emitting material is not placed within the patient. It does apply to radium or cobalt interstitial or intercavitary implants.

---

*1 mrem $\cong$ 1 mr due to x- or gamma radiation.
†This is a condition placed on all AEC licensees for therapeutic human use of by-product material; that is, patients containing larger amounts of radioactivity shall remain hospitalized until the residual activity is 30 mCi or less.

A point to be emphasized in the AEC regulations is that which relates to the exposure of 2 rems/hr. This means 2 rems in any one hour; it does not mean that one could receive 10 mrems in an hour and remove himself from the patient's room for the next four hours.

When the exposure rate exceeds 2 rems/hr, calculations must be performed to determine the length of time that visitors and nursing personnel can remain there. The following problem will demonstrate the point:

Problem

The survey meter measurement at the bedside of a recently treated patient indicates an intensity of 12 mr/hr. What is the length of time that a visitor or a nurse could remain at the point where the reading was taken?

Solution

According to the following calculation:

$$\frac{12 \text{ mr}}{60 \text{ min}} = \frac{2 \text{ mr}}{x}$$

Solve for x: when 2 mr is equal to the amount of exposure a nonoccupational personnel may receive in any one hour

$$12 \text{ mr } (x) = 2 \text{ mr } (60 \text{ min.})$$
$$x = \frac{2 \text{ mr } (60 \text{ min.})}{12 \text{ mr}}$$
$$x = 10 \text{ min}$$

If this reading of 12 mr/hr was taken at the bedside of the patient, by taking a reading 3 or 6 feet from the patient, the radiation dose rate would be decreased in accordance with the inverse square law, and the visitors would be allowed to remain longer. It might also be important to indicate that in some therapeutic applications of radiopharmaceuticals, this dose rate will decrease with time because of large eliminations via normal biologic processes. If such is the action of the therapeutic agent, readings taken at various times of the day could extend visitation privileges.

DOSIMETRY

Perhaps the major consideration in all studies in which radionuclides are administered to human beings is the amount of activity administered to a patient and its consequent radiation dose to vital organs. For the diagnostic utilizations of such drugs, this becomes the limiting factor. It is obvious that all of these problems of statistics, time involved in any given study, and so on, could be resolved immediately merely by increasing the amount of radioactivity administered. Nuclear medicine procedures are not like x-ray procedures in which millions of photons are available for a given study. Because of this fact, many radiographic techniques require only fractions of seconds to complete. The magnitude of photons from a nuclear medicine procedure are on the order of hundreds to thousands of photons and, therefore, minutes or hours are required to obtain enough counts to make a statistical evaluation of a study. In such studies the radioactive materials become lodged, pooled, or incorporated into selective organs and remain there for periods as short as seconds to as long as months or even years. While the radioactive material is in the organ or is being excreted by the body, it is irradiating the exposed tissues even after the study has been completed. X-rays, however, originate external to the body and produce effects only during the time that the body and/or organ is exposed to the x-ray unit.

Since this is the case, the radiopharmaceutical user must be able to give thoughtful consideration to the question of radiation dosage caused by the agent during the time that the body and its critical organs are being exposed. This is considered important by all three government bodies having at least some form of jurisdiction in the use of radiopharmaceuticals (Atomic Energy Commission, National Institutes of Health, and the Food and Drug Administration). The FDA has authority over all pharmaceutical preparations whereas the Atomic Energy Commission has authority in only by-products from a nuclear reactor, and the National Institutes of Health has control of blood derivatives.

Present knowledge of dosimetry is much too fragmentary to establish exact values of dosage to the body and critical organs as a result of the administration of a known amount of radionuclide. The prevailing compromise is to attempt to predict in the approximate order of magnitude the absorbed radiation dose (in rad units) to the whole body, target organ (organ in which the radionuclide is primarily collected), and the organs of elimination. Many assumptions are incorporated into such a calculation. In many cases when exact values are unknown, it has become customary to use pessimistic assumptions. In this way, the result represents an acceptable figure, but on the upper limit of the true value. If this value is adequate, the true value would represent an even smaller radiation dose.

The classic expressions of radiation dosimetry are as follows:

$$D_\beta = 73.8 \times C \times \bar{E}_\beta \times T_e$$
$$D_\gamma = 0.0346 \times C \times \Gamma \times \bar{g} \times T_e$$

D_β = dose in rads from beta radiation
D_γ = dose in rads from gamma radiation
C = initial concentration of radionuclide in $\mu Ci/gm$
$\bar{E}_\beta$ = mean energy of β radiations in mev ($\cong \frac{1}{3}E_{max}$)
Γ = gamma dose constant in r/mCi/hr at 1 cm distance
$\bar{g}$ = geometric factor to account for variations in shape, size, and volume of organ
T_e = effective half-life in days

The two constants, 73.8 and 0.0346, are conversion factors so that the product appears in rads. $\bar{E}_\beta$ and Γ are parameters which can be found in any handbook of radiation health and in many advanced texts. All other factors are variables. C is a variable since the number of microcuries and the gram weight would both vary among individuals. The adequate calculation of this parameter is compounded when radiopharmaceuticals are used for dynamic function studies, such as rose bengal and hippuran. T_e varies from person to person. The $\bar{g}$ values are available for a variety of standard geometrical configurations, but no human organ exactly resembles a sphere or a cylinder so this contributes to the value as something removed from the true value. Other complicating factors include unequal distribution of the radioactive material in the organ, energy of the emission (some gammas are so weak that they are betalike as far as dosimetry is concerned), and irradiation from adjacent organs (pancreas and liver) or companion organs (cross irradiation from one lung to the other or one kidney to the other).

Perhaps the most practical means of learning to utilize the dosimetry formulas is to present a well-known clinical situation and use the formula to calculate the radiation dose to the critical organ. For a liver scan, 100 μc of colloidal ^{198}Au could serve as an example. The calculations for liver dosimetry are as follows:

Assumptions:

1. 100% uptake by the liver with no excretion
2. Therefore, $T_e = T_p = 2.7$ days
3. $\Gamma = 2.35$ r/mCi/hr at 1 cm
4. $\bar{g} = 65$
5. $\bar{E}_\beta = 0.331$ mev
6. Weight = 1,700 gm, Dose = 100 μCi; therefore $C = \dfrac{100}{1,700}$

Calculations:

$$D_\beta = 73.8 \times \frac{100}{1,700} \times 0.331 \times 2.7 = 3.88 \text{ rads}$$

$$D_\gamma = 0.0346 \times \frac{100}{1,700} \times 2.35 \times 65 \times 2.7 = 0.84 \text{ rads}$$

Therefore $D_{\beta+\gamma} = 4.72$ rads (82% from the beta component)

Dosimetry is by no means an exact science, as the number of assumptions necessary to perform the calculation above indicates. At the present time, dosimetry calculations inform the user that the patient is receiving 1.0 rad, not 100 rad or 0.01 rad. Further, nuclear medicine techniques are in a constant state of flux. New procedures, new radiopharmaceuticals, and new instrumentation are constantly being advanced to try to reduce the radiation dose to the patient.

Chapter 7

Biologic effects of radiation

Some of the specific factors involved in radiation protection were discussed in the preceding chapter. The reason for various methods of radiation protection is obvious—to decrease the radiation dose to the human body. There is concern about radiation exposure to the human body because of its generally harmful biologic effect. Radiation acts on biologic tissue at the molecular level and, therefore, on the cell and its constituents. For this reason, exposure to ionizing radiations may result in changes in the highly organized molecular system, destruction of certain cellular elements, and, of greatest concern, altered function or death of the cell. In this chapter, theories about the action of radiation at the cellular level and the somatic and genetic effects of radiation on biologic systems and organs will be discussed.

RATIONALE
Discussion

Before proceeding into a discussion on the biologic effects of radiation, it should be said that the science of radiobiology is still in its infancy. For this reason, very few fundamental principles concerning it are known, and only a few general statements may be made regarding radiobiology. One thing is certain: when biologic material is irradiated, a long chain of events begins to occur, and the biologic material absorbs a certain amount of energy from the radiation. Exactly what occurs and exactly what causes the death of the cell is not completely known. There are several theories relating to the action of radiation on cells, the most prominent feature being that *profound changes or damage to the cells can result when a single charged particle passes through the cell nucleus.* This appears to be the case whether the cell is somatic or genetic in nature.

Somatic cells are those cells with paired chromosomes; *genetic* (germ) cells, by definition, are cells with unpaired chromosomes. The somatic cells constitute all the cells of an organism with the exception of the reproductive cells. The somatic cells are generally more resistant than genetic cells to the effects of ionizing radiation, although damage to these cells leads to organic damage, loss of function of tissues or organs, and may even result in death of the cell. When damaged, however, they cannot bring about genetic alterations in the organisms offspring. Mutations can occur in somatic cells, but they cannot be transmitted sexually and, therefore, they disappear when the cell dies. Damage to germ cells, however, can be transmitted to the offspring.

The chain of events leading to cell damage or change begins as an ionizing particle passes through the biologic material. Since charged particles have the capability of ionizing and/or exciting atoms and molecules, the charged particles leave a path of such matter in their wake. In ionizing or exciting an atom, energy is released from the particle as it passes. In this way, the particle loses its energy and eventually comes to rest, at which point it is no longer of radiobiologic significance. The spacing of the energy releases along this track is called the LET (linear energy transfer). Up to this point these energy releases have been referred to as specific ionization. The two terms, for all practical purposes, are synonymous. The LET is known to be a function of the charge and velocity of the ionizing particle. The greater the charge and the lower the velocity, the greater is the particle's LET. A comparative example would be that of alpha particles and beta particles. The alpha particle is of low velocity (because of its large mass) and it has a positive charge of $+2$. A beta particle is of high velocity (because of its insignificant mass) and it has a charge of -1. For these reasons, the LET of the alpha particle is much greater than that of the beta particle. There have been many investigations as to the importance of LET in radiobiology. In general, it can be said that as the LET increases (as the number of ionization events increases), the lethal effect of radiation also increases.

As the high velocity, charged particle enters matter, the LET is relatively small. The velocity is such that fewer ionization events occur. As each ionization event happens, the charged particle becomes reduced in energy and travels slower. In traveling slower, the possibility for an ionization event to occur is increased; therefore, the LET is increased. As the particle is reduced in energy, it loses more and more of its energy per unit path until it finally stops. Just prior to the particle reaching rest mass the LET increases tremendously.

Theories concerning the action of radiation on cells

At the present time, there are two theories regarding what occurs in a cell following the passage of a charged particle. These theories are the direct theory and the indirect theory.

Direct theory. Originally, it was theorized that changes in irradiated cells were the result of ionization of some of the essential molecules necessary for the survival of the cell. Another name for this theory is the direct hit theory. It has since been fairly well determined that the probability of destroying one essential molecule in millions of molecules is disproportionate to the amount of radiation necessary to cause total destruction. This theory was considered feasible when biologic systems were exposed to large quantities of radiation; however, relatively low doses of radiation also produced a great amount of damage to cells—more than was expected. For this reason, the direct hit theory did not suffice as an explanation. It would seem, according to the laws of probability, that if a known amount of radiation damaged a known number of cells, half that amount would damage half the number of cells. Actually, however, considerably more than one-half of the cells were damaged. As a result, the indirect theory is now accepted by most authorities.

Indirect theory. The indirect theory uses a number of physical and chemical events to describe the death of the cell. Since water is a major constituent of all biologic materials, water enters into the reaction which is believed to eventually cause the death of the cell following irradiation. The death of the cell by water is brought about by the formation of free radicals. The most important process following a series of complicated ionization events seems to be the dissociation of the water molecule into a free hydrogen radical (H·) and a free hydroxyl radical (OH·) according to the following formula:

$$H_2O \text{ ionization } H_2O^+ + e^- \longrightarrow H^· + OH^·$$

Note that the hydrogen and the hydroxyl groups are not ions but are short-lived and highly reactive radicals. The ionization event has broken the covalent bond, and these fragments possess unfilled electron shells. They carry no charge; therefore, they are not ions. They are neutral atoms in search of another atom with which to combine in order to fill their shells.

What happens to the hydrogen and the hydroxyl radicals following the breaking of the covalent bond is highly dependent upon the LET of the particle. Two reactions are possible. The hydrogen and the hydroxyl radical could recombine to form water:

$$H^· + OH^· \to H_2O$$

This result is always in competition with the possibility of two hydrogen atoms combining to form hydrogen gas, and two hydroxyl radicals combining to form hydrogen peroxide according to the following formulas:

$$H^· + H^· \to H_2$$
$$OH^· + OH^· \to H_2O_2$$

Primarily, the LET value determines which reaction or set of reactions takes place. If the LET value is low, the spacing of the ionization events will be far apart and the probability that recombination will occur to form water is increased. If the LET value is high, the ionization events are closer together and the possibility of the hydrogen radicals combining and the hydroxyl radicals combining is much greater. The resulting hydrogen peroxide is toxic to the cell and death of the cell can ensue.

RADIATION EFFECTS AT THE CELLULAR LEVEL

It can be generally stated that *no* living cells are completely resistant to radiation. Cell damage manifests itself in many different ways. The damage may vary from alteration of a single molecule, which can be repaired at once, to death of the cell. Which portion of the cell that is most sensitive and is directly responsible for the cellular damage has been a subject of debate for a long time. It is generally assumed that there is a significant difference between the radiosensitivity of the nucleus and of the cytoplasm of the cell. Nuclear structures, particularly the chromosomes at time of division, undergo dramatic changes as a result of radiation. The cytoplasm, however, does not appear to be as radiosensitive under the same radiation conditions.

Growth suppression. One of the most obvious effects on the cell from radiation is growth suppression. Cells decrease in number following radiation, because mitosis (the process responsible for cellular division) and, therefore, growth are interrupted.

It is generally agreed that cells with greater mitotic activity are more sensitive to radiation. This mitotic activity depends upon the number of cells entering mitosis and the length of time that each cell spends in mitosis. The statement does not imply that the cell must be actually in mitosis at the time of the radiation in order to be damaged, but only that it be mitotically active—one that will enter mitosis at some subsequent time.

This latent form of radiation damage manifests itself at the time of division. The cell loses the ability to divide successfully. This relationship between a mitotically active cell and radiation has a number of paradoxic exceptions. Some tumors, such as malignant melanoma and osteogenic sarcoma, are relatively radioresistant even though they show considerable mitotic activity. Conversely, seminomas and lymphocytes are radiosensitive although they show no mitotic activity (the lymphocyte is one of the most radiosensitive cells in the human body). Other radiation effects on cells are *restriction of motility, alterations in gland secretions,* and *inactivation of enzymes.*

Effect on chromosomes. Another readily demonstrable effect of radiation is the effect on chromosomes. Following irradiation, chromosomes become adherent. Varying amounts of radiation cause chromosome adhesions, nuclear clumping, and chromosome breakage. Chromosome breakage results in new arrangements of a higher general mortality in these groups of heavily irradiated people. There remain open, or they may unite with another chromosome. The genes of the chromosomes may be locked, duplicated, inverted, or moved to a new position on the same chromosome. Mutations may occur at the site of a chromosome break. Mutation-like changes may result from rearrangement of gene sequences. It is known that breakage can have a lethal effect on the cell. The hypothesis at this point in the science of radiobiology is that damage to chromosomes is the basis of lethal effects of radiation on dividing cells.

Giant cells. One of the outstanding effects of irradiation of cells is the production of the giant cell. This type of cell is produced in the radiation therapy of tumors. Cells may be damaged to the point where they are not capable of cell division, but the irradiated cell may not die immediately. It still may be able to carry on its metabolic activity. For this reason the cell becomes larger and larger. Since the cell can never divide, however, it ultimately dies.

Environmental factors. Environmental factors also play a role in the effect of radiation on living cells. The mechanism of action is not completely known, but oxygen content, temperature, and pressure can increase or decrease radiosensitivity. A general statement can be made regarding the three environmental factors. Radiosensitivity of a cell is directly proportional to the amount of *oxygen, temperature, and pressure.* As any of the environmental factors increases, so also does radiosensitivity; as it decreases, radiosensitivity decreases.

RADIATION EFFECTS ON BIOLOGIC SYSTEMS

The effects of radiation vary considerably from one organ system to another. The following discussion of some of the major systems will provide a basis for anticipating problems in a radiation accident.

Hematopoietic system

Organs that produce blood cells, such as the bone marrow, spleen, and lymph nodes, are extremely radiosensitive, as are the blood cells themselves. The mature circulating cells are relatively radioresistant in contrast to the blood cell precursors. The latter are highly radiosensitive, and this radiosensitivity is demonstrable within a few hours following irradiation by the effect on the subsequent circulating blood cells. The white blood cells (leukocytes) are the most radiosensitive and disappear from circulation first. The first type of white blood cell to disappear is the lymphocyte, followed by the granulocytes. The red blood cells (erythrocytes) disappear next, followed by the platelets.

The drop in lymphocytes, since they are the most radiosensitive components of the blood, becomes an irradiation indicator. If the lymphocyte count decreases to a level of 100 to 200/mm^3 within 12 to 24 hours, the radiation dose is probably lethal. (The normal average lymphocyte count is 2,100/mm^3.) A decrease to 500/mm^3 in the first 24 to 48 hrs is indicative of a questionable prognosis. If the count remains above 1,000/mm^3, the prognosis is good; if the count increases after the first week, recovery is almost assured. Death may occur with no measureable drop in the number of circulating red blood cells, since a drop in cellular components is due to nongeneration by the hematopoietic system. Lymphocytes disappear rapidly because they have a life-span of about 2 days, whereas, erythrocytes have a life-span of about 120 days, so radiation effects are not quite as observable.

Hemorrhage is directly related to the circulating blood platelet level and the effects of radiation on capillaries. Since radiation causes a decrease in platelet count, hemorrhage is a symptom of radiation exposure. Bleeding rarely becomes severe until the platelet count is less than 20,000/mm^3 (the normal average is 240,000/mm^3). A decreased platelet count is clinically observed as a reduced coagulation time. Hemorrhaging can lead to circulatory embarrassment and ultimate cardiac failure.

Blood plasma is highly radioresistant and there have been no predictable changes in its constituents to date. Further, there have been no functional changes in circulation observed, such as changes in cardiac output or blood pressure, until after several thousand roentgens of radiation have been administered to the whole body. Circulatory embarrassment has been known to occur with lesser amounts of radiation because of tissue destruction of the vascular bed, fragility of the vascular walls, and occlusion of the vessels.

Reproductive system

The gonads (the ovaries in the female and the testes in the male) are highly radiosensitive. Mutations and aberrations occur in the chromosome system in either the ova or the sperm following irradiation. Sterility is also known to be a radiation effect. The latter can be either permanent or temporary. Both degrees of sterility occur at lesser doses in the female of a species than in the male. Temporary sterility occurs in female mammals after exposure to doses less than 200 r; permanent sterility occurs after exposure to doses exceeding 300 r. In the case

111

of the male mammal, temporary sterility occurs when the testes are exposed to radiations exceeding 300 r; permanent sterility occurs after exposure to doses greater than 1,000 r. In the female mammal, the ova and precursor follicular cells are the highly radiosensitive elements. Spermatogonia are the most radiosensitive element in the male mammal; the spermatocytes, spermatids, and spermatozoa are highly resistant. In the male mammal, there is a noticeable loss of sperm motility and an increased incidence of sperm abnormalities following irradiation. One outstanding feature in male mammals, however, is the capacity for complete testicular regeneration following radiation exposure and the formation of functional spermatozoa.

Occupational radiation personnel and the radiation therapy patient are constantly worried about radiation causing sterility or impotency. Sometimes the two terms become confused and are used synonymously. They actually are two distinct entities. Sterility is defined as the involuntary, total inability to reproduce; potency is defined as the ability of the male to perform the sexual act. Radiation will affect sterility both on a temporary basis in low levels of radiation and on a permanent basis in higher levels of radiation exposure. Human potency, however, does not seem to be affected by radiation exposure except in lethal doses. Potency may be affected by fatigue accompanying radiation illness and by the psychologic factors that are always involved upon exposure to any degree of radiation. However, the radiation itself does not produce impotency. Radiation to the testes depresses or prevents spermatogenesis, but it does not affect hormonal secretion; therefore, potency is not affected.

Lymphatic system

The spleen, lymph nodes, and thymus all exhibit high degrees of radiosensitivity, since all of them are related to the lymphatic system. The spleen shows inhibition of mitosis in less than an hour following medium doses of radiation. This is followed shortly by severe damage to the lymphocytes. Another radiation effect on the spleen is loss of splenic weight. In fact, this weight loss becomes a sensitive indicator of the dose of radiation to which the organ has been exposed. A most profound observation in the function of a spleen exposed to radiation is the cessation of the production of both red blood cells and white blood cells. During this period, the precursor cells completely atrophy. If the radiation is such that hemorrhage occurs throughout the entire body, bleeding into the spleen becomes marked.

Lymph nodes and other lymphoid tissue are also highly radiosensitive at very low levels of radiation. Following radiation, lymph nodes initially decrease in size. Then, depending upon the amount of radiation, they either reconstitute themselves and regain their function or they become swollen, edematous, and hemorrhagic.

The thymus gland also shows a highly radiosensitive response caused by a large lymphocyte content. Special note is made of the thymus, since in the 1920's, many children were given x-ray treatments for enlarged thymus glands in order to reduce the glands' size and activity. There is evidence now that such treatment has increased the incidence of leukemia and thyroid cancer.

Gastrointestinal tract

The mucosal epithelium of the gastrointestinal tract is quite radiosensitive, but not as highly sensitive as that of the hematopoietic system and the gonads. The first change to be seen following irradiation is the cessation of mitosis, followed by edema, degeneration, and necrosis of the mucosal epithelial cell. These early changes are responsible for the gastrointestinal syndrome of radiation sickness. This syndrome exhibits itself through anorexia, nausea, vomiting, and diarrhea. There are also functional changes that include the depression of pepsin and acid secretion by the stomach, increased mucus production by the small intestine and the colon, and impaired intestinal absorption. Another common symptom is dryness of the mouth caused by a decrease in salivation. As the radiation dose increases, the intestine becomes inflamed and bizarre forms of mucosal cells are produced. The diarrhea produced by the gastrointestinal syndrome appears thin, mucoid, or bloody. The latter is usually controlled by drugs such as paregoric. Vomiting occurs after very low radiation doses and can be of diagnostic importance. Early onset of vomiting is usually an indication of heavy doses of radiation and it carries a poor prognosis. This symptom is also of diagnostic importance in ruling out psychosomatic causes and malingering. The vomiting can be controlled by anti-emetic drugs if it is not of psychosomatic origin.

Skin

The skin is a relatively radiosensitive tissue of about the same magnitude as that of the gastrointestinal tract. Radiation effects on the skin are usually exhibited by a redness (erythema) and changes in its appendages (hair and nails). Loss of hair (epilation) is noticeable at fairly low exposure doses. With higher dosages, depigmentation, ulcerations, and dermatitis occur. Treatment for skin contamination consists of prompt decontamination of the skin and hair with the use of detergents and copious amounts of water. Treatment of actual burn lesions is similar to the treatment of thermal burns. The burn is cleansed, itching and pain are reduced, and antibiotics are applied.

Eye

Protection of the eye has long been the concern of radiation workers. The most radiosensitive area of the eye is the lens. It is a well-known fact that opacities of the lens of the eye (cataracts) result from exposure to ionizing radiation. This fact is of primary concern to radiologists and x-ray technologists and is especially applicable to those working with fluoroscopic equipment. The protection of the eye is one of the primary considerations in the design of such equipment. Cataract formations have been noted on radiation workers who were involved in the development of the cyclotron and in Japanese survivors of the atomic bombing of Hiroshima and Nagasaki. The lens is such a simple structure from a histologic standpoint that cataract formations are the only lesions of radiobiologic significance. Inflammation of the cornea, increased photosensitivity, pain, and redness of the eye have been caused by radiation.

Central nervous system

The central nervous system is the most radioresistant organ system in mammals. Further, the brain is considered more radiosensitive than the spinal cord; however, this radiosensitivity exhibits itself only after exposure to thousands of roentgens. Radiation effects on the central nervous system are usually caused by localized radiation exposure, such as that used in therapy, not by exposure to the total body. Under conditions of localized exposure, radiation may permanently injure the blood vessels of the brain or spinal cord, resulting in a lack of blood supply (ischemia) to the brain. Several thousand roentgens of radiation have also been known to destroy certain elements in the central nervous system, causing a dysfunction of vital nerve centers, after which death ensues. In general, however, the central nervous system is a highly radioresistant organ system.

All other organs

All other organs, including the heart, kidney, liver, and pancreas, are extremely radioresistant. The only changes found in these organs are caused by high radiation doses. Such changes include hemorrhage, infarcts, necrosis, and edema.

RADIOSENSITIVITY

According to the above discussion of biologic systems, all organs can be placed in one of three rather ill-defined groups: radiosensitive, radioresponsive, and radioresistant. The radiosensitive category includes all blood-forming organs including the bone marrow and lymph organs, and the reproductive tissues. The radioresponsive group includes the epithelium of the gastrointestinal tract and the skin. The radioresistant group includes all other organs.

This division into the three categories of response to radiation is, at the present time, a qualitative rather than a quantitative categorization. It is not well understood why such a range of response exists. An even more difficult phenomenon to understand is the tremendous degree of species variation regarding the amount of radiation causing death. Familiar medical terminology involving dose to mortality is LD_{50}. This term refers to the lethal dose whereby 50% of a species die. A similar term, MLD/30 (sometimes written as $MLD_{50}/30$), is used to describe mortality caused by radiation. This term refers to the median lethal dose whereby 50% of those exposed die in 30 days. This tremendous species variation is exemplified by two extremes—the guinea pig and the bat. Guinea pigs have an MLD/30 of 250 rems, while the MLD/30 value for bats is 16,000 rems. The paramecium, one of the most radioresistant forms of life, has an MLD/30 value of 300,000 rems. In man, the MLD/30 value is 400 ± 100 rems. All other organisms have MLD/30 values that vary between that of the guinea pig and the paramecium.

Mammals seem to be more radiosensitive than birds, fish, and reptiles. The fact that they are *warmblooded* organisms may contribute to this increased sensitivity. *Age* is an extremely important factor in that the adult organism or the adult cell is much more resistant than the embryo or the newly formed cell. This is the rationale for radiation therapy of cancer. A cancer is an uncontrolled growth and is made up, therefore, of predominantly newly formed cells. Increases in *temperature, pressure,* and *oxygen* content also increase radiosensitivity. *Unicellular* organisms are generally more resistant to radiation than multicellular organisms. Those tissues that *proliferate cells* needed for maintenance and function of the organ seem to be the most susceptible to radiation. Such tissues include the blood-forming components, the gastrointestinal tract mucosa, the precursors of the germ cells, the skin, and the lens of the eye. Mature cells of cartilage, bone, muscle, and the central nervous system are relatively insensitive to radiation.

ACUTE SOMATIC EFFECTS OF RADIATION

When man is exposed to a large, single, short-term (from several minutes to a few hours) whole body dose of ionizing radiation, the resulting injury is expressed as a complex of clinical symptoms and laboratory findings. These are collectively termed the *acute radiation syndrome.* This syndrome represents a clinical expression of the damage to many important organs simultaneously by depletion of radio-sensitive cells resulting from their inability to reproduce themselves. From studies of survivors of nuclear bombing attacks, radiation therapy patients, and occupational radiation accident victims, the sequence of events following large whole body radiation exposure can be divided into four clinical stages:

1. Initial stage—0 to 48 hours following exposure
2. Latent stage—48 hours to 2 or 3 weeks following exposure
3. Severe illness stage—2 to 3 weeks to 6 to 8 weeks following exposure
4. Recovery stage—6 to 8 weeks to several months following exposure

The clinical findings in the initial stage include loss of appetite (anorexia), nausea, sweating, and fatigue. In the latent period, which begins about 2 days following exposure, these clinical findings may become normal and remain that way for 2 to 3 weeks. The severe illness stage may include fever, infection, sensitive scalp, loss of hair, hemorrhage, diarrhea, lethargy, disturbances in consciousness and perception, and cardiovascular collapse. These symptoms depend entirely upon the dose to which the human being was exposed.

Although responses of a patient of a given dose are difficult to itemize, Table 7-1 is presented to give some idea of what symptoms to expect in approximate dose ranges. According to this table, the first system to stop functioning is the highly radiosensitive hematopoietic system. If the radiation injury is more severe, gastrointestinal symptoms become predominate. Finally, as the radiation dose becomes extremely severe, damage to the relatively radioresistant central nervous system causes almost immediate death, although the exact cause of death is subject to controversy at the present time. The predominance of gastrointestinal symptomatology with doses of 600 rads and central nervous system complications after exposure to 3,000 rads does not indicate that severe hematologic damage has not taken place at these levels of exposure. These patients simply do not survive long enough to display the full manifestation of their hematologic injury. The information on this table is based primarily on cases of external radiation exposure. Similar manifestations of this acute radiation syndrome may accompany the administration of internal radiation emitters, such as gold 198 and phosphorus 32, when given

115

Table 7-1. Summary of the acute radiation syndrome

Group	Dose (rads)	Symptoms	Treatment	System involved	Time of death
I	100	Anorexia; nausea; vomiting	Antiemetics	(Leukemia?) Increased aging?	Approaches normal life span
II	200	Same as group I, plus slight anemia; infection; hemorrhage; conjunctivitis; sweating; purpura; scalp pain; hair loss; weight loss	Antiemetics; aseptic isolation (masked and gowned attendants); antibiotics and transfusions, if warranted	Same as above	Approaches normal life span
III	400	Same as groups I and II; plus disorientation; shock; coma	I.V. feeding (calories and electrolyte balance); transfusion of whole blood and platelets	Hematopoietic	10 to 30 days
IV	600	Increased shock; increased hemorrhage; severe infection; fever	I.V. feeding (blood diet); bone marrow transplant; steroids and vasopressors; Hemodialysis, if needed; antibiotics	Gastrointestinal	3 to 14 days
V	3,000	Immediate burning sensation over entire body; immediate vomiting and diarrhea; cyanosis; acute respiratory distress; papilledema; oliguria; WBC: 41,000 by 16 hours; lymphocytes disappear by 7 hours	I.V. fluids; steroids; pressor agents	Central nervous system (?)	Hours to 2 days after exposure

in very high doses. In general, however, the true acute radiation syndrome is not seen after exposure to internal emitters. The effects of internal emitters are usually chronic and occur after long-term, low-level exposure.

CHRONIC SOMATIC EFFECTS

Chronic somatic effects caused by exposure to radiation are more difficult to demonstrate with certainty. It was not until about 10 years after the discovery of the x-ray and of natural radioactivity that it was realized that somatic effects from overexposure to ionizing radiation might not be evident until years or decades following the event. The fact that radiation could have a chronic effect was based primarily on the changes in the skin. Burns and dermatitis, known to be a result from radiation exposure, progress eventually to cancer of the skin. Knowing the positive agent for the burns, it was hypothesized that not all of the effects of radiation were acute in nature, but that they could occur at some later time. This has since been supported by evidence from laboratory animal experiments. Other chronic effects of radiation are shortening of the life-span, early aging, increased incidence of leukemia, and increased incidence of benign and malignant tumors.

Shortening of the life-span. Animal experimentation has demonstrated very clearly that shortening of the life-span follows single or repeated doses of radiation exposure. There is not, however, conclusive evidence that this is a general manifestation of radiation exposure in man. It is known that there is an increased incidence of leukemias and malignancies following radiation, and these are obviously going to reduce the life-span of individuals having these diseases. The problem is further complicated because it is difficult to extrapolate results of animal experimentation to man. It is also difficult to obtain such information in human populations. At the present time, it can be generally stated that there is very little evidence of human life shortening from radiation exposure. Further, there are, as yet, no data for man that provide a satisfactory basis for quantitative estimation of overall life-shortening effects. The atomic bombing survivors (60,000 still living in 1950 including 7,000 who demonstrated the major symptoms of the acute radiation syndrome) have been and are being carefully studied. Thus far, there is no evidence of a higher general mortality in these groups of heavily irradiated people. There has been some controversial evidence presented that radiologists die 5.2 years earlier than physicians not occupationally exposed to radiation. With improvements in radiation safety practices and radiation safety devices in recent years, this deficit in life-span has been shown to decrease.

Early aging. Early aging, the enhancement of the physiologic aging process, has been associated with radiation exposure. It has been shown that following irradiation, fibrosis of the skin, heart muscle, lymphoid organs, and endocrine glands results. Chronic lung inflammation has been observed. Atrophy and defective development in the skin, lymphoid organs, bone marrow, and gonads have also been seen. There have been alterations in the pigment deposition in the skin and hair. These are all processes associated with aging. This whole concept of premature aging, however, is subject to controversy.

Leukemia. Increased incidence of leukemia has been reported in a number of groups of individuals exposed to radiation—radiologists, survivors of atomic bombing, children who were treated with x-rays for thymus gland abnormalities, persons who received intravenous Thorotrast, and persons who were treated by x-ray for rheumatoid arthritis of the spine. The body load of internal emitting radionuclides is kept to a minimum because of the possibility of their leukemogenic (leukemia-producing) effects in man.

Cancer. Development of cancer from radiation exposure has definitely been shown to be one of the chronic effects following total body irradiation. There seems to be very little evidence contrary to this conclusion. Carcinomas have been noted in several groups of occupational radiation workers, as well as that large group of people injected with Thorotrast. Cancer, since it was first observed as a skin lesion on pioneers of the x-ray, has appeared as lung carcinoma in miners of radioactive ores and as carcinoma of the mouth in some radium dial painters.

The radium dial painters were girls who painted luminous watch dials in New Jersey, Connecticut, and Illinois from 1914 to 1925. It was their habit to put a fine point on their brushes by shaping them with their lips. In so doing, they ingested the radium, and osteogenic sarcoma developed. Many of these radium dial painters (over 500 of the exposed have been studied) died with severe anemia and destructive lesions of the mouth and jaw. Of particular significance is the fact that no leukemia has been demonstrated in these cases of radium ingestion. It has been estimated that about 2,000 such luminous dial painters are still living, most of them in good health. It is known that about 50 have died as a result of this internal exposure to radiation. These cases have now become classic examples of the destructive effects of radioelements in humans.

Another source of information on the internal dose problem is the large group of persons who were injected with Thorotrast. This suspension of ThO_2 was injected for the purposes of diagnostic radiology from 1928 to 1945. In these patients, hepatic tumors seem to be the predominant neoplasm. There is a long induction period for cancer, ranging from 10 to 20 years.

GENETIC EFFECTS

Every human individual develops from a single cell formed by the fusion of two germ cells from the two parents. Each cell contains a number of microscopic, thread-like structures called chromosomes, which in turn contain genes. Genes constitute the material that determines the hereditary characteristics of the individual. The germ cell receives half of its genes from each parent, and these determine the family likenesses.

Occasionally, something happens to the gene and the likeness is altered. This alteration is called a mutation, and the characteristic which it governs may be changed in the offspring. These mutations may be of thermal or chemical origin, or they may be induced by ionizing radiation.

Some mutations are beneficial. The evolution of man is an example. Man has evolved to his present state through small changes from the average. Other mutations are harmful. Approximately 2% of all defects in the present population are of genetic origin; defects such as congenital malformations, idiocy, and so on. Some of the defects are undoubtedly caused by ionizing radiation, but the exact percentage is uncertain. There are two types of mutations—dominant and recessive. Dominant mutations change the characteristic in the next generation, if either parent develops the mutation. Recessive mutations change the characteristic only if both parents develop the mutation and pass it on to their offspring. Dominant mutations are much rarer than recessives, and the chance of passing the altered characteristic to the offspring is even more rare. The transmission of the more common recessive mutations becomes progressively less in subsequent generations. If both parents have the recessive trait, the probability is that 50% of the children would receive it, 25% of the grandchildren, and 12.5% of the great-grandchildren. It is well known that everyone carries his share of recessive mutations from his ancestors. This is one of the arguments against "blood" marriages—the chances that both parents would have the same recessive gene from their ancestors would increase the probability that their offspring would exhibit the recessive trait.

There are no accurate data as to the genetic effects of ionizing radiation in man. Much work has been done on insects and animals in this regard, but extrapolation to man must be done with caution. The survivors of the atomic bombings in Hiroshima and Nagasaki are being carefully studied, but very little information is available from these studies. Some general statements may be made, however, regarding the genetic effects of ionizing radiation:

1. Any amount of radiation can produce some mutation; there is no lower threshold.
2. The rate of mutation is proportional to the radiation exposure.
3. There is no recovery by the gene following its mutation.
4. Damage to genetic material is cumulative. Long continued exposure to low intensity radiation produces as much genetic damage as a single exposure to an equal dose of higher intensity. This is quite unlike somatic damage.
5. Radiation increases the frequency of gene mutation, but produces no new kinds of mutations.

Conclusions at the present time are that the genetic effects of radiation do not constitute a serious consideration in the production of damaging mutations. The studies of the Japanese bomb survivors reveal in one generation only a very few types of mutations. Further, everyone carries a large number of damaging mutations received from their ancestors. A few additional ones as a result of exposure to radiation will not alter the hereditary pattern significantly.

Chapter 8

Principles of radiation detection

Since ionizing radiations cannot be perceived by any of the human senses, it is advantageous to have some sensory device which can detect the presence of such ionizing radiations. Further, it is desirable to be able to quantitate the amount of ionizing radiation present, which is useful not only for radiation protection, but also for diagnostic and therapeutic applications. A large number of such devices are available and all have specific applications. These devices have been grouped into three main categories: gas detectors, scintillation detectors, and miscellaneous detectors.

GAS DETECTORS
Rationale

The counting function of a gas detector depends upon the collection of ion pairs produced in the gas volume by the passage of radiation to the detector. These ion pairs are collected by the walls of the gas chamber, which are electrically conductive. An external circuit consists of a DC voltage source in series with a sensitive current meter.

As ion pairs are produced by radiation passing through the enclosed volume of gas, the positive ions begin to migrate to the negative wall and the negative ions (electrons) begin to migrate to the positive wall of the detector, provided an external voltage is applied. The positive ion, which has a mass many thousand times greater than that of the electron, is accelerated toward the negative electrode at a slow rate compared to the rate at which the electron will travel to the positive electrode (anode) (Fig. 8-1).

The operation of gas detectors may best be explained through pulse heights. The number of ions collected at their respective poles is a function of voltage and is directly proportional to pulse height. A characteristic curve for gas detectors may be received by plotting pulse height versus voltage (Fig. 8-2). The figure outlines six regions defined by changes in pulse height response to changes in voltage. These areas are called the recombination, the ionization, the proportional, the nonproportional, the Geiger-Mueller, and the continuous discharge regions, respectively. The two curves, denoted by alpha and beta particles, are typical pulse height responses to these two particles. In Fig. 8-2, the alpha curve, because the alpha particle is more ionizing, corresponds to a level having 100 times the number of ion pairs initially produced by a beta particle. Each of the regions will be discussed individually. The kind of machine used is determined by the intensity of the radiation field and whether a specific particle is responsible for the intensity.

Recombination region. If no voltage is applied between the two electrodes, no

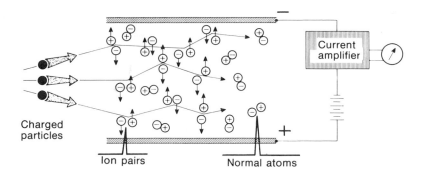

Incoming particles ionize atoms

Electrodes attract ions

Arrival of ions constitutes current

Current is measure of particles

Fig. 8-1. Diagram of a gas detector and its method of radiation detection by attracting the products of ionization events to oppositely charged electrodes. (Courtesy of the U.S. Atomic Energy Commission)

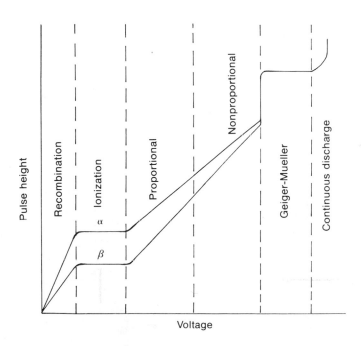

Fig. 8-2. Characteristic curve of gas detector responses to pulse height versus voltage. The curve demonstrates the response expected from two different particles passing through each of the three fundamental types of gas detectors: ionization, proportional and Geiger-Mueller.

direction is given to ion pairs produced by the passing radiation. With no voltage, no ions are collected by the respective poles and no pulse is produced. This is indicated by the curve beginning at the lower left-hand corner of Fig. 8-2. The initial application of a voltage permits the collection of some ion pairs; other ion pairs recombine. The latter will not affect the current and will not be observable on the meter. As the voltage is increased, the number of ion pairs collected increases rapidly, because, by increasing the voltage, the probability of an ion reaching an electrode before it combines with a positive ion also increases. This increase in pulse height continues until eventually the region of ionization is reached.

Ionization region. In the ionization region, the increase in pulse height as a function of voltage no longer exists. The curve flattens out. This area is called a *plateau* or *saturation voltage.* No increase in pulse height is seen because the voltage is sufficient to collect all ions produced by the passing radiation. There is no longer a probability of recombination. Once this region is reached, further increases in voltage serve only to collect the ionized particles more rapidly.

The device used to measure radiation in this region is called an *ionization chamber.* When it is operated at the proper voltage (saturation voltage) the current (flow of electrons) going through the meter is a direct measure of the total number of ion pairs produced per unit time in the enclosed volume of gas. It is, therefore, a measure of the ionization due to radiation.

The ionization chamber is used primarily in areas of high radiation intensity, such as measuring the output of an x-ray tube. Since one ion pair is produced and collected per ionization event, the pulses from single ionization events are much too small for even the most delicate electric meter to register. The proportional pulse heights of the alpha and beta curves allow differentiation between the types of emissions.

The ionization chamber may be a portable dose rate meter, such as the "Cutie Pie," which measures the intensity of radiation per unit time (r/hr); or it may be a dose meter, such as the condenser-r meter (a calibration instrument) or a pocket dosimeter (a personnel monitoring device).

Dose rate meter. The portable dose rate meter is an enclosed volume of gas with a sensitive current meter and a voltage usually supplied by dry cells. The dry cells are such that a few hundred volts are supplied to the system in order that the saturation voltage is reached. Although usually used in high intensity radiation fields, dose rate ionization meters that measure very low intensities are available. These are ordinarily very expensive and heavy. The usual ionization type survey meter is seen in Fig. 8-3, *A.*

Dose meters. Other ionization chambers are available which measure just the quantity (dose) of radiation rather than intensity (dose delivered over a certain unit of time).

An ionization chamber can be charged to a certain voltage and the voltage source disconnected. When this chamber is exposed to ionizing radiation, the ions are collected at their respective poles, and the collection decreases the voltage (discharges) proportionally. The discharge is measured on a voltage meter which is calibrated to read in units of radiation intensity.

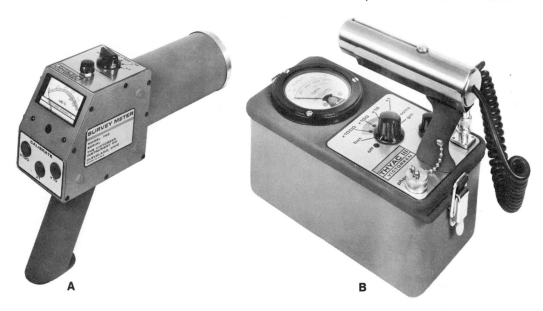

Fig. 8-3. A, Ionization type dose rate survey meter. **B,** Geiger-Mueller type dose rate survey meter. (Courtesy, Victoreen Instrument Co.)

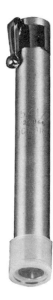

Fig. 8-4. Ionization type selfreading dose meter, commonly called a dosimeter. (Courtesy, Victoreen Instrument Co.)

The dose meter must be initially charged to predetermined voltage. This is accomplished by a charger. Some chambers require a separate reader, in which case the charger and reader are in a self-contained charger-reader unit. Other chambers (dosimeters, primarily) are self-reading. In this case, the chamber incorporates a quartz fiber voltage meter, which, when held up to the light, casts a shadow upon a scale calibrated in units of dose (Fig. 8-4).

Proportional region. As the voltage is increased beyond the saturation voltage,

123

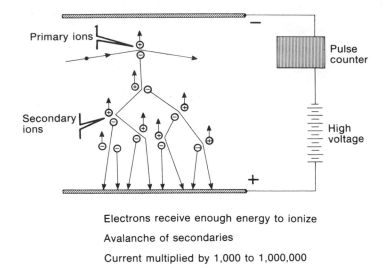

Electrons receive enough energy to ionize

Avalanche of secondaries

Current multiplied by 1,000 to 1,000,000

Fig. 8-5. Diagram of a gas detector illustrating the phenomenon of gas amplification which follows the primary ionization event. This occurs when the voltage between the electrodes is sufficiently high, which is the case in the area of proportional counting. (Courtesy, U.S. Atomic Energy Commission)

another rise in the number of ion pairs collected is seen. This area is called the region of proportionality. It has already been stated that in the ionization region, all ion pairs formed are collected. With additional voltage, however, there is an increase in the number of ion pairs collected (see Fig. 8-2). This increase in number of ion pairs collected cannot result from increased primary ion collections, since all have been accounted for in the region of ionization. The increase is caused by the phenomenon called gas amplification. At higher voltages, the increased speed or energy acquired by the ions during collection eventually gives them the capability of ionizing other gas atoms in their path to their collecting electrode (Fig. 8-5). The path of the electron as it makes its way to the positive electrode becomes tortuous, since it rebounds from one neutral molecule to another. If the electric field is sufficient, as it is in this proportional region, these electrons can obtain enough energy to ionize a neutral molecule on collision and thus create an additional ion pair, which in turn will be collected also. Because of this phenomenon, an amplification occurs whereby *more than one* ion is collected per ionizing event, in contrast to that which occurs in the ionization region. As the voltage increases in this region, the gas amplification phenomenon becomes even greater. The secondary ions also acquire enough energy to ionize other neutral atoms on their path to the positive electrode, thereby, creating other secondary ion pairs. This phenomenon is called an *avalanche.*

The device used in this region is called a *proportional counter.* Many have a continuous flow of gas through the detector. This counter has a distinct advantage over the ionization chamber in that the current pulse height produced by the passage of a single charged particle is large enough to be detected. Further, the pulse heights have maintained a proportionality, so that low intensity radiation can be detected as to alpha or beta emissions by the sorting of the pulses. A problem arises because, even though the current pulses are detectable, they are so small that only the most delicate and elaborate electronic devices are used. These are usually not used in a routine nuclear medicine laboratory. They are used for detecting low-level contamination of alpha particles, as in the case of a possible leak of a radium needle used in therapy.

Nonproportional region. Further increases in the voltage result in the two curves of Fig. 8-2 coming closer together. This region is called the region of nonproportionality. In this region true proportionality between primary ionization and the number of ions collected is no longer maintained. Instead, the pulse height becomes more and more a function of the applied voltage and less and less a function of the amount of initial ionization, as the curves in Fig. 8-2 come together and lose proportionality entirely. This region is not important from the standpoint of radiation detection.

Geiger-Mueller region. Further increases in voltage result in a sharp rise in the curve in Fig. 8-2. This is called the Geiger-Mueller region. In this region the pulse height shows no difference as to primary ionization events, so there is no distinction between ionizing particles. Gas amplification is so intense in this region that a limiting value has been reached. High acceleration in this region produces a catastrophic avalanche of ions delivering a mass of electrical pulses to the collecting electrode. The avalanche of ions results from the production of low energy photons due to Bremsstrahlung. The voltage in the region is so high and the energy acquired by the negative member of the ion pair (electron) is so great that they create Bremsstrahlung photons on their path to the positive electrode (anode). The photons have the ability of striking the negative electrode (cathode) and knocking off electrons from its surface. They traverse the entire gas volume on their way to the anode, creating more Bremsstrahlung and secondary ion pairs. In this way, ionization is spread throughout the entire gas volume.

The size of the pulse is no longer in proportion to the initiating event. This is called the Geiger effect. The voltage at which Geiger-type counting becomes established is called the threshold. It is followed by a *plateau,* over which the counting rate increases slowly. The device for measurement of radiation in this region is called the Geiger counter or G-M counter. The Geiger counter is applicable to areas of low intensity radiation such as determining the extent of a radioactive spill in a routine nuclear medicine laboratory, because a tremendous number of electrons are collected per single ionization event. This is in sharp contrast to the ionization chamber where only one electron is collected per single ionization event.

The Geiger counter (see Fig. 8-3, *B*) has some disadvantages. Since one ionization event spreads ionization through the entire gas volume, a second ionization event may go undetected. The time during which the counter cannot respond to another ionizing event is called its *dead time,* which makes the Geiger counter grossly inefficient. Another disadvantage is that proportionality is lost. The life of a counter is the number of counts which can be accumulated before deterioration of the gas takes place. The counting life of a G-M tube is ordinarily in the range of 1 billion to 10 billion counts. This means that in the usual applications of such a counter, the shelf life would be several years. As the tube ages, the plateau of the Geiger counter becomes shorter until eventually stable operation can no longer be maintained.

Continuous discharge region. If the voltage is raised significantly beyond the G-M region, a rapid rise in numbers of ions collected is seen. This is the region of continuous discharge. Up to this point the discussion has been devoted primarily to the collection of electrons at the anode. Meanwhile, however, the positive ions, because of their mass, move slowly toward the cathode where they are eventually neutralized.

As the positive ion approaches the negative electrode, it acquires an electron and is deionized. Since it requires energy to ionize the gas, energy must be released upon deionization. This energy is released in the form of ultraviolet light, which has sufficient energy to cause another electron to be ejected from the cathode. These additional free electrons enter the gas volume and proceed toward the anode just as did the initial electrons from the primary ionization event. Further, these electrons initiate avalanches on their path to the positive electrode just as did the primary ionization event. The collection of electrons from these events results in an increased number of ion collections, accounting for the sharp rise in the continuous discharge region. If this is allowed to continue, the electrode surfaces of the counter are damaged and the counter may even be destroyed. The continuous discharge can be stopped to a certain degree by a process called *quenching*. This process limits the discharge process. It can be done by momentarily reducing the voltage on the tube or by incorporating a suitable constituent in the counting gas.

SCINTILLATION DETECTORS
Rationale

Certain materials have the property of emitting a flash of light or scintillation when struck by ionizing radiation. A scintillation detector is a sensitive element used to detect ionizing radiation by observing the scintillation induced in the material. When a light-sensitive device is affixed to this special material, the flash of light can be changed into small electrical impulses. The electrical impulses are then amplified so they may be sorted and counted in order that the amount and nature of radiation striking the scintillating materials can be determined. Scintillators are used to determine the amount and/or distribution of radionuclides in one or more organs of a patient for diagnostic purposes.

The procedure of recording a scintillation involves several systems: the detector, the photomultiplier, a high voltage power supply, the preamplifier, the amplifier, gain controls, a pulse-height analyzer, and the display mode. All of these will be treated individually showing the sequential stages of the detection and recording process of a disintegration.

Detector. Two major types of scintillation detectors are currently being used: crystal and liquid. Since the liquid scintillation detector is not as common in routine nuclear medicine laboratories, it will be discussed only briefly.

Liquid detector. Scintillating solutions can be prepared so that when radioactive materials are added to the solution, the radiations are detected through light production. The light is detected and measured through a system of one or more photomultiplier tubes and ancillary electronic equipment to analyze and count the radiations. The liquid solution contains the material being counted, a solvent, and a scintillator. There is a variety of liquid scintillator materials, most of which are organic compounds. The solvents are primarily aromatic hydrocarbons, which efficiently transfer energy from the point of emission to the scintillator molecule. The use of liquid scintillation materials has its greatest advantage in its ability to detect β^- emissions or weak energy gamma rays, since the radioactive material is mixed with the scintillating material so that there is no loss of emissions by absorption before they reach the detector. Such absorption could be by the cover of the detector or by self-absorption.

Crystal detector. The most widely used scintillation detector is the solid type—a sodium iodide (NaI) crystal activated with thallium, commonly written NaI (Tl). Pure sodium iodide crystals do not scintillate at room temperature. If, however, impurities are added, such as thallium, centers of luminescence are produced which can be excited at room temperature by ionizing radiation.

Sodium iodide is hygroscopic (retains water) and must be kept in a moisture-free atmosphere. Consequently, the crystal is hermetically sealed. It is enclosed by an aluminum container on all sides except that side attached to the photomultiplier tube (see Fig. 8-6). A glass window protects it on this end. The inside surfaces of the container have reflective capabilities. More recently, the crystal and photo-multiplier have been produced as an integral assembly, eliminating the necessity for the glass shield, and the entire assembly is hermetically sealed. Should the crystal or the assembly become damaged so that there is a break in the seal and moisture enters, the crystal shows a yellow discoloration (probably due to free iodine).

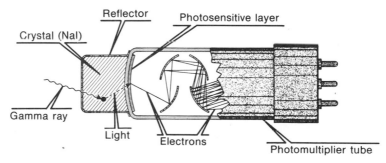

Total light to tube nearly proportional to gamma ray energy

If 1 electron ejects 5 from a dynode, 11 dynodes result in 5^{11}

or

about 50 million electrons output

Fig. 8-6. Crystal photomultiplier assembly illustrating the detection of a gamma ray by the crystal and its subsequent amplification through the photomultiplier tube. (Courtesy, U.S. Atomic Energy Commission)

The process of detection is initiated when an incident gamma ray enters the crystal. Under ideal conditions, the energy is eventually totally absorbed. This is usually accomplished through a series of Compton collisions with subsequent total absorption of the energy by a photoelectric collision. (Pair production is also possible if the incident gamma ray is greater than 1.02 mev of energy.) Each time such a Compton collision occurs, some of the energy of the incident gamma ray is transferred to an electron which will produce luminescent light in proportion to its energy. The light is in the form of small flashes following the interactions of the ejected electrons. If the energy of the incident gamma ray is high, many Compton collisions will occur before the energy is totally absorbed. The increased number of Compton collisions will produce more secondary electrons which will, in turn, produce more flashes of light. If the energy of the gamma ray is low, fewer collisions will occur before total absorption and, therefore, there will be fewer flashes of light. These small flashes of light, although emitted in a sequential manner, appear to the human eye or on the photomultiplier tube as a single flash or shower of light. The intensity of the light is directly proportional to the number of flashes of light. Since the number of flashes increases with energy of the gamma ray, it can be said that the intensity of the light is proportional to the energy of the incident gamma ray. This flash of light is eventually directed to the photomultiplier tube, either by reflection from the interior surface of the aluminum housing or by the direction in which it was emitted.

Photomultiplier. The photomultiplier is a light-sensitive device which is optically connected to the sodium iodide crystal. Its purpose is to convert the light energy from the crystal to electrical energy and amplify the resultant pulse of electricity. The photomultiplier tube consists of a photocathode and a series of 10 dynodes. The photocathode receives the flash of light from the crystal. The photocathode consists of a material that responds to waves of light energy, much like any atom responds to waves of gamma energy in the Compton effect; the incident light wave hits the atoms of the photocathode and causes electrons to be ejected. This is called *photoemission*. The principle of this operation is not unlike that which occurs in "electric eye" applications. The number of electrons released from the photocathode is directly proportional to the intensity of the light from the crystal.

As the electrons are emitted from the photocathode, they are drawn to the first of the 10 dynodes in the photomultiplier tube (see Fig. 8-6). They are drawn to the dynode because of an applied voltage between the photocathode and that dynode. This voltage accelerates the electron, impinging it on the dynode with such force that more than one electron is released from the dynode. This is called *secondary emission*. These electrons are then drawn to the second dynode by a similar increase in applied voltage, whereupon, secondary emission occurs again. This process continues throughout the entire photomultiplier tube. By the time the electrons have left the tenth dynode, the number of electrons released may be on the order of millions. The photomultiplier tube possesses the ability, therefore, to convert one flash of light to a burst of millions of electrons; hence the name, photomultiplier. The usual terminology to describe this burst of electrons is a voltage pulse and the number of electrons collected at the last dynode is proportional to the voltage pulse height.

A system of proportionality exists throughout the entire crystal photomultiplier assembly. This can be summarized by the following:

1. The pulse height is proportional to the number of electrons received at the last dynode which is, in turn, dependent on the number of electrons released by the photocathode.
2. The number of electrons released by the photocathode is directly proportional to the intensity of the light received from the crystal.
3. The intensity of the light received from the crystal is directly proportional to the energy of the incident gamma ray.
4. *The pulse height is directly proportional to the energy of the incident gamma ray.*

High voltage power supply. In any standard counting device (scaler or rate meter) almost invariably there is a separate voltage supply unit to provide high voltage to the photomultiplier tube. The total high voltage applied to the tube is divided among the various dynodes. For instance, if the voltage is 500 v, a 50 v potential difference exists between successive dynodes (voltage and potential difference are synonymous). If 1,000 v were applied to the photomultiplier tube, a potential difference of 100 v would exist between successive dynodes. The purpose of the high voltage power supply is to provide enough "attraction" of the electrode in order that secondary emission will occur each time an electron hits a dynode. It is important that this high voltage power supply be very stable. Instability of this voltage power supply is called "drift." It may be caused by temperature change, change in line voltage, and so on. The purpose for being concerned with drift, or rather the lack of it, is its effect upon secondary emission. The number of secondary electrons produced by each electron that strikes a dynode is directly dependent upon the voltage that exists between the two dynodes. Should the voltage at time of calibration be such that 5 electrons are released by secondary emission for each electron striking the dynode, then a drift in the voltage might cause only 4 electrons to be given off by secondary emission. This would alter the clinical results considerably. (This will become more clear during the discussion of pulse height analysis.)

The drift may occur upward as well. If it is sufficient, the voltage becomes so great that electrons are pulled off the dynodes without other electrons striking the dynode. This is referred to as *thermal emission* or "noise." This phenomenon is easily demonstrated by increasing the voltage without a source of radioactivity. Eventually a high count rate is received, caused by thermal emission.

Preamplifier. The preamplifier is generally found at the rear of the detector assembly. The word "preamplifier" is a misnomer, because it implies that the size of the voltage pulse is amplified in some manner. The actual result, however, is that it is usually a little less in amplitude, because of the phenomenon of transmission of electrical power known as impedance. This is a fairly complicated principle, the definition of which is not of particular importance to nuclear medicine personnel. Impedances between the photomultiplier tube and amplifier must

129

be matched in order that there is no loss of power. For this reason, a reduction in pulse height is sometimes necessary. The preamplifier also provides a driving force, characteristics of which are such that the pulse will not be lost in the several feet of cable connecting the detector to the main scaler chassis. The pulse is then fed into the amplifier.

Amplifier. The pulses that are fed into the amplifier have a wide variation in pulse height because there is a wide variation in energies of gamma rays striking the scintillation crystal. All of these pulses must be increased in amplitude by a constant factor so that the final pulse is still proportional to the energy lost by the gamma ray in the crystal. This is called linear amplification. Nonlinear amplification would defeat the purpose of pulse height analyzers (see p. 133), because all pulses, regardless of their size, would be amplified to the same height. The amplifier consists of four tubes or transistors in two successive sections. The voltage gains for the two sections are approximately 70 to 120, so that the overall amplification is something more than 8,000. The amplifier receives pulses on the order of millivolts. If 1 mv were sent through this amplifier, it would be increased to 8 v. The amplifier is capable of amplifying to 100 v or more with negligible distortion.

Gain control. Between the two sections of the amplifier there is a stepped gain control. This allows the operator to increase or decrease the amplification, as desired. In scalers there are usually five such positions represented in a variety of ways, depending upon the manufacturer of the detector. Gain control values are usually represented by the numbers 32, 16, 8, 4, and 2 or 4, 2, 1, 0.5, 0.25. Regardless of their value, they do the same thing. The five steps on the gain control represent full gain, one-half, one-quarter, one-eighth, and one-sixteenth of the maximum gain; at each step the amplification is one-half that of the next higher step. This type of gain is called an *inverse gain.*

The exact opposite is true in the utilization of gain settings on most scanners. These settings are represented by the numbers 1, 2, 5, and 10, which, rather than decreasing the amplification by factors of one-half, it actually increases the amplification by the factor indicated by the number. Therefore, a pulse of a certain height on a gain of 1 would be increased to twice the height on the gain of 2, five times the height on the gain of 5, and ten times the height on the gain of 10. This is called a *true gain.*

A simplified explanation of gain settings is shown in Fig. 8-7. The dark line (third from the top) represents the actual settings on the gain control. This is expressed as a range of 0 to 100 v, equivalent to 0 to 1,000 kev on that gain setting. The usual procedure is to calibrate on mid-gain (a value of 8 or 1, depending upon the settings available). By calibrating on this gain, the operator has essentially set each small division on the discriminator dials (which have 1,000 small divisions) to be equal to that number in kev. The gain setting essentially expands or contracts that scale depending upon the gain settings used. If the operator has amplified the pulse to 50 v (500 kev), by changing the gain setting to 16 (or 2) that same pulse would no longer be found at the 500 units setting, but would be found at approximately the 250 setting. If the settings are changed to 32 (or 4), that same pulse will now be found at a 125 value. The converse is also true. If, going

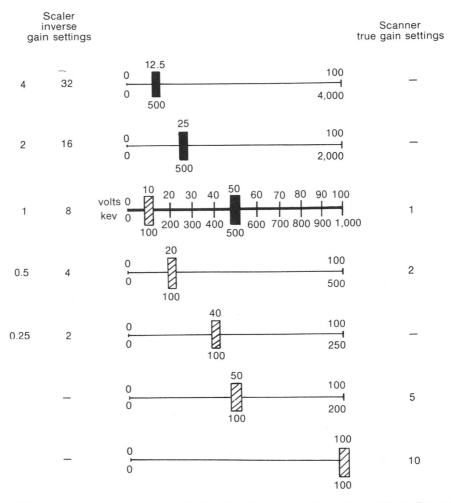

Fig. 8-7. Diagram demonstrating the principle of gain control, using various settings. The values to the left of the diagram represent the principle of inverse gain as seen on most scalers. The values to the right of the diagram represent the principle of true gain as seen on most scanners and other electronic equipment.

back to the gain settings of 8 (or 1), the operator is analyzing a 10 v pulse (100 kev) the pulse would be found at 100 kev. By changing the gain settings to 4 (or 0.5), the pulse will now be seen at a setting of 200 kev; or by changing the gain setting to 2 (or .25), that same pulse will be seen at 400 kev units. By increasing the numerical value of the gain setting, the pulse height has actually been decreased and, therefore, the operator must go down scale to receive it; conversely, by decreasing the gain settings, the pulse height has actually been increased and the operator must go up scale to receive the pulse.

In using the true gain settings as found on some scanners, the figures to the right on Fig. 8-7 apply. As the gain setting is increased, the pulse amplitude is also increased; therefore, the operator must go up in analyzer units to receive the pulse. A 100 kev pulse on range 1 would be found at 100 kev units; however, on range 2, the same pulse would be found at 200 kev units; on range 5 the same pulse would be found at 500 kev units; and on range 10 the same pulse would be found at 1,000 kev units.

Most linear amplifiers will only analyze pulses from 0 to 100 v high. This ability to analyze is most accurate from 10 or 15 v high to 100 v high. If low energy pulses are to be amplified correctly and subsequently analyzed, they must be amplified further by the gain settings. For example, if an operator were using mercury 197, which has 77 kev (7.7 v), inaccuracies would result if it were to be analyzed on gain settings of 8 (or 1) or on scanner settings of 1, since the pulse is not high enough to be analyzed correctly. The alternative is to change the gain settings to 4 (or 0.5), at which point the pulse would be seen at 154 kev units (15.4 v); a gain setting of 2 (or 0.25) would be even better since the pulse would be seen at approximately 308 kev units (30.8 v). The same is true for the scanner. For 770 kev units (77 v), a gain setting of 1 would be inadequate; however, a gain setting of 10 would be more accurate. By the judicious use of gain settings, low

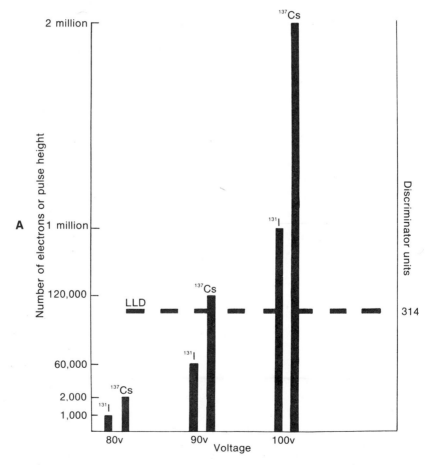

Fig. 8-8. Diagram demonstrating the principle of pulse height analysis. **A,** Lower level discrimination only. Only pulses rising above the LLD setting will be accepted and counted. **B,** Spectrometer. Only pulses that rise above the LLD and fall below the ULD will be accepted and counted.

energy electromagnetic radiations would not be all squeezed down into a range of a few volts where they are not discernible. The same is true of energy radiations greater than 1,000 kev. For example, cobalt 60 decays with a gamma emission having an energy of 1.17 and 1.33 mev. This is representative of 117 v and 133 v and is greater than the range of the analyzer. In this case, the pulse height will have to be decreased in order that it fall within the analyzer's capabilities. This could be accomplished on a scaler by changing the gain settings to 16 (or 2) or 32 (or 4). In this way the pulse height would be halved or quartered, respectively, for correct analysis.

It becomes clear that each spectrum to be investigated must be treated individually and the operator must choose the most advantageous gain setting in order that the radionuclide be utilized to its fullest advantage. Having chosen the appropriate gain settings and voltage settings, the pulse is now capable of being correctly analyzed.

Pulse height analyzer. The pulse height analyzer is an electronic device that

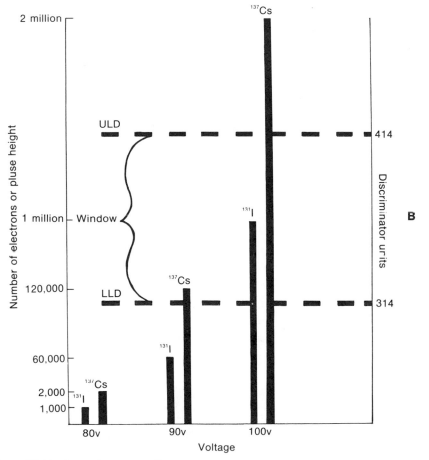

Fig. 8-8, cont'd. For legend see opposite page.

enables the operator to select pulses of a certain height and reject all pulses of a different height. There are two types of pulse height analyzers: lower level discriminators and spectrometers. The former do not recognize any pulse height below a predetermined level; the spectrometers do not recognize any pulse heights below one level and above another level, recognizing only those which fall between the two settings. A device that isolates only one set of pulses is called a single-channel analyzer. Most analyzers on instrumentation used in a routine nuclear medicine department are single channel analyzers. (A multichannel analyzer is a circuit combining two or more single-channel analyzers to provide simultaneous and sequential counting of radioactivity in more than one energy range or more than one pulse height.)

Since pulse heights are directly proportional to the number of electrons collected at the last dynode, a pulse height analyzer might best be described by comparing that number of electrons to the energy of incident gamma as a function of voltage (Fig. 8-8). Suppose a sample of activity is being used which contains two isotopes of varying energies, for example, iodine 131 (364 kev) and cesium 137 (662 kev). Assume total absorption in the crystal and that the intensity of the light was such that 1 photoelectron was emitted from the photocathode for ^{131}I and that 2 photoelectrons were emitted for ^{137}Cs. If a potential difference existed between each dynode of 80 v (800 v to the entire system), the attraction force of the dynode to the electron might provide sufficient energy to release 2 secondary electrons for each primary electron striking each dynode. Since there are ten dynodes, the number of electrons accumulated at the end of the photomultiplier tube would be 2^{10} or approximately 1,000 electrons. Similarly, if each of the 2 cesium 137 photoelectrons releases 2 electrons by secondary emission, the end result would be 2×2^{10} electrons or 2,000 electrons accumulated at the end of the photomultiplier tube. The pulse heights are represented in Fig. 8-8 above the units 80 v.

Should the voltage to the dynodes be increased so that a potential difference of 90 v exists between each dynode, the attraction force would be greater and the number of electrons released by secondary emission might increase to 3 electrons for each electron striking the dynode. The iodine 131 single electron from the photocathode would be multiplied to a factor of 3^{10} or 60,000 electrons and the cesium 137 would be 120,000, as seen in Fig. 8-8, above 90 v. Should the voltage be increased to 100 v per dynode, the number of electrons produced by secondary emission might increase to 4, therefore, 4^{10} or approximately 1,000,000 electrons for the iodine 131 absorption and 2,000,000 electrons for the cesium 137 absorption, as in Fig. 8-8 above 100 v.

Lower level discrimination. By arbitrarily setting a threshold to which a pulse must rise to or exceed in height to be counted, a lower level discriminator (LLD) has been established. In Fig. 8-8, *A,* at 80 v, neither iodine 131 nor cesium 137 would have been counted since neither pulse height attains the lower level discriminator setting. At 90 v, however, the cesium 137 pulse rises higher than the lower level discriminator setting, and therefore, it would be counted; the iodine 131 pulse would not. At 100 v, both the iodine 131 and the cesium 137 would be counted since both rise above this lower level discriminator setting.

It is important to note that the use of a lower level discriminator allows the separation of a higher energy radionuclide from a lower energy radionuclide, but the reverse is not true. At 90 v, only the pulses from ^{137}Cs are seen and counted and, therefore, are discriminated from ^{131}I pulses. There is no voltage setting, however, which will separate ^{131}I from ^{137}Cs. Any setting which includes the lower energy radionuclide must necessarily include the higher energy radionuclide too. This is termed *integral counting*.

Spectrometer. The spectrometer is an electronic device that enables the operator to reject any pulse whose height falls below one analyzer setting or above another. Should an upper level discriminator be introduced, as in Fig. 8-8, *B*, placed at a level higher than the lower setting, such a device has been electronically arranged. The lower level discriminator continues to reject any pulses that do not rise to that level and the upper level discriminator (ULD) will reject any pulses rising higher than its level. This is called *differential counting*. By using this two-level arrangement, both high energy radionuclides and low energy radionuclides can be separated from each other by varying the voltage. If 90 v are applied to each dynode, only the higher energy cesium 137 will be detected and recorded. If 100 v are applied, iodine 131 would be the only radionuclide to be counted. The area between the upper level and the lower level discriminators is called a *window*. Accordingly, pulse height analysis can be a function of voltage. This is not the usual use of a pulse height analyzer; however, in some scanners, this is the case. The windows are automatically preselected and the voltage is varied to accommodate the window.

The usual use of a pulse height analyzer is to predetermine the voltage setting and change the window to see the different pulses. This is accomplished by presetting the LLD and ULD, placing a source near the crystal, and adjusting the voltage until the highest count is reached. The dials governing the settings of the lower level and the upper level discriminators are usually ten-turn, 1,000 unit potentiometers. These are two main control dials listed as the lower level setting or base (E dial), and the window or the upper level setting (ΔE dial). The lower level dial is usually calibrated to read from 0 to 100 v (0 to 1,000 kev).* The upper level dial, if designated as window, is usually calibrated on scalers to read from 0 to 30 v (0 to 300 kev)* or, if ULD, to read from 0 to 100 v (0 to 1,000 kev).* (Window is found on scalers, ULD is found on scanners.) There are two different types of upper level discriminators, since on scalers, the upper level discriminator is dependent on the LLD and exists as a window riding on top of the lower level discriminator setting. For instance, it is known that cesium 137 (actually, barium 137m) has an gamma energy of 662 kev. If the machine was to be properly calibrated using this source, a suggested lower level discriminator setting would be 652 units on the 1,000 unit potentiometer and the window would be set at 20 units, meaning that the window would be from 652 to 672 units. In the case of most scanners, the upper level discriminator is completely independent of the lower level discriminator, in which case the LLD would read 652 units and the ULD would read 672 units to calibrate the same source. This calibration procedure

*This is true only with proper gain settings.

would be used on the scanners which have variable window control. Some scanners have preset windows set in arbitrary units and pulse height analysis is a function of varying voltage for each radionuclide.

It can be seen from Fig. 8-8 that by increasing the high voltage, the pulse height of any event which occurs in the sodium iodide crystal can also be increased. Rather than setting the window at arbitrary settings and varying the voltage, the usual procedure is to calibrate the voltage setting so that the 1,000 units on the ten-turn potentiometer become equivalent to kev units. Cesium 137 is the usual standardizing source because of its monoenergetic gamma at 662 kev. The procedure of calibration is to set the arbitrary units on the analyzer to 652 units and 672 units. If a ^{137}Cs source is placed near the crystal and the voltage is increased, eventually the pulse will be built up to such a point that it will be received by the preset window. The voltage at which the maximum count is received would be equivalent to seeing all energies between 652 and 672 kev. By increasing the voltage any further, the pulse heights will be driven above the upper level discriminator setting and rejected. That point at which the highest count is received is the proper operating voltage, for it has essentially calibrated the arbitrary units on the analyzer control dials to read in terms of kev and no longer in arbitrary units. It is important to point out that this is true only at the gain setting used at the time of calibration. Should the gain be changed, these units have a new meaning in energy units dependent upon that gain control.

Following the usual calibration procedure, each unit on the potentiometer is equal to 1 kev. Since the voltage has produced pulse heights proportional to the energy of the incident gamma ray, it is now possible to slide the window up-scale or down-scale in order to accept pulses from other radionuclides of different energies. By calibration, 662 potentiometer units have become 662 kev units; therefore, 364 potentiometer units are now 364 kev and pulses from ^{131}I will be recorded. Similarly, ^{198}Au will be recorded at 411 potentiometer units, ^{99m}Tc will be recorded at 140 units, and so on. This suggests a linearity between pulse height and voltage. This is generally true for all energies above 100 kev (10 v). Below that level, adjustments must be made either in gain, voltage, or window settings. This is often a cause of decreased count rate in the use of ^{197}Hg (77 kev) or ^{125}I (35 kev). The voltage determined for counting ^{137}Cs and all energies above 100 kev often does not apply to ^{197}Hg and ^{125}I. Either the voltage must be redetermined for these radionuclides, using the ^{137}Cs voltage as a base (the voltage, although representative of many lost counts, should only be slightly deviated from the value found for ^{137}Cs); or the window must be changed. Which of these procedures should be used is the subject of much controversy. Whatever the procedure, it should include gain since its use would be most advantageous in this situation.

Most commercially available pulse height analyzers provide the flexibility of using just the lower level discriminator or the spectrometer. These may be simply an "in-out" switch. The "out" position signifies just the lower level discriminator; the "in" position signifies a window. It may also be listed as "integral" and "differential," respectively. When the switch is in the "integral" or "out" position it essentially cuts out the operation of the upper level discriminator.

Gamma spectrum. A gamma spectrum is a linear graph of the number of counts received per unit(s) of kev. Another way of expressing a gamma spectrum is the number of times a pulse of a certain height occurs per unit of time. In Fig. 8-8, *B* the lower level discriminator may be designated as having units of 314 kev and the upper level discriminator as having units of 414 kev. At a voltage setting of 100 volts per dynode, the iodine 131 pulse height is exactly in the center of the window. Although this is theoretically correct, not all pulses of iodine 131 are represented by exactly 364 kev energy. Since the highest percentage of iodine 131 decays by the emission of a gamma ray of 364 kev, this should be the case. The fact is that most of these pulses are near the 364 kev energy peak, but do not always reach it exactly. Actually, they extend from approximately 314 to 414 kev.

The reasons for this are several. If the gamma ray was not totally absorbed in the crystal, which is possible, the intensity of the light emitted in the crystal and the pulse height would indicate this. These pulses would probably not occur anywhere near the main peak of iodine 131. They are referred to as scatter. Those that would occur near the main peak but which would represent a slight increase or a slight decrease in energy are primarily those that have been totally absorbed, but for some reason, the instrumentation has not faithfully reproduced them. A gamma ray that was totally absorbed near the outside edge of the crystal, for example, would have to pass its light all the way through the crystal in order for it to be seen by the photocathode. Consequently, some of the intensity of the light would be lost through transmission. This would appear to be slightly lower in energy than one that was totally absorbed in an area of the crystal immediately adjacent to the photocathode.

Another reason for pulse variation would be the dynodes. It is impossible to expect each dynode to faithfully multiply the number of electrons each time an electron strikes it. In some cases, if the voltage was such that 4 secondary electrons were supposed to be released and only 3 were, the pulse height would actually be lower, giving the illusion that the energy of the incident gamma ray was less. In other cases, the number of secondary electrons released from the dynode may be 5 instead of 4, at which point the pulse height would be increased, giving the illusion that the energy of the incident gamma ray was greater than 364 kev. If one more or one fewer electron were released at the first dynode, it would have considerably more effect than if this discrepancy existed on the last dynode; the deficiency or abundance of electrons would be changed by a power of 10 if it occurred on the first dynode, a power of nine on the second, and so on. For this reason, the end result is a variety of slightly different pulse heights; all represent valid counts from iodine 131 and should be used in the analysis of the radionuclide.

A sample of the variety of pulse heights is seen in Fig. 8-9. If the number of times a pulse height occurs were counted and plotted versus the representative energy of that pulse height, a graph would be produced similar to that shown in Fig. 8-10. This is exactly the case of the gamma spectrum. Rather than showing the gamma spectrum as just the main energy peak, it shows the numbers of pulses of energy from 0 to 1,000 kev, as seen in Fig. 8-11.

PLOTTING A GAMMA SPECTRUM. An analogy may be made between plotting a

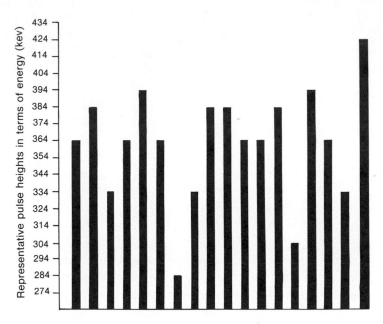

Fig. 8-9. Representative pulse heights in terms of energy. Variety of pulse heights that might be received from the interaction and complete absorption of 18 ^{131}I gamma photons with a crystal detector. Their absorption and subsequent amplification represent energies other than 364 kev even though every one of these pulses is from a 364 kev ^{131}I gamma photon.

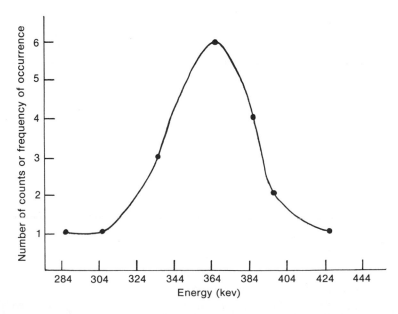

Fig. 8-10. Plot of number of pulses (counts) versus the representative energy of each pulse from Fig. 8-9.

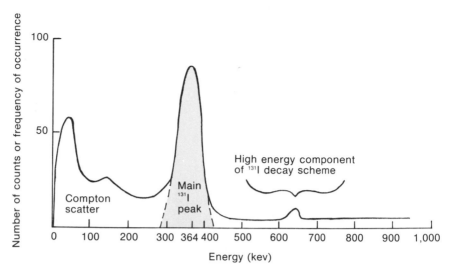

Fig. 8-11. Gamma spectrum of [131]I.

gamma spectrum and plotting the heights of a random sampling of 50 males. Of the 50 males, the heights may be as follows:

Height	Number of people
6'4''	1
6'2''	2
6'1''	6
6'	9
5'11''	13
5'10''	9
5'9''	7
5'8''	2
5'6''	1

By plotting number versus height, a curve would be received (as in Fig. 8-12) similar to the iodine 131 main energy peak.

The gamma spectrum can be plotted much like counting the number of men in the above example. The men would have been asked to line up according to increasing height, and then counted according to height. The same principle is applied in plotting a gamma spectrum. Using the proper voltage, a very narrow window is set. Only those gammas within the narrow window would have been counted for a predetermined period of time. The process is repeated changing only the window until the entire spectrum is displayed. Using Figs. 8-9 and 8-10, a window could have been set with an LLD at 324 and the window set at 20, therefore, counting a window of 324 to 344. In a preset period of time three counts would have registered and the number would be plotted in the center of the window (334). If the same window is retained but the LLD is increased to 354, the window would be reading all pulses having the height representative of 354 kev to 374 kev, at which point six counts would have registered and that number would be plotted in the middle of the spectrum (364). This would be continued until the entire spectrum is displayed. In actual practice, a smaller window is usually preferred,

139

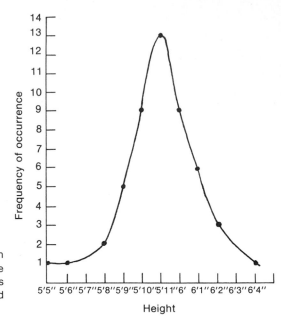

Fig. 8-12. Plot of heights of a sampling of the population versus frequency of occurrence. A graph of this nature is analogous to a gamma spectrum where pulse heights (representative of different energy levels) are plotted against frequency of occurrence.

and the LLD is usually increased in smaller increments than has been shown in this example. A typical peak may be run with a 10 kev window and increases in increments of two units.

Narrow windows used for calibration purposes are *not* the windows used for routine nuclear medicine procedures. Routine studies require a larger window. The reason for using a larger window is the stability of the lower level discriminator and the window width. This is very important for the accurate performance of the system. Narrow window counting requires the ultimate in stability. By increasing the window width to include most of the peak, two purposes are served— to increase the counting rate and therefore obtain better statistics and to reduce the effect of possible analyzer instability. According to the graph in Fig. 8-10, appropriate analyzer settings would be a LLD of 314 and a window of 100 (or ULD of 414). This determination of working window width should be performed on all scintillation detectors for each radionuclide and checked periodically. Although this is a relatively long procedure with a standard single-channel analyzer, a gamma spectrum can be accomplished very rapidly by using a single-channel analyzer in series with a count-rate meter, or by using a multichannel analyzer.

Multichannel analyzers. A multichannel analyzer is a circuit that combines two or more single-channel analyzers to provide simultaneous or sequential counting of radioactivity in more than one energy range. Gamma spectra are performed very quickly on the multichannel analyzer because each channel is analyzed individually but is recorded at the same time. This is quite unlike the single-channel analyzer which must be moved to each channel until the entire spectrum is seen, and then the results for each channel must be plotted.

Display modes. There are two types of display modes, the scaler and the count rate meter.

Scaler. A scaler is an electronic circuit which accepts signal pulses from a radiation detector and counts them. Scalers provide a unit for rapid counting of electrical pulses that result from light flashes from ionizing radiations interacting in the crystal. This method of counting is far superior to the dark-adapted eye. The scaler is usually electronically devised so that the operator has a choice between accepting a certain number of counts (preset count) or a predetermined period of time over which counts can be accumulated (preset time). With preset time, the scaling device will count the number of events that occur during a set interim of time and will then shut off automatically; the number of counts becomes the variable. With preset count, the predetermined number of counts are accumulated, after which the scaler is automatically shut off; time becomes the variable.

USE OF SCALER AS A COMPUTER. A scaler may be used as a computer provided it has both preset time and preset count accommodations. This can be accomplished by setting the scaler for a preset number of counts (10,000) and noting the time required to accumulate the preset number of counts. This is usually done with the standard sample. This time value is then used in the preset time section (preset count must be manually eliminated) and all unknowns are counted for that preset period of time. The answer can be read directly as percent by moving the decimal point over the required number of spaces. (In the case of 10,000, the decimal point must be moved two places to the left.)

Count rate meter. Another type of display mode is the count rate meter. This is a radiation detector connected to an indicator that continuously shows the average rate of counts coming from the detector per preselected time periods. Count rate meters have wide usage in survey meters and laboratory monitors, since their usual purpose is to promptly indicate increases in activity. The count rate meter also has extensive use for clinical work in dynamic studies where the accumulation and transportation of radiopharmaceuticals is followed by external detectors, such as renograms and cardiac outputs.

There are two types of rate meters currently in use: the analog rate meter and the digital rate meter. The fundamental difference between the two types is in the kind of memory used to store information from the incoming pulses. The analog rate meter stores a *charge* that is proportional to the number of pulses received per unit time. A digital rate meter stores the *count* in digital form much like the scaler. Since rate meters are so dependent on time constants, a discussion of time constants is warranted at this time.

TIME CONSTANT. The time constant is an electronic averaging property of the circuit for determining the time interval over which the summation of the incoming pulses is taken. Since the nature of radioactive decay is one of random events, fluctuations will be seen in the count rate meter. The degree of fluctuation is dependent upon the time constant and/or the count rate. It is similar to taking subsequent counts on a scaler and plotting them. If a radioactive source counted 10,000 cpm, variations between readings would not be appreciable; the counts will not vary by much more than 2% from the true count rate. Plotting the results of subsequent 1 minute counts would yield almost a straight line. The count rate meter with the time constant set for 1 minute performs this accumulation and

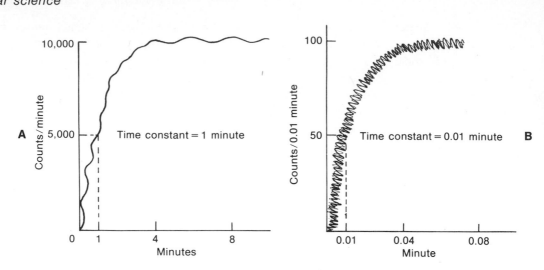

Fig. 8-13. A, Effect of a time constant on the response of a count rate meter. A long constant of 1 minute at the indicated count rate allows only slight deflection of the needle but it requires four times the time constant setting to achieve 100% value. **B,** Effect of a much shorter time constant but the same count rate. The vascillation of the needle is greater, but four times the time constant is still necessary to achieve the 100% value.

averaging automatically. When the meter is connected to a stripchart recorder, the results are graphed as in Fig. 8-13, *A*. Note that there is a delay in reaching the true count rate. Actually, the rise in count rate is an exponential function of time. For this reason, the rate meter reads only 50% of the true count rate value at the time indicated by the time constant; that is, the time constant is 1 minute, but at 1 minute only a count rate of 5,000 cpm is indicated. The true count rate (10,000 cpm) is not realized until after approximately 4 minutes (four times the time indicated by the time constant). With such a long time constant in this count-rate situation, statistical variations are not a factor.

By using the same source of radioactive material, but reducing the time constant to 0.01 minute (100 counts per 0.01 minute), a stripchart record similar to that in Fig. 8-13, *B,* will be obtained. The statistical fluctuation now becomes a real factor. Counts may vary from one averaging period to another by as much as 20% from the true count rate. Note that it still requires 4 times the time constant value to achieve the true reading; that only 50% of this value is received by the time indicated on the time constant setting, but at this setting the true value is required in $\frac{1}{100}$ the time.

Based on the above discussion, the setting of the time constant must be a compromise; a compromise between the response required of the particular study and the statistical accuracy of the resultant data. Longer time constants and higher count rates produce relatively less statistical uncertainty and therefore result in a more stable meter reading. Statistical accuracy takes precedence in a study where there is no appreciable change in count rate; an example would be a thyroid uptake study using a count rate meter, rather than a scaler. In this case, the operator would choose a time constant that demonstrates very little fluctuation, remembering the time required to achieve the true value. In situations where there is change in count rate, as a function of radionuclide clearance (renogram) or a moving detector over organs having inconsistent distribution of a radionuclide (scanning), both the selection of the time constant and count rate must enter into the decision. If the time constant is too long, the response to sudden increases or sudden decreases in count rate (both are exponential functions) will be too slow and the true clinical situation will perhaps be overlooked. If the time constant is too short, the statistical variations in count rate may present erroneous information.

ANALOG RATE METERS. Analog rate meters are the most common type of count rate meter. This rate meter allows a response that is directly proportional to the count rate. A delay is required, however, before an equilibrium state is reached, and this delay is a function of the time constant. This delay suggests a lag of the rate meter and therefore there is a distortion of the shape of curves, especially with dynamic function studies. Techniques are available to correct this, but in routine clinical studies, such techniques are not warranted. This type of rate meter is usually associated with a continuously moving graph paper (stripchart recorder) which plots the changes in activity (renograms).

DIGITAL RATE METERS. The digital rate meter is becoming more and more the rate meter of choice in nuclear medicine instrumentation because of the present clamor for digital information as well as the present trend for computer analysis of data. The use of a digital rate meter makes both of these possible.

The digital rate meter may be thought of as an automatic reset-scaling device in which the number of counts per unit time is continuously recorded. A standard scaler can be thought of as a simple digital rate meter. If the scaler continuously counted for a specified period, automatically recorded the count, and was then reset and allowed to count again, this would be the essence of a digital rate meter. On the digital rate meter, each time the entire process is recycled, the counts received during this predetermined counting period (which is adjustable) can be recorded on a visual display of numbers, printed or punched on tape, or graphed on a stripchart recorder as in the analog rate meter. There is a difference, however, in the appearance of the graph. It does not have a smooth curve as does the classic renogram, for example; it has a "stepped" appearance. This graph is called a *histogram*.

Magnetic storage tape. Storage of data on magnetic tape is a method of data accumulation. Tapes are useful in nuclear medicine because they are capable of storing all the information received from the detector. A strip of ferromagnetic material is magnetized by a current and this current represents information coming from the detector. The particularly useful feature of such materials is the permanence of the magnetization after the magnetizing field has been removed. Therefore, the information may be inspected and reinspected until the necessary information has been presented in the desired form. Another useful characteristic of magnetic tapes is that various tape speeds may be selected for recording data as well as playing back data. For this reason all the information may be stored during a long renogram procedure, for instance, but may be played back in its entirety in a fraction of the time it required to do the study. In this way, should incorrect parameters of a procedure be used, the study may continue and then be replayed following the procedure using the correct parameters. For example, if the operator of a renogram study uses a scale factor that is inadequate for the count rate, the pen will go off the chart paper. Without tape storage, the entire study would be invalid and would have to be repeated at some later time. With magnetic storage the study could be repeated with the correct scale factor after the patient has left the laboratory. Further, the tape may be rerun as many times as necessary to get the desired results. This is termed nondestructive storage, since the data will not be erased from the tape. Magnetic tape is also used for repeating a scan using different contrast values or repeating a study using different background subtraction. In this way the most useful information can be gained from the scan and the patient need not remain in the laboratory.

Modifications of scintillation detectors

The basic process of detecting and recording gamma rays is the same in all scintillation detectors, but there are modifications based upon use and the nuclear medicine procedure. The following is the discussion of a number of the most common modifications.

Probe. The scintillation detector in probe form is the common method of performing thyroid radioiodine uptake measurements (Fig. 8-14, *A*) and renal uptake measurements (Fig. 8-14, *B*). The present recommendations suggest that the sodium iodide crystal be not less than 1 inch in diameter with a thickness of not less than 1 inch, since about 70% of the iodine 131 gamma rays that enter the crystal are absorbed by 1 inch of sodium iodide. It has been determined that a thicker crystal would increase the counting efficiency, but the increase would be less than the increase in background count. The standard ^{131}I uptake probe contains a 1.5 inch diameter crystal by 1 inch in thickness. By increasing the diameter from 1 inch to 1.5 inches, both the background and the iodine 131 counting efficiencies are doubled. This becomes important from the standpoint of statistics in short counting periods. At the present time the larger diameter crystal seems preferred. Collimators* for an uptake probe are such that the entire thyroid gland is seen. This distance is usually between 20 to 30 cm for an adult thyroid gland. It should be emphasized that it is essential to see the entire gland. Since distance is constant to all patients, that distance must be such that all of the largest thyroid is included even if that would include greater amounts of nonthyroid tissue in patients with smaller thyroids. One exception to the constant distance might be in studies of children. In these cases, the distance may be shortened.

Well counter. A well counter is a scintillation crystal detector formed with a central well into which biologic samples (blood, urine, tissue) can be inserted and their radioactive emissions counted. The major advantage of this arrangement is the increased counting efficiency which results from surrounding the sample by

*A collimator is a device placed in front of a sodium iodide crystal for purposes of defining a region from which radiations are emitted to the exclusion of all other regions. A region could be as large as an entire organ (thyroid, kidney) or as small as a lesion within an organ (brain tumor). Many collimators are available for different purposes. (See Chapter 9, Collimation.)

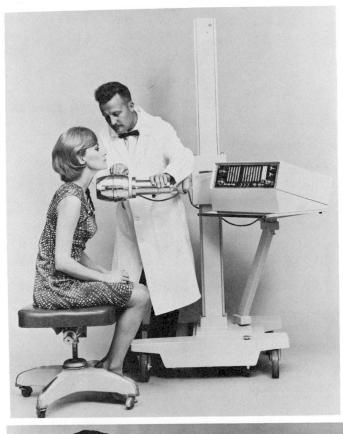

A

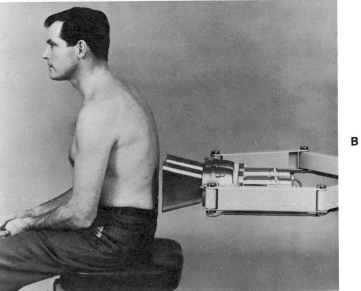

B

Fig. 8-14. A, Thyroid uptake probe and scaler. **B,** Renal uptake probes. (Courtesy, Nuclear-Chicago Corporation)

145

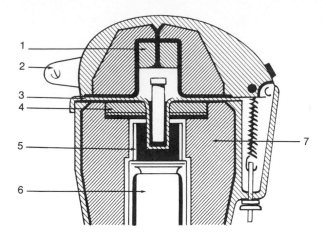

Fig. 8-15. Cross sectional view of Scintillation Well Detector. *1,* Removable lid plug; *2,* handle; *3,* splash guard; *4,* lead beaker plate; *5,* large well crystal; *6,* photomultiplier tube (6292); *7,* lead shield. (Courtesy, Picker Nuclear, White Plains, New York)

the detector. Most well counters presently in use employ sodium iodide crystals 1¾ inches in diameter and 2 inches in height; the well is ¾ inches in diameter and 1½ inches deep. Since the well is machined into the crystal itself, the well is surrounded by ½ inch of sodium iodide around the sides and at the bottom (Fig. 8-15). There are other sizes of crystals available which accommodate larger volumes or have a greater thickness of sodium iodide for greater counting efficiencies. The detection of pulses from this type of scintillation detector is the same as with any scintillation detector.

Organ imaging devices. In 1950 Cassen and his associates found that by using the newly developed scintillation counter, mounting it on an automatically moved carriage, and attaching a dot-producing mechanism which would respond to the electrical impulses from a scintillation counter, the spacial distribution of radioactive iodine in the thyroid gland could be printed mechanically. As a result, Cassen opened up a whole new area of isotope utilization in medicine. Until this discovery, the only means of scanning the organs of the body containing any radioactive material was manual scanning. A manual scan was performed by placing the probe as close to the skin as possible, moving in small increments over the gland or area to be scanned, and recording a count as each new area is surveyed. A "hot" or "cold" area would be indicated by an area with count rates which were increased or decreased respectively as compared to the count rates seen over the normal functioning areas of the organ. An anatomic map of the organ could be made by plotting the areas having the same count and by connecting these points by lines. These lines, called isocount lines, represented the shape of the organ and the distribution of the radioactivity. This procedure was long and painstaking.

Automatic scanners, called rectilinear scanners, were designed to perform this scanning procedure automatically, making a map of the location of radioactive materials in the patient's body. The scanner moves across the organ in one or more planes until the organ or the area in question has been completely surveyed by the scintillation counter. As it moves back and forth across the organ containing radioactivity, the scanning mechanism produces electrical impulses proportional to the amount of activity present in the area which, at that instant, is covered by the scintillation probe. It creates a picture by a number of read-out systems. Parameters are set for lateral movement and, through the use of microswitches, the detector head is automatically indexed upward or downward and begins again on its path across the body. In this way the entire organ can be visualized. The speed with which the detector moves laterally and the distance which it moves laterally or indexes up or down can be manually controlled.

Read-out systems. The map of the organ containing radioactivity can be presented as a visual display by several methods. One of these methods (and one of the first used) is a paper known as teledeltos. This paper is capable of electrical conductivity and is coated with a white, chalk-like substance. As the electrical impulse is received by the stylus of the dot-producing mechanism, this chalk-like compound is burned away by the electric current. This exposes a black material beneath producing a black dot on white paper. The paper is held stationary and the dot-producing mechanism moves synchronously with the detector head over the teledeltos paper.

Another device for the same purpose uses a solenoid-operated "tapper," which strikes the record paper through a carbon ribbon (much like a typewriter ribbon) to produce dots. The number of dots is proportional to the amount of radioactivity present in the area under the detector. As the radioactivity increases, the number of dots also increases.

Another type of visual display is the display on x-ray film. As in the dot mechanism, a small cathode tube moves synchronously with the scintillation detector over x-ray film. As scintillations are received, a collimated cathode light source produces a spot on the film, flashed on for a preset length of time. Upon completion of the scan, the x-ray film is developed in the usual manner. The developed x-ray film demonstrates the organ and its concentrations of radioactivity as dots or squares of darkening on the film. These film images are generally felt to be superior to teledeltos or tapper images because the image is produced by the overlapping of dots as well as density control of the dots. Consequently, variations in concentrations of activity can be seen as dots ranging from white (not seen on film) through shades of gray to black. The black areas represent high concentrations of radioactivity and the varied gray areas represent lesser concentrations of radioactivity. A variety of light sources has been used, including an incandescent lamp and a cathode tube. The latter has been used as the light source of choice because of its quick response.

Another display system found on some imaging devices is that of a color dot print-out. This displays a range of color from blue, indicating a cold area, through intermediate colors to red, indicating a hot area. It was designed because, theoretically, the ability to discern colors is much easier than variations in shades of gray. The color print-out is accomplished by a ribbon similar to a typewriter ribbon with several adjacent bands of different colors that move transversely under a fixed tapper. The position of the ribbon and, therefore, the color of the dot are

147

dependent upon the counting rate. If the count rate is low, the blue color band slides under the tapper. If the count rate is around 50% of the maximum, then the green band falls under the tapper; and if the count rate is the maximum count rate, then the red band falls under the tapper.

A more recent development in read-out systems is that of the Ektachrome color photo and the color Polaroid film. In each of these, the colors change in accordance with changes in concentrations of activity in an organ. The color Polaroid, seen on the Adams-Jaffe attachment to the imaging device, is regarded by some as being disadvantageous because of its small size and the difficulties involved in relating it to x-ray film. However, these difficulties are now less serious since many imaging devices now use black and white Polaroid film. The Ektachrome display system resolves this disadvantage because the representation of the organ on this read-out system is approximately equal to the true organ size. The latter, however, requires a special developing process. Other display systems range from oscilloscopes through black and white Polaroid films to magnetic storage tapes.

Types of organ imaging devices. There are several devices designed to show radionuclide distribution in the body and in the organs. One such device is the rectilinear scanner. Some of these scanners consist of one probe that moves back and forth across the organ; others have two probes that move back and forth synchronously, with the body or the organ positioned between the two probes. Other forms of organ imaging devices are stationary devices that visualize the entire organ at one time. These devices are of two types: (1) those which contain a single crystal (camera), and (2) those which contain multiple crystals (auto-fluoroscope), each of which is capable of visualizing the entire organ. Although these types differ considerably in construction, they all have many basic features in common. All imaging devices, whether rectilinear or stationary, have a collimator. In addition to this, they all have a detector unit, which, for scintillation imaging devices, consists of a crystal(s) and photomultiplier tube(s). They also have a linear amplifier, pulse height analyzer, and a scaler or rate meter or a combination of both.

Rectilinear imaging devices. There is a variety of factors that influence the results of the read-out system of a rectilinear imaging device, whether it is the dot record or the photographic record. It is important to realize that each patient presents a new set of variables for which the operator of the imaging device must supply a new set of factors to receive the optimum results. The imaging of organs is not an exact science by any means. Formulas are available to assist nuclear medicine personnel in producing an adequate image, but an element of art exists in the production of a better-than-adequate image. The establishment of such empirical values requires experience. The next section is included to provide the student of nuclear medicine with an understanding of the function of these various parameters in order that these empirical values might be learned with a minimum of experience.

PARAMETERS APPLICABLE TO BOTH PHOTO AND DOT RECORDINGS. There are four settings applicable to both the photo recording and the dot recording of a rectilinear image. These are the pulse height analyzer, speed, line spacing, and time constant. The pulse height analyzer has already been discussed and appropriate settings are necessary for the radionuclide being detected. The *speed control* is an adjustable potentiometer which controls the speed at which the detector traverses the organ. The speed is dependent upon the count rate determined from the area of highest activity, the line spacing, and desired information density (ID).* Speed can be calculated by the following formula:

$$\text{Scan speed} = \frac{\text{maximum counts per minute}}{\text{line space} \times \text{ID}}$$

The *line spacing* adjustment is a variable control that determines the distance the detector indexes before it attempts another sweep across the organ being visualized. The choice of line spacing is usually determined by the choice of light collimator on the cathode ray tube of the photo recording section. The usual procedure is to display as much information in as small an area as possible. This requires that the top of the spot on the film in one row be touching the bottom of the spot in the row above it. If they do not approximate each other in this manner, a line is produced with no information, referred to as the venetian blind effect, and in most cases, this interferes with interpretation. The standard small light collimator requires 0.2 cm spacing whereas the large light collimator requires from 0.35 to 0.4 line spacing. Some investigators have preferred square light collimators so that interpretation is not disturbed by the wavelike effect between the tops and bottoms of subsequent dots.

The *time constant* has already been discussed at some length with regard to rate meters, but its utilization in rectilinear scanning deserves special attention. It has been stated that the build-up of a rate meter is an exponential function so that there is a delay before the true count rate is indicated. There is also an exponential decrease in output of the count rate so that, should the detector move into an area containing no radionuclide, the reading on the rate meter is not immediately zero. This presents a unique problem in rectilinear scanning, because the increase or decrease in count rate must be quickly indicated or a possible lesion will be obscured. This is especially true in a scan which is performed on a long time constant setting. The value of rectilinear scanning lies in the fact that as the detector moves across the organ, it almost immediately presents the information consistent with the amount of activity in that area of the organ. However, this is not true if the time constant is too long, since the information will be presented from an area which was previously under the probe. Consequently, as the detector reaches the edge of an organ, the count rate does not decrease immediately. Information continues to be presented beyond the organ edge because of the exponential release of the higher count rate. As the detector indexes and begins to make another sweep across the organ, it does not present information until after it has gone some distance across the organ because of the exponential build-up. It continues across the organ displaying information from a previous scanning area. It continues to display beyond the other edge of the organ until the count rate decreases. This procedure continues throughout the entire scan. This defect of scanning produces an irregular outline of the organ and makes it appear

---

*ID = Number of observed events per cm^2 (see Chapter 9, pp. 180 to 183).

larger than it actually is. This defect is commonly referred to as *scalloping*. If there were a small lesion in the organ itself, the scalloping would tend to mask the lesion. Scalloping can also occur if the scan speed is too fast and, therefore, inconsistent with the time constant.

PARAMETERS APPLICABLE ONLY TO THE DOT RECORDING. There are two settings related to the dot recording: the dot factor and the background erase. The *dot factor* is a numbered dial that indicates the number of events seen by the detector to produce a dot. If the dot factor was 4, four events would have to be seen in order that one dot be produced; if the dot factor was 16, sixteen events would have to be seen to produce one dot. The choice of a dot factor is contingent upon the count rate at the area of highest radionuclide concentration, and it must be consistent with the response of the dot-producing mechanism and its subsequent record. The dot factor for teledeltos paper is always greater (more events per dot) than for the tapper systems. If a dot factor of 1 were used in the teledeltos system of recording, the record would be nothing but a straight line in areas of high activity with no difference in count rate suggested. Further, the dot pattern consists of lines of small dots. These are difficult to interpret because of the spaces between consecutive scan sweeps. Also, variations in dot density are difficult to recognize. The tapper systems are easier to interpret because these systems display a narrow vertical line which allows the lines to touch each other from one scan sweep to the other and the eye of the interpreter can distinguish differences more easily. Although graphs are available for this purpose, the dot factor can be mathematically determined by the following formula:

$$DF = \frac{\text{maximum counts per minute}}{\text{scan speed} \times 10}$$

Every scan includes areas where counts are received from areas other than the organ of interest (natural background or radioactivity in other portions of the body). Since these counts are not of primary interest and since they only disrupt the interpretive process, a technique of *background erase* is used to prevent any data recording of count rate below a preselected level. Lack of judicious use of this parameter can result in loss of valuable information. An example is a liver scan. The edges of the liver are very thin and the concentration of radioactivity approaches body background. If the background erase selector is set too high, the liver can actually be made to look smaller than it is because the liver edge is treated as background and is erased. Continual increases in background erase can cause the liver to appear to become continuously smaller.

Misuse of the background erase can also result in loss of information from different parts of an organ. The scanning of an autonomous thyroid nodule is an example. The area of highest concentration is not difficult to visualize in these clinical states, but visualization of the rest of the organ can present problems. The rest of the thyroid gland may have received some of the radionuclide, but the nodule acquired the major portion of the dose, resulting in the rest of the organ having activity levels only slightly greater than the surrounding extra-thyroidal tissue. Too much background erase will present the autonomous nodule as the only functioning tissue in the gland.

PARAMETERS APPLICABLE ONLY TO PHOTO RECORDING. The photo record has in general become the record of choice. The photo record displays the information as dots varying in density from white, through an infinite number of shades of gray to black. The variations in density reflect the variations in concentration of the radionuclide in the organ being studied. The interpreter of the photo record is usually better able to distinguish variations in shades of gray than the dot record which is black or white.

The photo record frequently employs a cathode ray tube (CRT). The CRT flashes a beam of light directly onto an x-ray film which, upon developing, is displayed as a dark area on the film. The size of the dark area is controlled by a light collimating device. The amount of film darkening can also be controlled. It can be accomplished by several methods: (1) by varying the brightness of the light flash, (2) by varying the "on" time of the cathode ray tube, or (3) by a combination of both. Further, the degree of darkening is dependent upon the scan speed and the count rate.

Parameters used to regulate the record on the x-ray film include the density, the range differential, the light source voltage (as opposed to the photomultiplier voltage), and the rate meter range. Some of these parameters are automatically adjusted on some instruments, some are manually adjusted on other instruments, and some instruments can be adjusted either manually or automatically. In any of these cases, the principles are not altered, and a basic understanding of their function will help the nuclear medicine student understand their use.

The *density control* indicates the duration of time the cathode ray tube is on per detected pulse. It, therefore, determines the length of time that the x-ray film is exposed. The longer the film is exposed, the darker the area on the film becomes. Further, a density setting which would produce a black dot if the cathode ray tube were stationary, would produce a less intense dot (gray) if the cathode ray tube were moving. The light rays would be superimposed on each other in the former instance but not perfectly superimposed in the latter. The same reasoning prevails if a scan is performed at a predetermined scan speed and density setting and is repeated at a faster speed. In order that the *film density* be duplicated, the density setting must be increased proportionally; to double the scan speed, the density must also be doubled. (Note: *density control* and *film density* are two separate entities. Density control relates only to the duration of the light flash. Film density relates to the degree of darkening of the film, which is governed by several factors, including the density control, the count rate, the scan speed, and the size of the light collimating device.)

The density is an automatically controlled device in some instruments. Graphs are available to determine the adjustment of this parameter in manually controlled instruments, or the value can be calculated as follows:

$$\text{Density} = \frac{\text{Scan speed} \times \text{light collimator conversion factor}}{\text{Maximum counts per minute}}$$

Conversion factor for small light collimator = 4,000
Conversion factor for large light collimator = 2,500

X-ray film, regardless of the type, possesses a known useful film density range.

This is the range from white to black, beyond which the dot does not become darker. It is generally considered desirable to manipulate the various parameters so that the maximum count rate area is represented by maximum film density (black) and background be represented by minimum film density (white). In this way, intermediate count rate areas will be represented by intermediate shades of gray. This is called the *range differential.* To accomplish this, the percentage of full scale deflection from maximum to minimum count rate must be ascertained. If the maximum count rate showed as 80% of the entire scale and minimum count rate showed as 20% of the entire scale (background representing 0-20%), the differential between the two extremes would be 60%. This value becomes the range differential. Note that the range differential becomes a background erase mechanism for the photo record. If more background is desired, the range differential value may be increased. By erroneously calculating the range differential, information can be lost, just as in the background erase for the dot record. Range differential is calculated by the following:

$$RD = \% \text{ maximum deflection} - \% \text{ minimum deflection}$$

The use of this parameter is a form of *contrast enhancement.* Just as the name implies, contrast (from white to black) is enhanced as the range differential is reduced. It requires less of a change in the count rate to proceed from the white to the black range, with fewer gradations of gray.

The *light source voltage* is a parameter which adjusts the brightness of each light flash to the output of the count rate meter. The voltage is adjusted so that the area of maximum count rate provides maximum film density as well. This parameter must be determined after the range differential has been calculated.

Using the range differential example of 60 with no light source voltage applied, this value could represent a range of 0 to 60, 10 to 70, 20 to 80, 30 to 90, or 40 to 100. The purpose of the light source voltage is to ensure that the range differential of 60 represents the deflection of the count rate needle from 20 to 80% of the full scale.

Another parameter in setting up a scan is the use of the *count rate meter range* adjustment, which must be selected prior to calculation of the range differential. This parameter has a variety of selections, which change the values of the scaled units. The same position on the scale could represent 1,000, 10,000 or 100,000 counts per minute, dependent upon the range switch value. Further, some units have an ancillary switch separate from the range selector control, which expands the scale by a factor of 2. Therefore, a maximum count rate of 10,000 cpm could be represented on the meter as 10,000 on the standard scale (meaning 10,000 cpm) or 5,000 on the expanded scale (meaning $5,000 \times 2 = 10,000$ cpm). The former would represent 100% full scale deflection on the appropriate scale and the latter would represent 50% full scale deflection on the same scale, expanded. This would mean that the range differential could be no greater than 100% on the standard scale, whereas the range differential could be no greater than 50% on the expanded scale.

CONTRAST ENHANCEMENT. It has been shown that contrast enhancement can be produced by varying the range differential. The phenomenon of contrast enhancement is generally considered to be of less and less significance as instrumentation and radiopharmaceuticals are improved. Contrast enhancement has been used in the past to accentuate areas with changes in count rate, which, because of the lack of statistics, actually represented very little change in count rate at all. It is currently believed that all information should be recorded, with few exceptions, and the contrast enhancing techniques be performed post-factum. (There is a certain degree of innate contrast enhancement in x-ray film, oscilloscopes, and so on, provided the information presented falls within a good statistical range.) Post-factum contrast enhancement is accomplished in a variety of ways. It can be performed by the use of ancillary equipment as expensive as computers and closed circuit television or as inexpensive as a piece of ordinary nonglare glass, the type used in picture frames.

The reason why contrast enhancement has fallen into disrepute can be exemplified in pulmonary imaging. A pulmonary scan demonstrating *decreased* perfusion is suggestive of pulmonary embolism whereas *no* perfusion suggests tumor. Since contrast enhancement demands a decision before the image is realized, an erroneous setting by the technologist may result in an erroneous interpretation by the physician.

Single crystal rectilinear imaging device. A single crystal rectilinear scanner is shown in Fig. 8-16. It consists of a centrally located chassis containing most of the

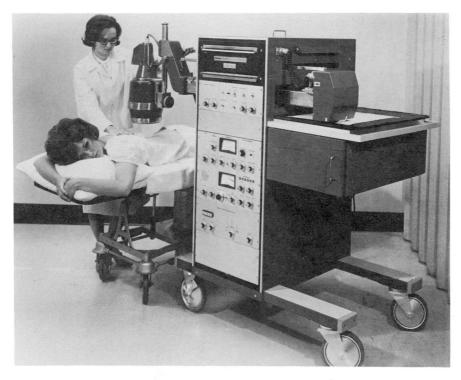

Fig. 8-16. Single crystal rectilinear imaging device (Magnascanner). (Courtesy, Picker Nuclear, White Plains, New York)

153

electronic components and the photo recording unit. All the controls for the parameters just discussed are also found in this central section. The detector assembly is mounted on one arm of the unit and the dot recording mechanism is mounted on the other arm above a platform upon which the required paper is placed.

The detector arm continually moves back and forth parallel with the front of the scanner and indexes stepwise in a direction perpendicular to the front of the scanner until the entire organ has been visualized. The person under study lies on a patient cart under the detector head.

Multiple crystal rectilinear imaging devices. There are two multiple crystal probes at the present time that are being used most extensively. These are the dual probe, dual crystal rectilinear imaging device and the single probe, ten crystal rectilinear imaging device. Both of these are similar in operation to the single probe, single crystal scanner. Both types have advantages over the single probe, single crystal device.

DUAL PROBE SCANNER. The dual probe scanner, as the name implies, is a scanner that has two scintillation detectors instead of one (Fig. 8-17). The scintillation detectors are opposite one another so as to view opposite sides of the same subject. The usual method of operation is to have the patient lie on a table. One detector traverses over the table and the other traverses under it. The patient, therefore, lies between the two detectors. This system offers the obvious advantage of obtaining two scans during the same time required to obtain one. There is very little difference in the operation of the dual probe scanner from the single probe. Each detector has its own system of detection, amplification, pulse height analysis,

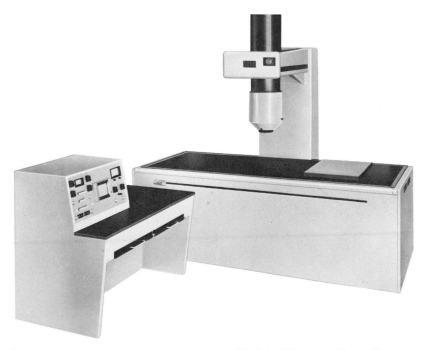

Fig. 8-17. Dual probe rectilinear imaging device (Model 84FD Dual Five). (Courtesy, Ohio-Nuclear, Inc.)

and read-out devices. The only difference is that both probes are linked mechanically so that they share the same mechanical moving facilities and therefore move in synchrony.

There are several features of using a dual scanner that deserve special mention. Commercially available dual probe scanners have a feature of minifaction by changing the gear ratio of the motors. Consequently, an image can be reduced by one-fifth. In using this feature, a 14 by 17 inch x-ray film, ordinarily just large enough to include a lung scan, is able to display an entire body scan. Another feature of dual probe scanners is that they allow the summation of all the events from both detectors to yield one image. This is especially applicable to scans involving low concentrations of radionuclides, such as bone scans. Another feature is that a dual probe scanner allows the subtraction technique. The subtraction technique is used to delineate organs which accumulate only one of two injected radionuclides from superimposed organs which accumulate both radionuclides. An example is the pancreas. Selenium 75-labeled selenomethionine localizes in both the liver and the pancreas, whereas, colloidal gold 198 localizes only in the liver. The concentration of selenium 75 in the pancreas can be visualized by subtracting any areas that contain both selenium 75 and gold 198. In this manner a liver-

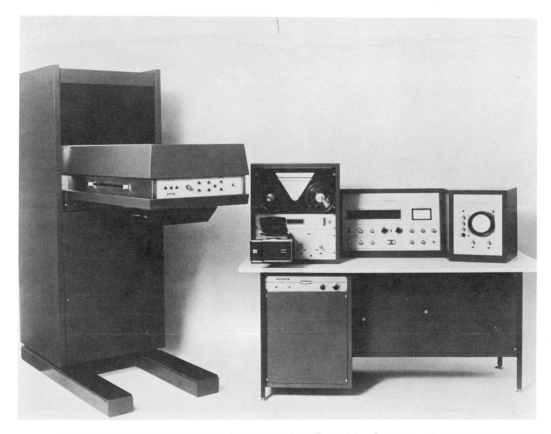

Fig. 8-18. Ten crystal rectilinear imaging device (Dynapix). (Courtesy, Picker Nuclear, White Plains, New York)

pancreas scan can be performed where the liver will be subtracted and the pancreas will be visualized. Another advantage to the dual probe scanner is the possibility of using the opposing heads to detect positron emissions. In this utilization a coincidence mode must be used so that only those pulses detected simultaneously (namely, the two gamma rays resulting from annihilation reactions) will be recorded.

TEN CRYSTAL RECTILINEAR IMAGING DEVICE. The single probe, ten crystal rectilinear scanner (Fig. 8-18) operates similarly to other types of rectilinear scanners, except that with ten crystals, the time required to visualize an entire organ is decreased tremendously. The detector of this imaging device contains ten parallel sodium iodide crystals. Each crystal has its own focused collimator and its own photomultiplier tube. The detector consists of ten adjacent parallel crystals each 6 inches long, 2 inches thick, and ⅞ inches wide. Since each crystal has its own photomultiplier tube and electronics, each crystal counts at the rate of a single detector. With ten such units, the whole assembly can count ten times as fast as a single detector. The entire ten detector assembly moves over the patient in a continuous traversing motion, much like that of a single probe rectilinear scanner. On each pass the detector assembly sees and records ten lines (Fig. 8-19). The second pass across the organ results in twenty lines, and so on. The entire organ can be seen as a rough scan in four passes (forty lines). If a more detailed picture is required, the detector assembly can be regulated automatically so that four more passes (40 more lines) can be interspersed between the first forty lines. If an even more detailed image is required, the detector can pass eight more times across the

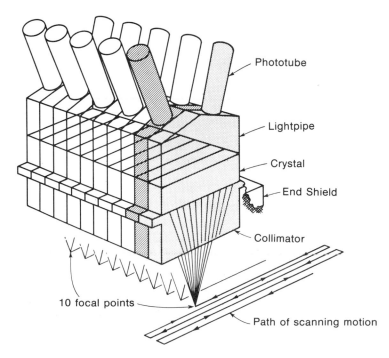

Fig. 8-19. Detector and collimator assembly of the ten crystal rectilinear scanner (Dynapix). (Courtesy, Picker Nuclear, White Plains, New York)

organ interspersing recording of ionization events between the lines already produced. Data read-out is provided through a television screen, a Polaroid camera viewing an oscilloscope, a magnetic tape recorder, and a scaler. The outstanding advantage of such a system is the decrease in time required for each organ examination. Other features include relative ease of operation, high resolution, and tomographic effects with the short focused collimator.

Single crystal stationary imaging devices. The single crystal stationary imaging device, commonly called the scintillation camera or Anger camera, is a device that views all parts of the radiation field continuously, rather than scanning the subject point by point. One commercially available scintillation camera (Fig. 8-20) employs a single sodium iodide crystal measuring 11 inches in diameter by ½ inch thick as the detector unit. This crystal is viewed by a bank of nineteen photomultiplier tubes.

In the single crystal stationary device, gamma rays pass through the holes of the collimator and are totally absorbed in the scintillation crystal. The light that is produced is emitted in all directions and is seen by all the photomultiplier tubes. The closest photomultiplier tube to any given scintillation event receives the most light. Since it receives the most light, that photomultiplier tube also produces the largest pulse, in comparison to the surrounding photomultiplier tubes (which also produce a pulse but of decreasing height). The circuit adds and subtracts the amplitudes of these pulses in such a way that three output signals are obtained. Two of the signals are used for positioning on an x-y coordinate and the third signal, z, is a summation of the amplitudes of all the pulses of the nineteen photomultiplier tubes so that that event can be accepted or rejected through pulse height analysis. By using the x-y coordinates, the exact location at which the event occurred can be localized and the individual scintillation in the crystal is reproduced as a flash on the oscilloscope at the appropriate position. The flashes on the oscilloscope screen can then be photographed, usually by Polaroid camera.

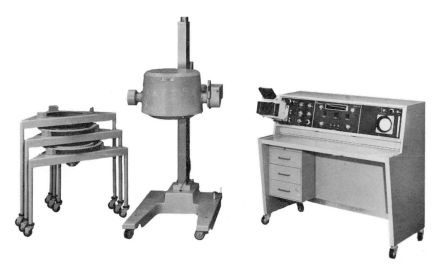

Fig. 8-20. Single crystal stationary imaging device ("camera"). (Courtesy, Nuclear-Chicago Corp.)

The image of the organ can be visualized after accumulating thousands or hundreds of thousands of these scintillations on the oscilloscope face. The ideal gamma energy for use with the scintillation camera is about 150 kev. This energy range allows a high percentage of absorption by the comparatively thin sodium iodide crystal. Higher energetic gammas are much less efficient because of the inability to stop the gamma within ½ inch of sodium iodide.

The scintillation camera also acts as a dual detector and rate meter since it possesses an ability to electronically split the crystal into two different parts. In this way, since the two parts of the crystal can be attached to the count rate meter and stripchart recorder, individual records can be made of the activity in each part of the crystal as a function of time. This has application, for instance, in renal function studies. The scintillation camera can also be adapted so that the information can be converted from analog to digital information for use in computer analysis. Unlike rectilinear scanners, the camera can also act as a dynamic function detection unit since it can view the entire organ continuously. Cerebral blood flows and cardiac function studies have been visualized using this camera.

Multiple crystal stationary imaging device. The multiple crystal stationary imaging device, commonly called the Autofluoroscope (Fig. 8-21), is an instrument with multiple crystals on the detector assembly. The detector head is made up of a matrix, measuring 6 by 9 inches and consisting of 294 separate scintillation crystals

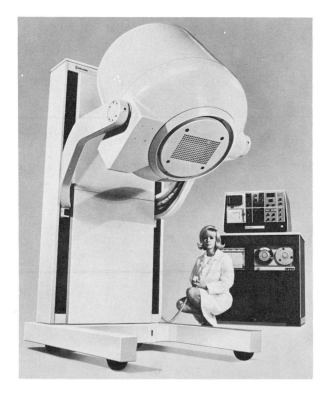

Fig. 8-21. Multiple crystal stationary imaging device. (Courtesy, Baird-Atomic, Inc.)

that form a grid of 14 by 21 crystals (Fig. 8-22). Each crystal is $\frac{7}{16}$ inches wide and 1½ inches thick. These crystals are mounted in a mosaic pattern and are separated from one another by lead. These lead separators help to stop gamma and light rays from crossing into adjacent crystals. This "cross-talk" is further reduced by the use of a multihole collimator having 294 tapered holes. Each hole corresponds to each crystal element in the mosaic. The electronic circuit and image read-out system are similar to those in the scintillation camera. The purpose of the thick mosaic scintillator is to obtain high detection efficiency for medium and high energy gamma rays, which is not possible with the scintillation camera.

Each of the 294 crystals in the 9 by 6 inch mosaic is optically connected by a pair of Lucite lightpipes to two of the bank of thirty-five photomultiplier tubes. One lightpipe goes to the x axis and the other lightpipe goes to the y axis. In this way, simultaneous pulses from the two photomultiplier tubes identify the crystal element in which the scintillation occurred. A light is then produced on the recording oscilloscope face corresponding to the original location of a gamma ray or scintillation of light resulting from the gamma ray. An anticoincidence circuit eliminates gamma rays scattered between one crystal and another in the mosaic. This technique eliminates scintillations caused by both the original gamma ray and the scattered gamma ray. As in the Anger camera, the signals from the two photomultiplier tubes are summed and fed to a pulse height analyzer for acceptance or rejection.

The nature of this detection system lends itself to obtaining digital data by a unique "flagging" technique. The areas of interest that are to be selected are addressed by means of a photocell light pen, called a "wand." The photocell generates control signals synchronized to the memory timing system. This synchronized signal generates a "flag" that keeps track of the selected memory locations and upon command, displays the stored information as a digital presentation.

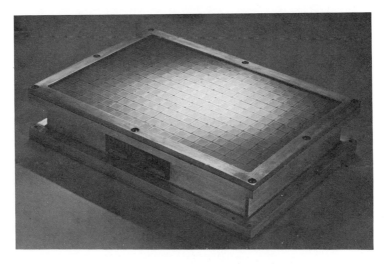

Fig. 8-22. Detector head of the multiple crystal stationary imaging device. (Courtesy, Harshaw Chemical Co.)

Miscellaneous detectors

In addition to the gas detectors and the scintillation detectors there are other detectors that do not use either of these operating principles. Radiation may be detected by image intensification similar to that used in radiographic instrumentation. Another type of radiation detector is a spark chamber (spintharicon), which is unique in its properties to detect radiation. Thermoluminescent dosimetry and radiologic film detection are two other possibilities. Each will be discussed separately.

Image intensification. An image intensifier tube has been used for a number of years with x-ray equipment. A similar system, used as a stationary imaging device, has also been established (Fig. 8-23). This system uses the Terpogossian camera principle. The gamma-sensitive image tube views an area up to 9 inches in diameter; this field of view is covered instantaneously. Consequently, static and dynamic isotope distributions for entire organs can be studied. By coupling the image tube to a television monitor, both dynamic and some static studies can be displayed. Film recordings can be made from television-type kinescope recorders or from video tape accessory equipment. Video tape recorders allow the information obtained during an examination to be captured and stored exactly as it occurred.

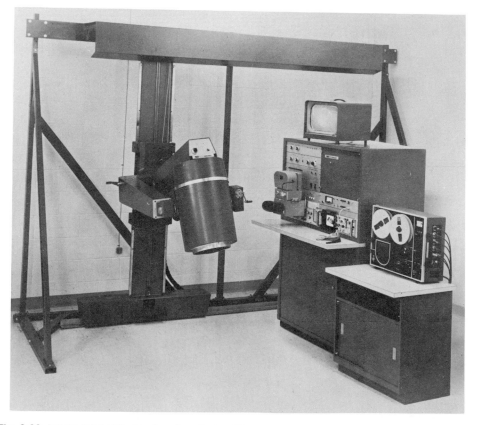

Fig. 8-23. Image intensification imaging device (Magnacamera). (Courtesy, Picker Nuclear, White Plains, New York, and Sony Corporation of America, New York)

The system consists of five parts: The basic blocks are:
1. Collimator, for radiation imaging
2. Image tube, for detection of the gamma rays
3. Low light level orthicon tube, for televising the radiation scenes
4. Television generator and target storage controls
5. Display and data storage devices

Several collimators have been commonly used with the camera. These are the multiple parallel hole type. Basic hexagonal units with cell sizes from ⅛ inch to ¼ inch across and 1 inch to 2 inches deep have been used in the parallel hole configuration.

Image tube. The image tube is a type of radiation detector that employs a scintillator, photocathode, anode cone, and output screen. The main problem in building a nuclear image tube is the problem of detecting and amplifying a picture formed by a low gamma flux level. The input screen must be thicker, optically clearer, and generally more efficient at a given input energy level than the conventional type of x-ray image tube.

Operation of the image tube is basically as follows (Fig. 8-24). Photoelectrons are generated in the photocathode that is stimulated by a scintillation from an absorbed gamma ray that has passed through the collimator. These electrons are accelerated to the anode cone under the influence of a very high voltage field. The electron image is then converted to a visible light image at the 1 inch diameter phosphor screen. The image consists of low level light flashes corresponding to

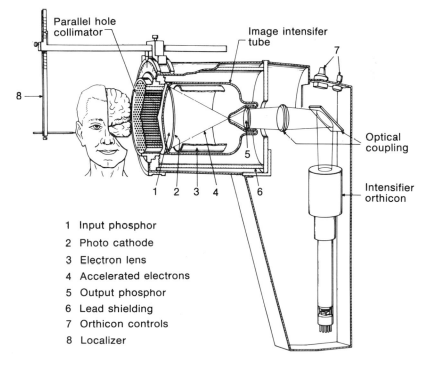

1 Input phosphor
2 Photo cathode
3 Electron lens
4 Accelerated electrons
5 Output phosphor
6 Lead shielding
7 Orthicon controls
8 Localizer

Fig. 8-24. Cut-away diagram of the image intensification imaging device (Magnacamera). (Courtesy, Picker Nuclear, White Plains, New York)

gamma rays being absorbed in the scintillator at the front of the image tube. These flashes are then sent through a conventional fast lens and mirror optical system to the next component in the chain (the image orthicon television camera tube).

Orthicon tube. The image intensifier orthicon camera is used to amplify the image. The flash image from the intensifier tube is applied to the orthicon photo-cathode, where it again becomes an electron image. The electrons from the image are then accelerated to the target section of the orthicon. In this section, the charge image can be read off by a scanning electron beam. The number of times per second that the information can be read off the orthicon target can be varied. This is important because the number of gammas per second may be insufficient to present a good, usable picture. During the time between the scans of the electron beam, the information is not lost, but it is integrated or piled up (stored) upon the target. This storage time can be controlled to allow the collection of the optimum amount of information on the target in the form of charge. In this manner the statistics of the gamma picture can be improved by storing for longer periods of time. This is especially valuable if the information rate from the patient is low, as in the usual static study. In a dynamic study, this storage may be cut to $\frac{1}{30}$ second for top read-out speed, because the information rate from the patient is high.

Television generator and controls. Normally, a television system completely scans the pickup tube target with an electron beam 30 times each second to permit fast motion and low flicker. Control circuitry is provided in this system to slow down this scan rate and make it intermittent, so that the orthicon reads the statistical information only as often as desired. The read-out of the integrated target charge is still read off in $\frac{1}{30}$ second, but the storage time (between read-outs) is varied to suit the picture content.

Display and data storage. One display system is a Polaroid camera of conventional design, which views a flat-face oscilloscope tube. The oscilloscope chassis can also be designed to display on a television monitor.

Data storage for both dynamic and static studies can be handled through video tape recordings. In this way the information is faithfully recorded as the study occurs. There is no danger of losing the study due to incorrectly exposed movie films. The examination can be played back and photographed carefully as many times as necessary. Also, information can be played back and photographed in pieces, using the still frame capabilities of the recorder.

Spark chamber camera. The spark chamber camera employs the spark chamber as the detector and is used for low energy emitters. The diameter of the spark chamber is about 8 inches, and it is filled with argon or xenon gas. A potential of several thousand volts is maintained between the cathode and the grid. When gamma rays or x-rays strike the gas between the cathode and the first grid, electrons are produced, which eventually, because of the high voltage process system, cause additional free electrons and ions to be produced until an avalanche occurs. The charged particles travel to the second part of the chamber, where they form the path for a visible spark. The sparks are then photographed by a camera through a glass end of the chamber. This spark chamber camera is used for iodine 125 thyroid studies.

Film badges. The film badge is probably the most commonly used radiation detection device today. It provides a reasonably accurate means of determining dosages from beta, gamma and x-radiation. Most film badges consist of a plastic holder containing radiation-sensitive film, usually of dental film size. The film badge also contains a variety of filters used to absorb certain radiations of varying energies. The variety of filters placed at different points on the film badge allows identification of a specified type of radiation. The use of these absorbers gives an indication of the penetration and energy of the radiation producing the exposure. There is also an area on the film badge that has no filter and that is not covered by even the plastic holder. Beta as well as very weak energy gamma radiation can be detected in this area.

Films are developed and then evaluated by measuring the density of the blackening on the film. These measurements are compared to standard films which have been exposed to known radiation doses. Generally, film badges are capable of measuring dosages from 50 milliroentgens to 500 roentgens.

The film badges are worn on the pocket or the belt of nuclear medicine personnel. The same film may be worn for a week to, usually, a month. The length of time depends upon the sensitivity of the film and the amount of radiation to which the radiation worker is exposed. Since nuclear medicine personnel are usually exposed to very low levels of radiation, the longer the film is worn, the greater will be the accuracy of the measurement. The film badge is not sensitive to radiation exposures much below 50 mr. It is suggested that nuclear medicine personnel wear their film badge for periods of one month at a time in order that the radiation level will fall into the sensitive area.

With the advent of radionuclide generator systems the Atomic Energy Commission has suggested that the radiation worker use finger or wrist badges as well. Since the hands come into closer contact with the radiation-emitting substances than the rest of the body, it is suggested that the wrist or finger badge be returned for evaluation on a weekly or biweekly basis.

Film badges have an advantage over other types of monitoring devices in that they provide a reasonably accurate record at a low cost. Further, since the film badges are not developed, evaluated, or recorded in the nuclear medicine laboratory, the film badges provide a permanent unbiased record of exposure. The disadvantage of a film badge is that since the mailing, evaluation, and return of the report requires approximately three weeks, an immediate record of exposure is not available. Other disadvantages would include the fact that film badges may become darkened if improperly handled. The latter would include such problems as leaving the film badge on a radiator or leaving the film badge on clothes that are sent to the laundry.

Thermoluminescent dosimetry. Thermoluminescent dosimetry is a method of radiation detection which is rapidly gaining acceptance as a personnel monitoring device. Materials used for the thermoluminescence are primarily calcium fluoride and lithium fluoride. These materials, when exposed to ionizing radiation, absorb the energies released in the material. This energy is liberated only on subsequent heating of the material. As the temperature reaches a characteristic value, the energy is released in the form of light and this light is analyzed for exposure intensities; hence, the name thermoluminescence.

Thermoluminescent dosimetry offers a variety of uses in the radiation medicine field. In addition to personnel monitoring applications, it is used in the measurement of dosages in tissues surrounding a therapeutic tissue implant source. The thermoluminescent method appears to be much more sensitive than the film badge.

Chapter 9

Considerations of
counting and imaging

The detection and subsequent count rate obtained from a radioactive source is governed by many factors. These factors include the operating voltage, resolving time, the geometric relationship between the source and the counter, scatter, absorption, background radiation, the efficiency of the counter, collimation, and the use of statistics. All of these factors are dependent upon the detector itself, the counter, the source of radiation, and the material surrounding the source.

OPERATING VOLTAGE

The count rate obtained from a given source with a Geiger or scintillation detector is highly dependent upon the voltage applied to the detector. This has been already discussed at great length, and in this chapter it will be assumed that the proper operating voltage has been determined.

RESOLVING TIME

Every counting system involving a detector and scaler requires a certain recovery period following the detection of a pulse before the system is capable of counting a second pulse. This time interval during which the counter is dead to any other pulses is called the resolving time of the system.

The resolving time varies with the type of detector and electronics involved. A Geiger detector, for example, has a resolving time of about 10^{-4} seconds. In the discussion of G-M tubes, it was stated that following an ionization event, the electrons travel quickly to the anode, but the positive ions travel at a much slower rate to the cathode. During the travel time of the positive ions, any other ionization events will not be seen by the detector. Any such event occurring during this time period is known as coincidence and the inability to detect the event is referred to as *coincidence loss.*

Scintillation detectors have resolving times from 10^{-5} to 10^{-6} seconds, and the scaler has a resolving time of 10^{-5} seconds. In the case of a scintillation crystal, it is often the scaler that is the limiting component in the system, rather than the detector.

As a result of the phenomenon of coincidence loss, the observed counting rate is always less than the true counting rate. There is a certain probability that one or more pulses will follow a detected event within the interval of the resolving time and will not be counted. As the counting rate increases or the resolving time increases, this probability will become greater. If the counting rate and resolving time are known, the number of events which are lost can be predicted, and the observed counting rate can be corrected.

GEOMETRY

The geometric relationship between source and counter has a profound influence upon the count rate obtained for a given activity. The count rate is particularly sensitive to the size and shape of the source and detector, and to the distance between the source and detector.

The inverse square law (discussed in detail in Chapter 6) has a profound influence on count rate. Using a point source, the counting rate is decreased by one-fourth if the distance is doubled, and is increased by a factor of 4 if the distance is halved. In the case of a source of activity that is not a point source, this relationship does not hold exactly, but the relationship between count rate and distance is still profound.

This principle is important in routine nuclear medicine procedures such as the thyroid uptake study and the renogram. An uptake study, for instance, that does not use the same distance between detector and thyroid as between the detector and the standard will represent a gross change in count rate and, therefore, the results will be erroneous.

Perhaps the greatest disregard for proper geometry considerations is not in the correct use of a probe, but in counting samples in a well detector. Distance and inverse square are not so readily recognized in this type of detection procedure. A common problem is comparing the counts from a 4 ml standard to a 2 ml unknown, where it was possible to collect only 2 ml of serum. In order to obtain a correct count, the *geometry must be identical,* unless a correction factor is known. This means that the technologist cannot compare the two samples by counting the 2 ml sample and multiplying by 2. The 2 ml sample must be diluted with an activity-free solution to 4 ml, then the count multiplied by 2, since more of the emissions from the 2 ml sample are being exposed to the detector than from the 4 ml sample (Fig. 9-1). The gray area in Fig. 9-1 represents percentage of counts that are not exposed to the detector from the 4 ml sample, but are exposed from the 2 ml sample. Since more of the emissions are allowed to go undetected by the 4 ml sample, the count could not be accurately compared to a 2 ml count.

This principle is dramatically proved by taking a count of a 1 ml sample, then making several 1 ml additions of water and counting after each addition. As the water is added (the water is activity-free), the count rate decreases until the level of the liquid reaches the top of the crystal. After that point, the changes are not as great.

Errors in well counting can occur in comparing two sources in unlike containers. A 4 ml sample counted in a narrow test tube and compared to a 4 ml sample counted in a wide test tube will represent a considerable error for the same reason as different volumes.

The size and shape of the detector also influence the count rate. For example, some counters, called 4π counters, completely surround the source and are geometrically able to count all radiations emitted. Two π counters detect only 50% of the radiation emitted, since they surround only half of the source. Probe type detectors count only a small fraction of the emitted radiations, and well type detectors, by partially surrounding the source, can detect 50% or more.

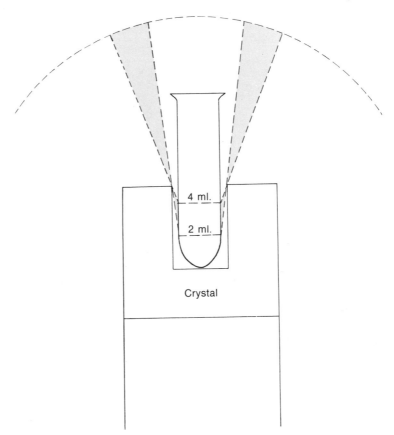

Fig. 9-1. Diagram illustrating the importance of geometry considerations in well counting. A 2 ml sample will have greater than one-half the count rate of a 4 ml sample of the same material because a greater number of photons will go undetected (gray area) from the 4 ml specimen.

SCATTER

Scatter is the term applied to radiation which is diverted from its original path by some type of collision. Radiation is emitted in all directions from its source. Those radiations emitted directly toward the detector may be counted. Those radiations that are emitted in any direction other than directly into the detector may be deflected in such a way that they will eventually strike the detector and also be counted. Since a collision of some sort was necessary, these emissions are reduced in energy. Barring pulse height analysis, this type of scatter would *increase* the count rate. The degree of scatter is influenced by the atomic number and the thickness of the backing material. Scatter will increase as either of these factors increases. Beta particles can be deflected by heavy nuclei through angles greater than 90 degrees and, therefore, can increase the count rate. Gamma ray backscatter is caused either by Compton collision, resulting in a photon of lower energy traveling in a different direction from the primary gamma, or by pair production, wherein two 0.51 mev photons are ultimately produced. This scatter phenomenon is extremely important in understanding the principles of collimators. Scatter can

167

reduce the count rate if it occurs in the material between the source and detector when gamma rays or charged particles are deflected out of the beam.

ABSORPTION

Absorption of radiation differs from scatter in that the total energy of the radiation is dissipated in the absorbing material. Three sites of absorption exist in any counting situation; the source itself, the media between the source and detector, and the detector. All influence the resultant count rate.

Absorption occurring in the source, called *self-absorption,* reduces the count rate. This can be very significant in particle counting. In some cases, self-absorption limits the number of counts that can be detected from a source material. As more radioactive material is added, the added material absorbs as many radiations as it emits. Gamma-ray detection does not usually involve problems with self-absorption. However, if the gamma ray energy is less than 0.1 mev or if the source is large, such as a human body or an organ, then self-absorption must be considered.

Absorption of radiation occurring in the media between the source and detector also reduces the count rate. An example would be the air and the window of the detector in beta or alpha particle detection. For gamma ray detection it is usually unnecessary to take into account those gamma rays absorbed by the air or the detector window. However, a material of high density may absorb many of the gamma rays.

The final site of absorption occurs in the detecting medium. The detection of radiation depends upon the absorption of, or transfer of, energy from the radiations to the detector. Particulate radiations will, in general, be absorbed by the detector if they have sufficient energy to penetrate into the detecting medium. Therefore, precautions must be taken not to allow the particles to be absorbed before they reach the sensitive volume of the detector. This is the rationale behind liquid scintillation counting. With gamma rays the problem is different. It is possible for a gamma ray to travel through a detector without interacting and, therefore, go undetected. The chance of this happening decreases as the mass or density of the detector increases. Therefore, gaseous detectors, such as Geiger tubes, stop only a few gamma rays, while scintillation detectors stop many more.

BACKGROUND

All counters will record some activity without a source present. This activity is known as room background activity. It is caused both by radiation from natural radioisotopes and cosmic rays entering the detector and by instrument noise. The *gross count* of a source also includes background counts. Thus, to obtain the *net count* from the source alone, the background count rate must be determined and subtracted from the gross count rate.

Many times the room background activity does not represent a significant change in the count, in which case it is a waste of time to consider it at all. In most of the recently developed instruments, background count rate never exceeds 100 counts per minute. Generally, any background count less than the square root of the total count can be disregarded, as it will not introduce a significant amount of error into the procedure. For example, if the count rate was 10,000 cpm, a background count rate less than 100 dpm would be considered insignificant ($\sqrt{10,000} = 100$).

The primary purpose of a background determination is assurance that the instrument is operating properly. A room background count is performed *daily* by determining the proper operating voltage and allowing the unit to count for a predetermined unit of time without a source of activity near or in the detector. Background counts should be taken in the approximate clinical situation. For instance, the background count for the thyroid uptake probe should be taken with the probe pointing in the same direction as it would if it were being used for a patient count; the room background count of a well detector should be taken with the lid closed (if this is the way it is being used with patient samples) or with the lid of the well open (if the clinical use of the unit dictates this procedure).

EFFICIENCY OF COUNTING

The above factors are all a part of counting efficiency. The efficiency of any system is loosely defined as that which is obtained from the system divided by that which is put into the system. It can also be expressed as a formula:

$$\text{Efficiency} = \frac{\text{counts/unit time}}{\text{disintegrations/unit time}}$$

To determine the efficiency of a well counter, it is possible to purchase a calibrated solution (iodine 131, for example) in which the disintegrations per second are known. For example, 1.0 μCi of a calibrated solution of iodine 131 can be used to determine the efficiency of counting. A microcurie has already been defined as 2.22×10^6 dpm, but this sample has been counted and determined to be only 222,000 (2.22×10^5) cpm. The efficiency can be determined by:

$$\text{Efficiency} = \frac{2.22 \times 10^5}{2.22 \times 10^6} = 1.0 \times 10^{-1} = 0.1 \text{ or } 10\%$$

This result would indicate that the unit was capable of counting only 10% of all disintegrations and, therefore, was only 10% efficient. It is important to realize that the measurement of any radionuclide in a given sample need not be determined as its absolute value of disintegrations per unit time. In a routine nuclear medicine department, the only concern is usually for relative values—the relative comparison of the activity in one sample with the relative value of the activity in another sample. The physician need not have the absolute value to make a valid diagnosis. The point can be demonstrated by the following examples.

A blood sample having an *absolute* value of 200 cpm was obtained from an injected dose having an absolute value of 20,000 cpm, representing 1% in the sample. The same samples counted on an entirely different instrument may represent *relative* values of 100 cpm from an injected dose having a relative value of 10,000 cpm—also 1% in the sample.

In both examples, whether using absolute or relative values, the percentage of administered dose recovered in the blood sample is the same. The factors which influence the count received are presented in this discussion in an effort to make

169

the technologist aware of these influencing factors so that in using relative values, these factors are kept constant. In this way, the relative comparisons reflect a true comparison.

COLLIMATION

Electromagnetic radiation of longer wavelengths, such as light, can be focused by bending rays through lenses or by reflection from polished surfaces. Electromagnetic radiations of shorter wavelengths, however, will not respond to such mechanical manipulations. The only way a gamma ray can be removed from its path is by absorption or scatter of the ray. Therefore, a device must be used which can eliminate from detection all gamma rays except those of interest. This device is called a *collimator*. The collimator is generally constructed of lead and usually extends in front of the scintillation detector. The lead is arranged in a configuration that allows it to perform the desired function. In the usual nuclear medicine laboratory, two types of collimators are used, the flat-field collimator and the multihole collimator. There are two types of multihole collimators—focused and parallel hole. Each of these types of collimators has different characteristics, since each is used for a different purpose. In addition, there are straight hole collimators and pinhole collimators.

Perhaps the most informative method of demonstrating the characteristics of these collimators is by the use of isocount lines (Fig. 9-2).

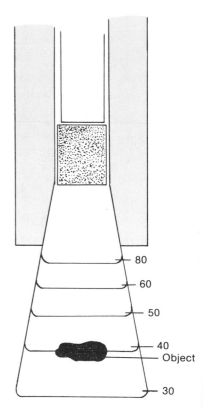

Fig. 9-2. Flat field collimator whose characteristic is demonstrated by the construction of isocount lines, indicating uniform "vision" through organ under investigation.

170

Flat-field collimator

In the event that a whole organ, such as a thyroid or a kidney, is to be seen by the detector, the collimators must be designed to eliminate not only a portion of the background radiation, but also radiation coming from other parts of the patient's body. The collimator chosen for this use must be able to detect radiations coming from any part of the organ of interest. A flat-field collimator would be used since a flat response is received at a certain distance from the face of the collimator (Fig. 9-2). In Fig. 9-2 the isocount (same count) or isoresponse is demonstrated as having a flat portion, which increases in diameter as the distance from the face of the collimator is increased. A point source lying anywhere along such a line would result in the same number of counts. A line drawn directly across the face of the collimator with the point source centrally placed would represent 100%, the maximum count detectable. The same source located anywhere on the 80% isocount line would give a count equal to 80% of the maximum count.

In using this collimator to visualize a whole organ, the distance that the collimator is placed away from the organ must be great enough to enable the detector to see the whole organ and to have a relatively uniform sensitivity to the entire organ. The flat-field collimator serves the uniform sensitivity criterion very well because of its flat response. The distance required to see the entire organ depends upon the collimator and the diameter of the detector. For example, a 1.5 inch diameter detector requires a 36 degree collimator to include a large thyroid at a distance of 20 cm. At a distance of 35 cm the same detector requires a 20 degree collimator.

Straight bore collimator. In other nuclear medicine applications, it is more desirable not to view the entire organ as a whole, but to study particular segments of an organ independently from the rest of it. This would require a detector that would view only a small area at a time. This requires a special collimator.

The collimator used to view small areas of an organ is one that can also distinguish between small areas of differing count rates. Such a collimator is rated by *resolution.* Resolution is the minimum distance between two radioactive objects that can still be distinguished as two distinct sources by the collimator. The degree of resolution varies with the physical design and material of the collimator, as well as with the energy of the gamma rays being counted. A collimator is chosen according to the requirements of a specific application. In general, one with good resolution should be used for studies of small organs and one with poorer resolution can be used for larger organs.

One of the first collimators used for viewing small areas of an organ was the straight bore collimator (Fig. 9-3). The straight bore collimator is nothing more than a large piece of lead with a small hole bored through it. The piece of lead is attached to the face of the scintillation detector. The resolution of the collimator is influenced by the diameter and the length of the hole; the smaller the bore and the longer the collimator, the greater is its resolution. Fig. 9-3 displays in a simple manner the effect of collimator length and bore size to resolution. All radiations emitted in the direction of the crystal and within the dotted lines will be detected

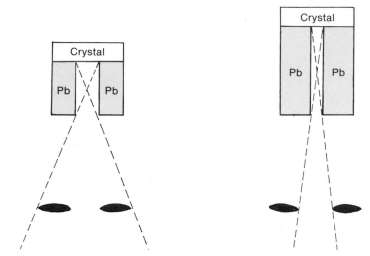

Fig. 9-3. Straight bore (single hole, single channel) collimator illustrating the effects of size of hole and depth of hole on resolution.

in their pure energy state. Both detectors are aimed at two ⅝ inch areas of activity situated ⅝ inch apart and at a depth of 3 inches from the face of the collimator. The first detector, which has a shorter collimator with a larger bore size, is unable to differentiate between the two lesions because the *solid angle of inclusion* encompasses both lesions. This detector would have very poor resolution. The second detector has a collimator which is increased in length and decreased in bore size. The same two areas of activity, situated identically with respect to each other and to the collimator, would be resolved as the detector unit passes over them. Emissions from the two areas of activity would not be detected in their pure energy state if the detector were situated as depicted. As the detector moves to the right or to the left, pure emissions would be seen only from the right or left areas of activity, respectively. Resolution would then be greatly enhanced and the system could be expressed as having a resolution of ⅝ inch. Another very important fact regarding resolution is that as resolution increases, statistics suffer. The collimator excludes more and more ionization events as resolution increases.

These principles of resolution are basic to understanding the influencing factors of any collimator, be it single bore, focused, or parallel hole. These principles are easy to understand in the straight bore collimator, but they often seem more complex when extended to the multibore or multichannel type collimator. However, there is no difference. The principles are the same, only the number of holes has changed.

Multihole collimators

Characteristics. The *number of holes* in a collimator is determined by the crystal size of the detector and the required septal thickness. In general, it can be stated that the number of holes for any given size crystal increases as the resolution increases. A decrease in number of holes suggests either nonutilization of the entire crystal, larger holes, or thicker septa.

The holes are usually hexagonal in shape and are arranged in a hexagonal array; or they may be round and arranged in a circular pattern. A hexagonal hole ensures that the thickness of the septa between holes is uniform. If the holes are round and large enough to circumscribe the hexagonal hole of a similar collimator, the minimum septal thickness may be less than the septal thickness of hexagonal holes. In this case, there is more penetration of the gamma rays if round holes are used than if the hexagonal are used. If the round holes of a collimator are such that they inscribe the hexagonal holes of another collimator, then the septal penetration in the collimator with the round holes is less than that of the hexagonal hole. In this case, the gamma ray penetration is less, but so also is the crystal sensitivity, since the area of the crystal which is exposed is reduced.

There are both low energy collimators and high energy collimators available today. As gamma rays increase in energy, the ability of the collimator to absorb or deflect them becomes less. Higher energy gamma rays require greater septal thickness than do low energy gamma rays. This reduces sensitivity because the greater the thickness of lead, the smaller the area of crystal utilization. Consequently, two types of collimators are available based solely on their septal thicknesses: (1) a low energy collimator, which is designed for all radionuclides having gamma energies less than 150 kev and (2) a high energy collimator for all radionuclides having energies greater than 150 kev. High energy collimators can be used for imaging an organ containing a low energy radionuclide, but the reverse is not true. Sensitivity, of course, would be much less with the high energy collimator and a low energy radionuclide than with a low energy collimator and a low energy radionuclide.

Multibore focused collimators. Although the straight bore collimator, as originally designed, had good resolution between two distinct lesions, tremendous amounts of radioactivity had to be administered to the patient in order for the count to be statistically adequate. For this reason, there had to be an increase in the number of events detected while limiting the detection area in order that the resolution did not suffer tremendously. Such a compromise led to the production of a multibore focused collimator.

This collimator consists of a series of holes in a piece of lead which are angled in such a way that their holes are aimed at approximately the same spot. This spot is called the focal point and represents the 100% isocount area. Unlike the other collimators discussed, the 100% area is not at the face of the collimator, but at a point distant to the face. Another feature of the focused collimator is that the diameter of the holes is tapered; the larger end is closest to the crystal in order to increase the detection efficiency. The isocount lines proceed in a somewhat circular fashion around the focal point as indicated in Fig. 9-4.

The same two factors of collimator length and bore size affect the resolution of the focused collimator. In addition, special consideration must be extended to the energy of the emission. The resolving ability of the collimator decreases as the energy of the gamma ray increases. As the resolution decreases a gamma ray is allowed to begin its path up one channel toward the detector, to pass through the lead septa without its energy being altered appreciably, and to enter into another

173

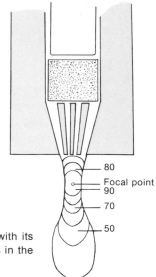

80
Focal point
90
70
50

Fig. 9-4. Multibore (multihole, multichannel) focused collimator with its isocount lines indicating focal distance, the point where all holes in the collimator converge.

channel where it strikes the crystal and is counted. This crossing into another channel is called "cross talk." Since that gamma ray did not come from the area toward which that hole was aimed, the collimator did not do its job in defining the area from which the gamma ray came. This represents erroneous information and, in effect, reduces the resolving power of the system. Therefore, the more energetic the gamma, the more absorbing material (usually lead) required between the holes to stop all the gamma rays.

Cross-talk is not permitted if a collimator is effective. The principle behind collimators and their use is to either absorb or scatter gamma rays in such a fashion that they either go undetected or are scattered to such a degree that the detection event will not be accepted (a function of pulse height analysis). Scatter is represented by gamma rays emitted from some other area of the organ not immediately under the view of the collimator; therefore, these rays do not have a clear path to the scintillation detector. In coming in from an angle, they must pass through lead before reaching one of the holes. The resultant secondary gamma is one of decreased energy and changed in direction (Compton effect). The direction may be such that the gamma ray is directed up the hole of the collimator. In such instances, the correct utilization of pulse height analysis will reject the detection event because the gamma ray is no longer of sufficient energy to produce an acceptable pulse height. It is for this reason that the operator of any imaging device must understand and correctly use pulse height analysis. If the pulse height analyzer is arranged is such a manner that the detection unit would accept and count this secondary gamma coming from an area not in the view of the collimator, it is possible to mask a cold lesion, for example.

It can be argued that pulse height analysis is not quite as important in well detection systems because the percentage of gammas from Compton collisions (scatter) remains as a constant percentage of the pure gammas emitted. This argument cannot be extended to any other utilization of radionuclides. Correct pulse height analysis in studies such as thyroid uptakes, renal studies, and imaging techniques is extremely important to the value of the study.

Focal depth is a variable with focused collimators. The focal depth is the distance from the face of the collimator to the point where all the holes converge. Standard focal depths are 3 inches and 5 inches. The focal depth cannot exceed the diameter of the scintillation crystal. Therefore, 3-inch diameter crystals have only 3-inch focal depth collimators; 5-inch diameter crystals have collimators available in both 3-inch and 5-inch focal depths; and 8-inch diameter crystals have collimators with 3-, 5-, and 8-inch focal depths.

The terms *coarse focus* and *fine focus* are used to qualitatively describe the degree of resolution that can be expected from the use of a collimator. These terms describe the isoresponse of a collimator. A fine focused collimator is one in which the isocount curves are shortened both in width and in length and are used primarily for definition of very small lesions in small organs. The coarse (or broad) focused collimator is one in which the isocount curve is larger both in length and in width and, therefore, does not have as high a resolving power. These are generally used on large organ imaging techniques in which the definition of small lesions is not quite so rigid. The fine focused collimator usually has a larger number of small holes. A coarse focused collimator usually has a smaller number of large holes. The names of the collimators describe their function.

Multichannel parallel hole collimators. A multichannel parallel hole collimator, as used in a stationary imaging device ("camera"), consists of a lead plate with hundreds or thousands of channels that are parallel to one another. Each channel accepts only vertically oriented gamma rays from one specific area. A gamma ray image of the subject is projected on the scintillation crystal detector. In normal use, the subject is positioned as close as possible to the face of the collimator. The reason is that the resolution is best for organs or parts of organs closest to the collimator. Resolution decreases with increasing distance from the collimator. By comparison a focused collimator has the best resolution along the plane of focal depth and the resolution decreases with increasing distance from the focal plane. In most clinical uses of the camera, the resolution of the system is limited mostly by the collimator, not by the inherent resolution of the image detector. Collimators with higher degrees of resolution are possible from an engineering standpoint, but with a loss of count rate. Other features, such as length of the parallel hole, number of holes, size of holes, and shape of holes, all affect the image, as they do in a focused collimator. The only difference is that, theoretically, the resolution is somewhat less than in a focused collimator. The holes do not converge upon one area at a fixed distance, but are aimed through the organ and through the body, at an infinite distance. The advantage to such a collimator is that the predetermination of the focal depth is not necessary, and the possibility of error from an improperly calculated focal depth is eliminated.

Pinhole collimator

The pinhole collimator operates on the old-fashioned box camera principle (Fig. 9-5). It consists of a single, small aperture at the end of a lead shield. The collimator is so designed that x-rays entering at any angle through the pinhole

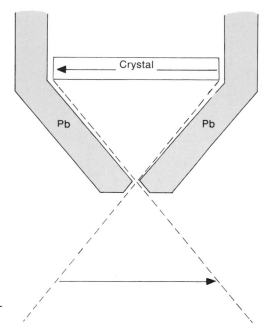

Fig. 9-5. Pinhole collimator. Diagram illustrating its principle of action.

will be seen by the scintillation detector. This is unlike the single bore collimator, in which the gamma ray must enter at an angle perpendicular to the face of the crystal in order to be detected. Pinhole collimators provide the best combination of sensitivity and resolution for small subjects that are positioned a short distance from the aperture. They can also be used to take pictures of very large organs by positioning the subject a greater distance from the aperture. This principle has been used for entire lung fields, liver imaging, and so on. The pinhole collimator has greater resolution than parallel hole collimators, but sensitivity is decreased. Unlike with the parallel hole type, the image size becomes smaller as the distance between the subject and the collimator increases.

STATISTICS

When a source of radioactivity is designated as having a certain number of microcuries or millicuries, it is, in effect, designated as having a certain number of disintegrations per unit time taking place, since units of activity are defined as the number of disintegrations per unit time (see Table 6-2). When such a source is designated as having a certain number of disintegrations per unit time, it is only an average, and is not a constantly reproducible number. The disintegration of a radioactive atom is a *random* event; therefore, the number of disintegrations is a random variable. It is impossible to predict exactly which atom is going to decay next and exactly how many will disintegrate per unit time; it is possible only to determine an average.

For this reason, a very basic knowledge of statistics is indispensable to both the technologist and the physician for correct utilization of radionuclides and the interpretation of the results of counting or imaging procedures. The physician must use statistical knowledge in evaluating the precision and accuracy* of the counting data. Decisions must be made as to the number of counts to be accumulated (preset count) or the time necessary to accumulate a certain number of counts (preset time), the minimum dose which should be administered, and the travel speed of a rectilinear imaging device. The likelihood that a difference between counts of two different samples or two different areas on an organ image represents a significant difference rather than the random variability between two identical samples or areas must also be determined.

This section on statistics will treat the statistics of sample counting and the statistics of imaging as two separate entities, because they are not easily related to one another. In both cases, however, the number of events recorded (counts) must be *adequate* to be certain that major differences in the results are not a function of poor statistics.

Statistics of sample counting

Since the number of disintegrations per unit time is a variable, it is to be expected that the counts from the same sample for the same period of time will not be identical. In fact, they can vary considerably, depending upon the number of counts accumulated. *As the number of counts increases, the variation between subsequent counts on the same sample also increases; but the percent error between subsequent counts decreases.*

An explanation of this statement requires a discussion of the Poisson distribution principle, a principle which is applicable to the observation of random events. The Poisson distribution principle states that the standard deviation is proportional to the square root of the number of observed events. This can be expressed as a formula as follows:

$$\sigma = \sqrt{N}$$

σ = standard deviation or standard error
N = number of observed events (counts)

If the number of counts is 100, one standard deviation is $\sqrt{100}$, or 10 counts. (Note that the 100 counts is a quantity, not intensity. It makes no difference as to the length of time required to accumulate that 100 counts.) This is usually expressed as plus or minus one standard deviation, or ±10 counts from the true count of 100. Further, it is an accepted principle from the Poisson distribution that 68% of all counts will fall within this range of 90 to 110 counts (Fig. 9-6). In other words, if a count was taken 100 times on a sample that emitted 100 counts, 68 of the counts would fall somewhere within a range of 90 to 110 counts, and 32 of those counts would fall outside that range. Another way of expressing this relationship is that if a sample was counted only long enough to accumulate 100 counts, the observer could be confident that 68% of the time (approximately two-thirds of the time) that count would be within ±10 counts.

---

*Precision and accuracy are two entirely different entities. A practiced rifleman can shoot a target four times in a row in almost the exact same spot, but outside the bull's-eye; precise but not accurate. Another rifleman may possess enough experience to have all four shots hit the bull's-eye; precise and accurate.

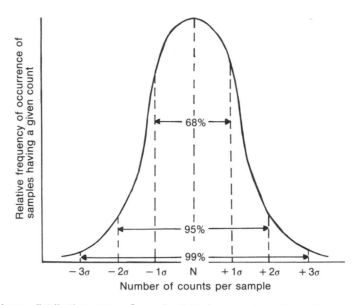

Fig. 9-6. Poisson distribution curve. Curve is plotted as number of counts per sample versus number of times that sample count occurs. In a series of 100 like samples (or the same sample counted 100 times), a 10,000 count sample would result in the largest number of counts having a value of 10,000 per predetermined time period. However, not all counts in this time period would be 10,000, because of the phenomenon of random decay. Some will be larger, some smaller. The above figure predicts that 68 of the 100 counts will fall within $\pm 1\sigma$ (9,900 to 10,000), 95 between $\pm 2\sigma$, and 99 between $\pm 3\sigma$.

Further, if $1\sigma = \pm 10$ counts, then $2\sigma = \pm 20$ counts and $3\sigma = \pm 30$ counts. The Poisson distribution principle also states that 95% of all counts will fall within $\pm 2\sigma$, and 99% of all counts will fall within $\pm 3\sigma$. In this case, 95 of the 100 counts would fall within a range of 80 to 120 counts, and only one of the counts would fall outside the range of 70 to 130 counts. Accordingly, the observer could be 95% confident that any count on a 100-count sample would be within ± 20 counts of the true value and 99% confident that it would be within ± 30 counts. These relationships are depicted in Fig. 9-6, where $\pm 1\sigma$ is the 68% confidence level, $\pm 2\sigma$ is the 95% confidence level, and $\pm 3\sigma$ is the 99% confidence level.

The value of the material just presented lies in the percent error that a certain number of counts is likely to introduce into the study. For instance, the 100 counts used in the example above shows that the observer is only 68% sure that the count that is received is within ± 10 counts of the true value. This is not many counts per se, but it represents a $\pm 10\%$ error. This is totally unacceptable as far as the results are concerned. To go to the higher confidence levels of 95% or 99% introduces an error of $\pm 20\%$ and $\pm 30\%$ error respectively, which is even worse.

To correct this problem, and since the whole area of statistics is based on the number of counts, the situation could be helped by counting $\sqrt{1,000}$ events instead of 100. In this situation, $\sigma = $ 1,000 or 32. Therefore, 68% of all counts would be within a range of 968 to 1,032 which represents an error of $\pm 3.2\%$. Notice that by increasing the number of counts, the range has increased (from 20 to 64 for $\pm 1\sigma$),

Table 9-1. Summary of relationship of counts to percent error

Number of counts	1σ (68%)	Range	Percent error
100	± 10	90 to 110	±10.0%
1,000	± 32	968 to 1,032	± 3.2%
10,000	±100	9,900 to 10,100	± 1.0%
100,000	±317	99,683 to 100,317	± 0.3%

but the percent error has decreased. Further, a count of 10,000 would present a standard deviation of ±100, but would represent a percent error of only ±1%. These relationships are summarized in Table 9-1.

In routine nuclear medicine work, the decision must be made by the observer as to how many counts must be accumulated to have reasonable confidence that the count is within an acceptable degree of error. A common solution to the problem is to accumulate enough counts that the observer is 95% confident that the count received is within ±2% error. Table 9-1 shows that a count of 10,000 represents a 68% chance of being within ±1% error. Since 2σ represents the 95% confidence level, the continuation of the table would read:

Number of counts	2σ (95%)	Range	Percent error
10,000	±200	9,800 to 10,200	±2%

Accordingly, if the operator accumulated 10,000 counts, he would be 95% certain that any such count would be within ±2% of the true value. This is reasonably good statistics for routine nuclear medicine procedures, and is the rationale behind the rule-of-thumb that *regardless of the time required, 10,000 counts should always be accumulated.*

The relationships between the number of counts and percent error, as related to the desired confidence level, can be expressed mathematically as follows:

$$\text{For 68\% confidence level: } N = \frac{10,000}{V^2}$$

$$\text{For 95\% confidence level: } N = \frac{40,000}{V^2}$$

$$\text{For 99\% confidence level: } N = \frac{90,000}{V^2}$$

$$N = \text{number of counts}$$
$$V = \text{\% error}$$

The 68% confidence level is usually used for preliminary studies when an approximate statistical evaluation is warranted. The 95% confidence level is used for routine work, and the 99% confidence level is used for research work.

A research project might require the best statistics possible without sacrificing too much time in counting. This would generally mean a statistical accuracy of ±1% error 99% of the time (99% confidence level). The question of how many counts must be accumulated would be solved as follows:

$$N = \frac{90,000}{V^2} = \frac{90,000}{(1)^2} = \frac{90,000}{1} = 90,000 \text{ counts}$$

This formula could also be used to substantiate the 10,000 counts rule-of-thumb, which states that by accumulating 10,000 counts, the result has a 95% chance of being within ±2% of the true value. Using the 95% confidence level formula and substituting 2% for the percent error, the number of counts to be accumulated is as follows:

$$N = \frac{40,000}{V^2} = \frac{40,000}{(2)^2} = \frac{40,000}{4} = 10,000 \text{ counts}$$

In some studies, such as Schillings test, it may take as long as 25 to 30 minutes to accumulate 10,000 counts.

Background counts must also be considered when making the final decision of how much time to allow for the count or how many counts must be accumulated for a statistically valid result. There are methods to mathematically calculate the background count value, but they are not practical to use. As mentioned previously, if the total count is at least the square of the background count, background need not be considered statistically (background must be considered when using net counts per minute). In most clinical situations, the background is never that high. If it is, the background count is subtracted from the gross counts and counting is continued until 10,000 *net* counts are received.

Statistics of imaging

Statistics also play a major role in imaging techniques with the use of either the rectilinear scanners or stationary cameras. The importance of statistics in both imaging techniques is similar to its importance in sample counting, since an adequate number of events must be recorded to be certain that the lack of a statistical count does not influence the results (diagnosis). The exact number of counts varies in both instances from the rule-of-thumb value of 10,000 used in sample counting.

Rectilinear imaging techniques. There are three parameters on a rectilinear scanner which influence the statistical evaluation of an imaging technique. They are: (1) maximum count rate, (2) the speed at which the detection device moves over the organ, and (3) the space that the detection unit indexes after making one complete pass (line spacing). The count rate has the same relationship to the final evaluation of an image as the number of observed events has to a counting study; that is, the higher the count rate, the better the statistics. However, if the speed is such that the detector unit is not over the area long enough to detect a predetermined number of counts, or if the line spacing is such that a lack of continuity exists, then an ideal maximum count rate becomes less than adequate. The position that the operator of the rectilinear imaging device must take is to accumulate and display a predetermined number of counts as quickly as possible, for the comfort of the patient. If the maximum count rate is high, a faster speed can be used; if the maximum count rate is low, the speed must be reduced to allow the detection unit to remain over any given area for a longer period of time. Line spacing is largely a matter of esthetics.

The predetermined number of counts has become known as *information density* (I.D.). The best quality scan from the standpoint of statistical evaluation is one in

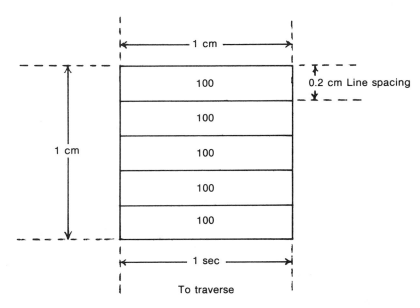

Fig. 9-7. Enlargement of one square centimeter of a scan with an information density of 500 to illustrate the effects of line spacing, speed, and the count rate on the quality of the scan. Line spacing = 0.2 cm; speed = 60 cm/min (1 cm/second); count rate = 6,000.

which the I.D. value is 800. I.D. 800 indicates that there are 800 events (counts) detected per square centimeter. Scans having an I.D. of less than 800 are poor in quality. Scans having an I.D. greater than 800 tend to be too dark, and clinical detail is often lost. This can be corrected, however, by adjusting the light intensity. Fig. 9-7 illustrates the effects of count rate, speed, and line spacing in statistical evaluation of a scan. In the example in Fig. 9-7, the detector unit would have to make five passes of 0.2 cm distance each. A speed of 60 cm/min would indicate that one pass would require one second. The count rate at the area of highest concentration (hot spot) is 6,000 counts per minute (or 100 counts per second). Since one pass requires one second, it would detect 100 events per pass. In five passes, 500 events would be detected and this technique would net an I.D. value of 500.

Since an I.D. of 500 is considered inadequate statistically, one of the three parameters must be altered: the line spacing must be decreased, the speed must be decreased, or the counts must be increased. The easiest solution would be to decrease the speed so that 160 events would be detected per pass over the one square centimeter area. This can be found by using graphs available from instrument companies or solving for speed with the following formula:

$$\text{I.D.} = \frac{\text{maximum cpm}}{\text{speed (cm/min} \times \text{line spacing (cm)}}$$

$$800 = \frac{6,000}{(x)\ 0.2}, \text{ where } x = \text{speed in cm/min}$$

$$0.2x = \frac{6,000}{800}$$

$$0.2x = 7.5$$

$$x = 37.5 \text{ cm/min}$$

Accordingly, the speed of the detector will have to be decreased from 60 cm/min to 37.5 cm/min in order to achieve an I.D. value of 800.

From the above formula, it is apparent that damage to statistical values would occur if the line spacing were increased to 0.4 cm, as some techniques suggest, and the count and speed settings remained the same. Increasing the line spacing would decrease the I.D. by one-half. The only compensatory move is to also decrease the speed by one-half. Therefore, by choosing a larger line spacing the time re-

A. 1,000 counts B. 2,000 counts C. 5,000 counts

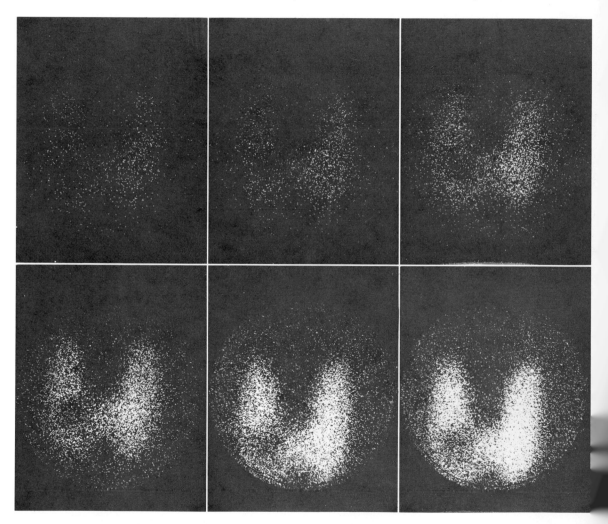

D. 10,000 counts E. 20,000 counts F. 30,000 counts

Fig. 9-8. Effect of statistics using a stationary imaging device. As the number of accumulated counts increases, the image becomes more informative and diagnosis is easier. A point can be reached, as evidenced by views **E** and **F,** where too many counts are accumulated, the detection device becomes saturated, and information is lost. This could be corrected to a degree by reducing the intensity.

quired to complete the imaging study is not decreased, as many might think. It becomes a matter of the type of scan the physician is trained to interpret.

Stationary imaging techniques. The statistics involved in stationary imaging techniques are entirely different from those used for rectilinear scanners or sample counting. The purpose of stationary imaging is to detect and record a certain number of events for an entire organ, rather than a segment of an organ, although one can easily be related to the other.

A predetermined number of counts (thousands or hundreds of thousands of counts) is agreed upon prior to a study. Each type of organ study varies as to the number of counts necessary to be accumulated to effect a study of diagnostic value. Three different parameters are of concern in establishing such a value: saturation effects, background cut-off, and dot size.

The saturation effects come into play when two flashes of light occur at the same place. If the detection device has reached a state of saturation, the second event, which becomes superimposed upon the first, is not displayed as a change in the intensity of the dot. Since under usual conditions the intensity would become brighter if two flashes occurred at the same place (suggesting a greater concentration in that area), information is lost if the saturation point has been reached.

Background erase (cut-off or suppression) also affects the image quality. This parameter is usually used to intentionally prevent recording from areas of an organ in which the concentrations of activity are no more than background level. This device is usually used to reduce the interpretive complications of background radiation. However, if the setting of the background erase is too high, more counts than desired are lost.

The size of the dot on the image is also important, and is directly dependent on the number of counts to be accumulated. As the accumulation increases, the size of the dot decreases and vice versa. Small density differences in the dots become more difficult to detect if the dots are small with large spaces between them. Conversely, large dots result in the loss of resolution.

These three factors must be taken into consideration when arriving at a statistical value. It has been stressed throughout this entire section on statistics that statistical accuracy increases with increased number of observed events. This is true only to a point with a stationary imaging device. Eventually, principles such as saturation and coincidence loss reduce the image quality and efficiency of detection, and, as a result, the study suffers.

Fig. 9-8 is a study with a thyroid phantom showing how too few or too many counts affects the image. Too few counts results in a very poor image, if any at all. As the counts are increased, the quality of the image also increases. Eventually, saturation occurs, and image quality is lost.

Chapter 10 *Radiation health safety*

In Chapter 6, the principles of radiation protection are discussed. The actual implementation of these principles depends on the caliber of radiation health safety programs employed in the individual departments of nuclear medicine. Procedures, such as monitoring, record keeping, and waste disposal, all place a burden on the nuclear medicine personnel involved. These procedures are time consuming and tedious, but they are very important to both the safety of occupational and nonoccupational personnel.

MONITORING

One of the most important health safety procedures is monitoring both the personnel and the work area. The purposes of monitoring are several: (1) to detect radioactive contamination, (2) to evaluate shielding arrangements, and (3) to measure personnel exposure.

Personnel monitoring

Personnel monitoring is usually performed through the use of film badges whereby the cumulative exposure of an individual is determined over a period of time. Other types of personnel monitoring devices are pocket dosimeters and thermoluminescent dosimeters. All three types have been previously discussed. Whatever the method used, monitoring records must be continuously maintained and preserved for a period of 5 years.

Exposure records. Title 10 of the Code of Federal Regulations, Part 20, outlines the procedures for the maintenance of exposure records. This has been discussed in detail in Chapter 6. Title 10CFR20 also stipulates that:

> . . . at the request of a former employee, each licensee shall furnish to the former employee a report of the former employee's exposure to radiation as shown in records maintained by the licensee. Such reports shall be furnished within 30 days from the time the request is made; shall cover each calendar quarter of the individual's employment involving exposure to radiation; or such lesser period as may be requested by the employee. The report shall also include the results of any calculations and analyses of radioactive material deposited in the body of the employee. The report shall be in writing and contain the following statement: "This report is furnished to you under the provisions of the Atomic Energy Commission Regulations entitled 'Standards for Protection Against Radiation' (10CRF Part 20). You should preserve this report for future reference."

The former employee's request should include appropriate identifying data such as Social Security number and dates and locations of employment.

Overexposures. A summary of the AEC regulations regarding notification proceedings of radiation incidents (10CFR20.402 and 10CFR20.403) is seen in Table 10-1. The regulations further stipulate that in addition to the notifications listed

Table 10-1. Summary of Atomic Energy Commission regulations regarding notification of incidents

Conditions of notification	Person(s) notified	Time element	Mode of notification	Remarks
Theft of radioactive materials	Manager of nearest AEC Operations Office	Immediately	Telephone *and* telegraph	If substantial hazard may result to persons in unrestricted areas
Loss of radioactive materials	Manager of nearest AEC Operations Office	Immediately	Telephone *and* telegraph	If substantial hazard may result to persons in unrestricted areas
Large overexposure	Manager of appropriate AEC Operations Office	Immediately	Telephone *and* telegraph	Whole body—>25 rems; skin of whole body—>150 rems; hands, forearms, feet, ankles—>375 rems
Release of highly concentrated radioactive materials	Manager of appropriate AEC Operations Office	Immediately	Telephone *and* telegraph	Concentrations >5,000 times the limits in Appendix B, Table II of 10CFR20, averaged over a 24-hour period
Large operational shut-down	Manager of appropriate AEC Operations Office	Immediately	Telephone *and* telegraph	Loss of one working week or more of the operation of any facilities affected
Large property damage	Manager of appropriate AEC Operations Office	Immediately	Telephone *and* telegraph	Loss in excess of $100,000
Small overexposure	Manager of appropriate AEC Operations Office	Within 24 hours	Telephone *and* telegraph	Whole body—>5 rems; skin of whole body—>30 rems; hands, forearms, feet, ankles—>75 rems
Release of moderately concentrated radioactive materials	Manager of appropriate AEC Operations Office	Within 24 hours	Telephone *and* telegraph	Concentrations >500 times the limits in Appendix B, Table II of 10CFR20, averaged over a 24-hour period
Small operational shut-down	Manager of appropriate AEC Operations Office	Within 24 hours	Telephone *and* telegraph	Loss of one working day or more of the operation of any facilities affected
Small property damage	Manager of appropriate AEC Operations Office	Within 24 hours	Telephone *and* telegraph	Loss in excess of $1,000

in the summary, the licensee will submit a written report within 30 days of each personnel overexposure, and/or any incident listed in Table 10-1 as to extent of overexposure, levels of radiation and concentrations of radioactive material involved, cause, and corrective action. This report will be sent to:

1. Director, Division of Licensing and Regulation, U.S.A.E.C., Washington, D.C.
2. Manager of appropriate AEC Operations Office
3. Any individual exposed to the radiation as to the concentrations of radioactive materials

Upon request, each licensee shall advise any employee annually of the employee's exposure record.

Area monitoring

Another important aspect of radiation health safety in a nuclear medicine department is the performance of environmental surveys in each working area. These working areas should include the injection preparation area, the "hot" sink, the storage area, the radioactive waste disposal area, and all surfaces where radioactive material is being used. The usual instrument used in this type of an area survey is a Geiger-Mueller survey meter.

The regulations for surveys are covered in Title 10 of the Code of Federal Regulations, Part 20.201.

A "survey" means an evaluation of the radiation hazard incident to the production, use, release, disposal, or presence of radioactive materials or other sources of radiation under a specific set of conditions. When appropriate, such evaluation includes a physical survey of the location of materials and equipment and measurements of levels of radiation or concentrations of radioactive materials present. Each licensee shall make or cause to be made such surveys as may be necessary for him to comply with the regulations in this part.

Weekly surveys are recommended for all laboratories and other areas in which radioactive materials are handled routinely. Any surface or article reading in excess of background radiation (usually considered to be 0.1 mr/hr) is considered contaminated and should be treated as such. Readings in excess of this value may be received when the reading is taken in proximity to areas containing large quantities of radioactive materials.* The surveyor cannot assume this to be the case, however, since such an area would mask an area of contamination. The latter can easily be ruled out by a "wipe" test in which the area is wiped with a piece of paper toweling and the toweling is subjected to the survey meter in an area where there are not large amounts of radioactivity.

DECONTAMINATION
Personnel decontamination

Nuclear medicine personnel contaminated by radioactive material must be quickly decontaminated because of the obvious dangers from radiation to the individual. There are two reasons for immediate decontamination. One is to prevent the possible transfer of radioactivity to internal organs either by absorption through the skin or ingestion; the other is to prevent spread of the contamination to other persons or to the environment.

Some general considerations to be used in determining the extent and immediacy of the decontamination process are as follows. If there is a break in the skin, decontamination must be prompt because radiation can be absorbed immediately into the body. If there is bleeding associated with the break in the skin, the bleeding should be encouraged while rinsing the skin with water. All contaminated clothing should be removed at once. (This is the reason for wearing long lab coats in the nuclear medicine department.) Decontamination is of secondary importance if the contaminated material is strongly acid or strongly basic. Concern for chemical burns to the skin would take precedence in this case. Steps should be taken

*In these cases, the value should not exceed 2 mr/hr.

immediately to neutralize the skin with an appropriate neutralizing agent; then, skin decontamination should be undertaken.

Decontamination of the skin is effectively carried out by the use of plenty of soap and water. The soap should not be of an abrasive nature or highly alkaline. It is best to use warm water, rather than hot, because the latter encourages increased blood flow to the area and, therefore, increased absorption of the contaminating material. Any materials and clothing that are contaminated or involved in the decontamination process should be checked with appropriate survey meters and treated according to the radiation level. If the radiation level is greater than the accepted level, the materials should be labeled and transferred to the radioactive waste storage area until the radiation decays to acceptable levels.

Equipment and working area decontamination

Decontamination of equipment or the working area is initiated with the use of absorbent material to remove as much of the liquid contaminant that has spilled as possible. The contaminated area is then scrubbed with soap and water until acceptable radiation levels are reached. A simple, but effective, procedure is to tape a piece of paper over the area to remind people that it is contaminated and to discourage people walking on the area, which would transfer the radioactivity to other parts of the laboratory.

A serious contamination problem occurs if the patient vomits or urinates in the bed following a therapeutic application of radionuclides. The patient must be immediately bathed; bed linen, rubber sheets, and so on must be collected carefully to reduce further contamination to the area and to personnel; contaminated materials are transferred to the waste storage area for decay to safe levels.

RADIATION AREAS

Since the use of radioactive materials represents a possible radiation hazard, laboratories, work areas, and storage areas must be labeled appropriately to aid individuals in minimizing their exposure to radiation. There are three signs approved by the United States Atomic Energy Commission as warnings. The type of sign indicates the dose rate of the area. All three signs use the conventional three bladed design. The design is purple or magenta on a yellow background. The three signs are as follows:

1. *Caution—Radioactive Materials* is a warning sign used in each area or room in which the concentration of radioactive materials is such that the radiation intensity would be from 0.6 to 5.0 mr in any one hour. It is best to use this sign wherever even lesser amounts of radioactivity exist.
2. *Caution—Radiation Area* is a warning sign to be placed in the room or area in which the concentration of radioactive materials is such that the radiation intensity would be from 5.0 to 100 mr in any one hour.
3. *Caution—High Radiation Area* is a warning sign used in areas in which the radiation intensity would be in excess of 100 mr in any one hour.

Each container in which licensed material is transported, stored, or used, and contains a greater quantity of radioactive material than that specified in Appendix

C of 10CFR20 shall bear a clearly visible label bearing the radiation caution symbol, the appropriate words, the name of the radionuclide, the activity, and the date. A label is not required if the concentrations of the material in the container does not exceed that specified in Appendix B, Table 1, Column 2 of Title 10CFR20. Further labels are not necessary for laboratory containers such as beakers, flasks, and test tubes used transiently in laboratory procedures when the user is present.

One exception to the above posting regulations concerns radioactive materials packaged for shipment. These materials are packaged and labeled in accordance with the regulations of the Interstate Commerce Commission. The ICC stipulates that shipment of radioactive materials should provide enough protection so that the radiation intensity is no greater than 200 mr/hr at the surface of the package or 10 mr/hr at a distance of 1 meter from the surface of the package. The ICC regulations further state that the radiation intensity should be expressed in units in which 1 unit is equal to the radiation intensity in millirems per hour at a distance of 1 meter from the surface of the package. The shipment should be labeled as to the principal radionuclide and the activity of the contents.

STORAGE OF RADIOACTIVE MATERIALS

When radioactive materials are not being used, they should be stored in an area such that radiation levels are reduced to a minimum for the occupational personnel. Another consideration for storage is that these radionuclides be stored in such a manner as to discourage the inadvertent exposure of individuals to their emissions. Provision of adequately shielded storage locations is a necessity to good radiation health safety. These areas should be designated by the appropriate caution signs and access to the area should be limited to those individuals who work with the materials. This may mean that a lock be provided to prevent deliberate or inadvertent entry into the area, if that area is not constantly supervised. A lock is not necessary if entrance into the area is controlled.

Perhaps the easiest approach to the shielding of stored sources of radioactivity is the use of lead bricks. If the lead bricks are placed on a counter top abutting one another two or three bricks high (a standard brick is 2 inches by 4 inches by 6 inches) adequate protection is provided for the whole body. A top or bottom shield is not necessary under these circumstances, because the radiation personnel are always working in the "shadow" of the lead bricks. The only time that protection would not be maintained is when the radiation worker would have to search for one of these stored radionuclides for use. This would not present a radiation hazard in the usual nuclear medicine laboratory. Radiation limits are kept to an intensity of 2 mr/hr outside the lead storage area, which is not at all difficult in the usual nuclear medicine department with the use of standard size lead bricks. The design of the storage area should be such that adequate space is available for storing the radionuclides, and even more important, that identification and ready accessibility is provided for each source.

ISOTOPE DISPOSITION RECORDS

Another important series of records is an inventory of all radioactive material, which lists activity received, activity used, and activity disposed.

Single dose disposition forms

There are a number of ways to keep disposition records (ledgers, loose-leaf notebook, or file cards). Any one of these forms must contain information similar to the table below if the sources are packaged in single dose amounts (such as uptake capsules).

Lab no.	Patient's name	Date and hour	Number on hand	Number adminis.	Test performed	Results

As soon as a shipment of radioactivity is received, the shipment should be checked to ascertain whether everything that was ordered has been received. Immediately, information should be recorded as to date received, invoice number, and number of doses received. One of the labels attached to various inclusions in the package should be attached to record sheet as proof of shipment. The packing slip is an A.E.C. record and is filed chronologically. When the radiopharmaceutical is given, the patient's name, date of administration, number of doses on hand, number administered, and type of test are recorded. The results can be recorded upon completion of the test if desired. The latter sometimes serves as a quick reference should a question arise at a later date. At this point, the record is complete until the next patient is considered. This process is continued until the sources are all used or outdated. If used, the record is complete. If outdated, the remaining sources are candidates for disposal. The number disposed, the date of disposal, and the disposal method are recorded. The card is then filed for future reference and/or checked by the officials of the Atomic Energy Commission. Records should be kept on file for 5 years.

Multiple dose disposition forms

In multiple dose packaging of a radiopharmaceutical (such as, mercury 197, gold 198, rose bengal) another form of record is used, as shown on the following page.

Upon receipt of an order from a radiopharmaceutical supplier, information is listed as before; the shipment is checked, receipt date and invoice number are noted, a label is attached to the use record, and invoice is filed chronologically. Upon receipt of a request for a study, the patient's name and the date are recorded.

The first consideration is to determine how much activity is on hand. Should the time of use be something different than the precalibration date, the activity on hand is calculated by the formula:

$$\text{Activity on hand} = \text{Original activity} \times \text{decay factor}$$

189

Lab no.	Patient's name	Date and hour	Activity on hand (UC)*	Volume on hand (ML)	Activity adminis. (UC)	Volume adminis. (ML)†	Activity remain. (UC)	Volume remain. (ML)	Purpose of administration

*Activity remaining × decay factor.
†Volume on hand × activity administered ÷ activity on hand.

The initial entry under volume would be identical to that on the label. Activity administered is predetermined depending on the patient and the desired study, and this predetermined amount of activity is entered in the space provided. The volume representing this predetermined activity must then be calculated. This is calculated by the following formula:

$$\text{Volume injected} = \frac{\text{Volume on hand} \times \text{activity administered}}{\text{Activity on hand}}$$

After the activity and volume to be administered has been determined, the record is completed for this patient by subtracting activity administered from activity on hand to receive the activity remaining; the volume administered is subtracted from the volume on hand to determine the volume remaining.

A second request would be handled exactly the same way with the exception that the activity on hand would be calculated by the activity remaining from the first patient, multiplied by the decay factor (which represents the time interval between the time the first source was used and the time the second source was to be used). The volume on hand for the second patient would be the same as the volume remaining from the first patient. This process is continued until the source is depleted or considered unusable. At that time, the number of microcuries disposed of, date of disposal, and the disposal method are recorded on the record. The card is now completed and filed under the appropriate heading for future reference and/or AEC checking methods.

A system such as this covers every aspect of records to be kept by a nuclear medicine department regarding receipt and disposition of radiopharmaceuticals.

DISPOSAL

There are two philosophies concerning waste disposal: *concentrate and contain* or *dilute and disperse.* Because of the nature of most medical radioisotope departments and the quantity of radiopharmaceuticals used, the latter philosophy is the usual maxim.

Sewer system

Radioactive wastes may be disposed by any of the several methods, depending upon the quantity, concentration, type of radiation and half-life. They may be flushed directly into the drain, emptied into an effluent pond or a retention basin to be held for decay, drained into hold-up tanks for decay and then flushed into the sewer, or put into special shielded containers for delivery to a chemical processing plant.

These alternatives have been listed in order of increasing radioactivity of the disposal products. Most waste can be disposed of by flushing it directly into the drain.

Title 10CFR20.303 states that no licensee shall discharge licensed material into a sanitary sewerage system unless (1) it is readily soluble or dispersible in water and (2) unless the quantity of any licensed or other radioactive material released into the system by the licensee in any one day does not exceed either of the following quantities:

1. Ten times the quantity listed in Appendix C of Title 10CFR20 (for example, iodine 131 = 10 μCi, therefore, 100 μCi of iodine 131 could be disposed of in a sanitary sewer system).
2. The quantity which, if diluted by the average daily quantity of sewerage released into the sewer by the licensee, will result in an average concentration equal to the limits specified in Appendix B, Table 1, Column 2 of Title 10CFR20 (for example, iodine 131 = 6×10^{-5} μCi/ml).

The average water flow for a hospital in the United States is about 1,000 liters per day per bed. Calculations for the disposal of iodine 131 for a 100 bed hospital would proceed as follows:

$$\text{Water flow} = 1,000 \text{ liters} \times 100 \text{ beds} \times 1 \text{ day} = 10^6 \times 10^2 \times 1$$
$$= 10^8 \text{ ml water flow}$$
$$\text{Therefore:} \quad 6 \times 10^{-5} \text{ } \mu\text{Ci/ml} \times 10^8 \text{ ml/day} = 6 \times 10^3 \text{ } \mu\text{Ci/day}$$
$$= 6,000 \text{ } \mu\text{Ci/day}$$
$$= 6 \text{ mCi/day}$$

Accordingly, a 100 bed institution could discard 6 mCi of iodine 131 into the sewer system in any one day.

The Code of Federal Regulations further states that the quantity of any licensed or other radioactive material released in any one month, if diluted by the average monthly quantity of water released by the licensee, will not result in an average concentration exceeding the limits specified in Appendix B, Table 1, Column 2 (6×10^{-5} of iodine 131). It has already been shown that sewerage flow is equal to 10^8 ml/day. Therefore, for iodine 131 the monthly rate would be:

$$6 \times 10^{-5} \text{ } \mu\text{Ci/ml} \times 30 \times 10^8 \text{ ml/month}$$
$$= 180 \times 10^3 \text{ } \mu\text{Ci/month} = 180 \text{ mCi/month}$$

191

Accordingly, the total amount of iodine 131 discarded during any one month cannot exceed 180 mCi.

The Code of Federal Regulations further stipulates that the gross quantity of licensed or other radioactive material released into the sewerage system by the licensee cannot exceed 1 curie per year. This section of the regulations qualifies all the others. If 180 mCi were discarded per month as calculated above, this would be 2,160 mCi or 2.16 Ci per year of iodine 131. Although the daily and monthly amounts have not been exceeded, the governing clause is 1 Ci per year. Further, if it were desirable to dispose of 180 mCi in one day, the 180 mCi per month value has not been exceeded (providing nothing else was discarded during that month), but the 6 mCi per day value would be exceeded.

If it is necessary to dispose of a combination of radionuclides, the limit for each radionuclide is determined as follows. For each radionuclide in the combination the ratio between the quantity present and the limit for the nuclide as stated in Title 10CFR20 is determined. The sum of the ratios for all the radionuclides in the combination cannot exceed 1. For example, if a batch contains 2,000 μCi of gold 198 and 25,000 μCi of carbon 14, not more than 3,000 μCi of iodine 131 can be included. This value was derived as follows:

$$\frac{2,000 \ \mu\text{Ci} \ ^{198}\text{Au}}{10,000 \ \mu\text{Ci}} + \frac{25,000 \ \mu\text{Ci} \ ^{14}\text{C}}{50,000 \ \mu\text{Ci}} + \frac{3,000 \ \mu\text{Ci} \ ^{131}\text{I}}{10,000 \ \mu\text{Ci}} = 1$$

(The denominator in each ratio is obtained by multiplying the value in Appendix C by 1,000 as stated in Title 10CFR20.)

These are all exaggerated examples to point out how *all* facets of the AEC regulations must be known and adhered to. A hospital should never discard 6 mCi of iodine 131 in one day.

Another alternative and perhaps the most practical method for disposal of material is to allow the radioactive material to decay ten half-lives. At that time, it can be released into the sewerage or subjected to incineration. Any source of radioactivity undergoing ten half-lives is essentially reduced to background radiation.

A very important addendum to this regulation is "Excreta from individuals undergoing medical diagnosis or therapy with radioactive materials shall be exempt from any limitations contained in this section."

Incineration

According to Title 10CFR20.305, no licensee shall treat or dispose of licensed material by incineration except as specifically approved by the Atomic Energy Commission. To obtain such approval, a special application is required which should include an analysis and evaluation of pertinent information as to the nature of the environment, usage of ground and surface waters in the general area, nature and location of other potentially affected facilities, and procedures to be observed to minimize the risk of unexpected or hazardous exposures.

The only basis by which an incinerator can be used without adherence to these regulations is to incinerate material that is equal to background radiation measured at contact with the Geiger-Mueller probe. The value generally accepted to be background or approaching background is 0.1 mr/hr, at which point, the material would be treated as uncontaminated and incinerated in the usual manner.

Transfer to authorized recipient

Title 10CFR20.301 allows the transfer of radioactive wastes to an authorized recipient, thereby obviating many of the details of records regarding storage, disposal, and so on. Several companies offer this service. The Commission will not approve any application for a licensee to receive licensed material from other persons for disposal on land not owned by the federal government or by the state governments.

Burial

The only other alternative for disposal of radioactive material is through burial methods. This method may be used provided:
1. The amount per burial does not exceed 1,000 times the amounts shown in Appendix C of Title 10CFR20 (For iodine 131, the value given is 10 μCi; therefore, 10 mCi of iodine 131 can be buried)
2. The material is buried at a minimum depth of 4 feet
3. Burials are spaced not less than 6 feet apart
4. Burials are limited to twelve per year in any one area. Larger amounts may be approved on application to the AEC, supplying full details

REGULATIONS FOR NUCLEAR MEDICINE LABORATORY PERSONNEL

The following are regulations which must be followed by all laboratory personnel.
1. Good housekeeping must be maintained at all times. The laboratory must be kept neat, glassware must be washed regularly, and waste or contaminated materials must not be allowed to accumulate.
2. No food may be eaten or stored in the radioisotope unit.
3. No smoking is allowed while handling radioactivity.
4. Protective outer garments, such as laboratory coats and rubber gloves, should be worn while handling radioactive materials.
5. All possible set-ups will be made on easily cleanable trays.
6. All trays and all other work surfaces will be covered with disposable absorbent paper.
7. All containers of radioactive materials must be labeled stating the kind, the quantity of isotope, dose of assay, and the radiation symbol.
8. Some monitoring device, such as a film badge, should always be worn by occupational personnel while working in the unit. This should include a monitoring device for whole body dose as well as dose to hands and forearms for personnel using a generator.
9. Pipetting by mouth is not allowed; an automatic pipette must always be used.
10. All work areas will be monitored regularly and results of surveys recorded.

Bibliography

Blahd, W. H.: Nuclear medicine, New York, 1965, McGraw-Hill Book Co.

Brucer, M.: Vignettes in nuclear medicine, St. Louis, 1967, Mallinckrodt/Nuclear.

Chase, G. D., and Rabinowitz, J. L.: Principles of radioisotope methodology, ed. 3, Minneapolis, 1967, Burgess Publishing Co.

Hine, G. J.: Instrumentation in nuclear medicine, vol. 1, New York, 1967, Academic Press, Inc.

Johns, H. E.: The Physics of Radiology, ed. 2, revised second printing, Springfield, Illinois, 1964, Charles C Thomas, Publisher.

King, E. R., and Mitchell, T. G.: A manual for nuclear medicine, Springfield, Illinois, 1961, Charles C Thomas, Publisher.

Morgan, K. Z., and Turner, J. E.: Principles of radiation protection, New York, 1967, John Wiley & Sons, Inc.

Quimby, E. H., and Feitelberg, S.: Radioactive isotopes in medicine and biology, ed. 2, Philadelphia, 1963, Lea & Febiger.

Quinn, J. L., III: Scintillation scanning in clinical medicine, Philadelphia, 1964, W. B. Saunders Co.

Shilling, C. W.: Atomic energy encyclopedia in the life sciences, Philadelphia, 1964, W. B. Saunders Co.

Silver, S.: Radioactive nuclides in medicine and biology, ed. 3, Philadelphia, 1968, Lea & Febiger.

Wagner, H. N.: Principles of nuclear medicine, Philadelphia, 1968, W. B. Saunders Co.

U. S. Department of Health, Education and Welfare, Radiological health handbook, revised edition, September, 1960, Washington, D. C., U. S. Department of Commerce Clearinghouse for Federal Scientific and Technical Information.

Wang, C. H., and Willis, D. L.: Radiotracer methodology in biological science, Englewood Cliffs, New Jersey, 1965, Prentice-Hall, Inc.

Glossary

Absorption: The process by which radiation imparts some or all of its energy to any material through which it passes. (See **Compton effect, Photoelectric effect,** and **Pair production**)

Absorption coefficient: The fractional decrease in the intensity of a beam of radiation per unit thickness (linear absorption coefficient), per unit mass (mass absorption coefficient), or per atom (atomic absorption coefficient) of absorber.

Activation analysis: A method of chemical analysis especially for small traces of material, based on the detection of characteristic radionuclides following nuclear bombardment.

Activity; *see* **Radioactivity.**

Acute exposure: Term used to denote radiation exposure of short duration.

Alpha particle: A helium nucleus, consisting of 2 protons and 2 neutrons; it has a double positive charge and posseses a mass of 4.00278 atomic mass units (amu).

Amplification: As related to radiation detection instruments, the process (either gas or electronic, or both) by which ionization effects are magnified to a degree suitable for measurement.

Anemia: Deficiency of blood as a whole, or deficiency of hemoglobin or in the number of red blood cells.

Angstrom unit (Å): 10^{-8} cm. Used to measure the wavelength of electromagnetic radiations.

Anion: Negatively charged ion.

Annihilation radiation: The photons produced when an electron and a positron unite and then cease to exist. The annihilation of a positron-electron pair results in the production of 2 photons; each has an energy of 0.51 mev.

Anode: A positive electrode; the electrode to which negative ions (anions) are attracted.

Anoxia: Oxygen deficiency; a condition that results from a diminished supply of oxygen to the tissues.

Antibiotic: A substance, of biologic origin, that inhibits the growth of or kills microorganisms. Common examples are penicillin, streptomycin, and aureomycin.

Anticoincidence circuit: A circuit with two input terminals that delivers an output pulse if one input terminal receives a pulse, but not if both input terminals receive a pulse simultaneously, or within predetermined time interval. A principle used in pulse height analysis.

Atom: The smallest particle of an element that is capable of entering into a chemical reaction.

Atomic mass unit: Unit of mass equal to $1/12$ the arbitary mass assigned to carbon 12. 1 amu is equivalent to 931.2 mev of energy.

Atomic number: Symbol: Z. The number of protons in the nucleus; therefore, the number of positive charges in the nucleus. The atomic number also reflects the number of electrons outside the nucleus of a neutral atom.

Atomic weight: The relative weight of the atom of an element compared with the weight of one atom of oxygen taken as 16.

Attenuation: The process by which radiation is reduced in intensity when passing through some material. This is a combination of absorption and scattering processes.

Atrophy: The wasting-away or diminution in the size of cell, tissue, organ, or part from defect or from failure of nutrition.

Autoradiograph: The record of radiation from radioactive material in an object that is made by placing its surface in close proximity to a photographic emulsion.

Avalanche: The multiplicative process in which a single charged particle, accelerated by a strong electric field, produces additional charged particles through collision with neutral gas molecules.

Average life (mean life): The average of the individual lives of all the atoms of a particular radioactive substance. This average is 1.443 times the radioactive half-life of the substance.

Avogadro's number: The number of molecules in a gram molecular weight of any substance (6.03×10^{23} molecules); also, the number of atoms in a gram atomic weight of any element.

Background radiation: Radiation due to cosmic rays, to radioactive materials in the vicinity, and to a slight radioactive contamination of the materials of which the instrument is made.

Back-scattering: The process of scattering or deflecting into the sensitive volume of a measuring instrument radiations that originally had no motion in that direction. The process is dependent on the nature of the mounting material, the nature of the sample, the type and energy of the radiations, and the particular geometric arrangement.

Barrier: Shields of radiation-absorbing material, such as lead and concrete.

Beta particle: A charged particle emitted from the nucleus of an atom. Its mass and charge are equal in magnitude to those of the electron.

Betatron: A device for accelerating electrons by means of magnetic induction.

Binary scaler: A scaler in which the scaling factor is 2 per stage; *see* **Scaler.**

Binding energy: The energy represented by the difference in mass between the actual mass of the nucleus and the sum of the component parts.

Biologic half-life: The time required for the body to eliminate one-half of an administered dose of any substance by regular processes of elimination. This time is approximately the same for both stable and radioactive isotopes of a particular element.

Bone marrow: The soft material that fills the cavity in most bones and manufactures most of the formed elements of the blood.

Bremsstrahlung: The secondary photon radiation produced by the deceleration of charged particles as they pass through matter.

Cancer: The popular terminology for any malignant neoplasm.

Capillary: A small thin-walled blood vessel connecting an artery to a vein.

Carcinogenic: Cancer-producing.

Carcinoma: Malignant neoplasm composed of epithelial cells.

Carrier: (1) A quantity of an element that may be mixed with its radioisotopes to give enough of a quantity to facilitate chemical operations. (2) A substance that, when associated with a trace of another substance, will carry the trace with it through a chemical or physical process.

Carrier-free: An adjective applied to radioisotopes undiluted with stable isotope carrier.

Cataract: A clouding of the lens of the eye that obstructs the passage of light.

Cathode: A negative electrode; the electrode that attracts positive ions.

Cation: A positively charged ion.

Cell: The fundamental unit of structure and function in living organisms.

Chain reaction: Any chemical or nuclear process in which some of the products of the process, including energy, are instrumental in the continuation or magnification of the process.

Characteristic radiation: Radiation originating from an atom following the removal of an electron or excitation of the nucleus.

Chronic exposure: The term used to denote radiation exposure of long duration.

Cloud chamber: A device for observing the paths of ionizing particles that is based on the principle that supersaturated vapor condenses readily on ions.

Coincidence: The occurrence of one or more ionizing events in one or more detectors simultaneously or within an assignable time interval.

Coincidence circuit: A circuit with two input terminals that delivers an output pulse only when both input terminals receive pulses simultaneously or within a predetermined time interval. A principle used in the detection of positron emitters.

Collimator: A device for confining the elements of a beam within an assigned solid angle.

Compton effect: An absorption effect observed for x- and gamma radiation in which the incident photon interacts with an orbital electron on the absorber atom to produce a recoil electron and a photon of energy less than the incident photon.

Conservation of mass-energy: Energy and mass are interchangeable, as evidenced by the equation $E = mc^2$, where E is energy, m is mass and c is velocity of light.

Contamination, radioactive: The deposition of radioactive material in any place where its presence may be harmful. The harm may be in invalidating the experiment or procedure, or in actually being a source of danger to personnel.

Cosmic rays: Radiation, both particulate and electromagnetic, that originates outside the earth's atmosphere.

Count (radiation measurements): The external indication of a device designed to enumerate ionizing events. It may refer to a single detected event or to the total number that is registered in a given period of time.

Count rate meter: A device which gives a continuous indication of the average rate of ionizing events.

Cumulative dose (radiation): The total dose resulting from repeated exposures. This may be radiation to the same region or to the whole body.

Curie: That quantity of a radioactive material having associated with it 3.7×10^{10} disintegrations per second.

Cyclotron: A device for accelerating charged particles in a spiral fashion to high energies by means of an alternating electric field between electrodes placed in a constant magnetic field.

Daughter: A synonym for a product of decay.

Decade scaler: A scaler that has a power of 10 for a scaling factor.

Decay, radioactive: The disintegration of the nucleus of an unstable atom by the spontaneous emission of charged particles and/or photons.

Decay constant: The fraction of the number of atoms of a radionuclide that decay in unit time.

Decay curve: A curve showing the relative amount of radioactive substance remaining after any given time.

Densitometer: An instrument utilizing the photoelectric principle to determine the degree of darkening of developed photographic film.

Density: A term used to denote the degree of darkening of photographic film.

Deuterium ($^2_1$H): A heavy isotope of hydrogen having 1 proton and 1 neutron in the nucleus. It is sometimes called "heavy hydrogen."

Deuteron: The nucleus of a deuterium atom, containing 1 proton, 1 neutron and no orbital electrons.

Disintegration, nuclear: A spontaneous nuclear transformation (radioactivity) characterized by the emission of energy and/or mass from the nucleus.

Disintegration constant: The fraction of the number of atoms of a radionuclide that decay per unit time.

Dose (dosage): According to current usage, the radiation delivered to the whole body or to a specified area or volume.

Dose rate: Radiation dose delivered in unit of time.

Dose rate meter: Any instrument which measures dose rate.

Dosimeter: An instrument used to detect and measure an accumulated dosage of radiation. In common usage, it is a pencil-sized ionization chamber, with or without a built-in, self-reading electrometer used for personnel monitoring.

Dot scan: A display, on paper, of equi-dense dots in a manner that reproduces the spatial distribution of radioactivity in the area desired to be visualized.

Effective half-life: The time required for a radionuclide introduced into a biologic system to be reduced to one-half as a result of the combined action of radioactive decay and biologic elimination.

Efficiency (of counters): A measure of the probability that a count will be recorded when radiation is "seen" by a detector.

Electrode: Either terminal of an electric source.

Electron: A negatively charged particle that is a constituent of every neutral atom. A unit of negative electricity equal to 4.80×10^{-10} electrostatic units. It has a mass of 0.000549 atomic mass units (amu).

Electron capture: A method of radioactive decay involving the capture of an orbital electron by its nucleus.

Electron volt (ev): The amount of energy gained by an electron as it passes through a potential difference of 1 volt.

Electroscope: An instrument for detecting electric charges by the deflection of charged bodies.

Element: A pure substance consisting of atoms of the same atomic number.

Elution: The process for the extraction of the adsorbed substance from the solid adsorbing medium. Special reference in nuclear medicine to the removal of ions from an ion exchange medium.

Energy: The capacity to do work. Potential energy is the energy inherent in mass because of its position with reference to other masses. Kinetic energy is the energy possessed by mass because of its motion.

Enriched material: Material in which the relative amount of one or more forms of an element has been increased.

Epidermis: The outer layer of the skin.

Epilation: The temporary or permanent loss of hair.

Epithelium: The cells lining all canals and surfaces having communication with external air; cells specialized for secretion in certain glands.

erg: The unit of work done by a force of 1 dyne acting through a distance of 1 cm. The unit of energy that can exert a force of 1 dyne through a distance of 1 cm.

Erythema: An abnormal redness of the skin caused by the distension of capillaries with blood. It can be caused by such different agents as heat, ultraviolet rays, or ionizing radiation.

Film badge: The photographic film used for the approximate measurement of radiation exposure for personnel monitoring purposes.

Fission: The splitting of a nucleus into two or more parts with the subsequent release of enormous amounts of energy.

Fission products: The elements resulting from fission.

Flat field collimator: A collimator constructed so as to permit a broad area to be visualized by a radiation detector. It is usually made of lead with a single aperture that is either cylindrical or slightly conical in shape.

Focused collimator: A collimator constructed so as to permit only a restricted area to be visualized at one time. It is usually made of lead with holes arranged in a honeycomb fashion and converging at some point distant to the face of the collimator.

Fusion: The act of combining two or more nuclei into one nucleus.

Gamma ray: A short wavelength, electromagnetic radiation of nuclear origin with a range of wavelengths from 10^{-9} to 10^{-12} cm, emitted from the nucleus.

Gas amplification: The release of additional ions from neutral atoms caused by collisions of electrons that are set free in response to the paths of ionizing radiation and which have acquired high energies as a result of an increased electrical field. A phenomenon seen in proportional counters.

Gas-flow counter: A radiation detector in which an appropriate atmosphere is maintained in the counter tube by allowing a suitable gas to flow slowly through the sensitive volume.

Geiger-Mueller (G-M) counter tube: A highly sensitive, gas-filled, radiation-measuring device that operates at voltages in the region of avalanche ionization.

Geiger region: An ionization radiation detector whose operating voltage interval in which the charge collected per ionizing event is essentially independent of the number of primary ions produced in the initial ionizing event.

Geiger threshold: The minimum voltage at which a Geiger-Mueller tube operates in the Geiger region.

Genetic effect of radiation: Inheritable changes (mutations) produced by the absorption of ionizing radiations.

Germ cells (genetic cells): The cells of an organism whose function is to reproduce its kind. These cells are characteristically haploid.

Half-value layer (half-thickness): The thickness of any material required to reduce the intensity of an x-ray or gamma-ray beam to one-half its original value.

Induced radioactivity: That activity produced in a substance after bombardment with neutrons or other particles.

Integrating circuit: An electronic circuit that records, at any time, an average value for the number of ionization events occurring per unit time; or an electrical circuit that records the total number of ions collected in a given time.

Internal conversion: A method of radioactive decay in which the gamma rays from excited nuclei cause the ejection of orbital electrons from the atom.

Ion: An atomic particle; an atom or chemical radical bearing an electrical charge that is either positive or negative.

Ion pair: Two particles of opposite charge; usually refers to the electron and positive atomic or molecular residue resulting after the interaction of radiation with the orbital electrons of atoms.

Ionization: The process or the result of any process by which a neutral atom or molecule acquires a charge, either positive or negative.

Ionization chamber: An instrument designed to measure the quantity of ionizing radiation in terms of the charge of electricity associated with ions that are produced within a defined volume.

Ionization potential: The potential necessary to separate one electron from an atom, resulting in the formation of an ion pair.

Ionizing energy: The average energy lost by ionizing radiation for the production of an ion pair in air—about 34 electron volts (ev).

Ionizing event: Any process whereby an ion or group of ions is produced.

Ionizing radiation: Any electromagnetic or particulate radiation capable of direct or indirect ion production in its passage through matter.

Irradiation: Any exposure of matter to radiation.

Isobar: One of two or more different nuclides having the same mass number.

Isocount curves: Curves showing the distribution of radiation in a medium by means of lines or surfaces drawn through points receiving equal doses.

Isomer: One of several nuclides having the same number of neutrons and protons, but capable of existing for a measurable time in different energy states. Usually, the isomer of higher energy decays to one with lower energy by the process of isomeric transition.

Isomeric transition (IT): The process by which a nuclide decays to an isomeric nuclide of lower energy state. Isomeric transitions proceed by gamma ray and/or internal conversion electron emission.

Isoresponse curves; *see* **Isocount curves**

Isotone: One of several nuclides having the same number of neutrons in their nuclei.

Isotope: One of several different nuclides having the same number of protons in their nuclei and, therefore, the same atomic number. However, they differ in the number of neutrons and, hence, in the mass number. Isotopes have almost identical chemical properties.

K capture: A colloquialism for K-electron capture; also, loosely used to designate any orbital electron capture process.

kev: One thousand electron volts (10^3 ev).

Labeled compound: A compound consisting, in part, of labeled molecules. By observations of radioactivity or isotopic composition, this compound or its fragments can be followed through various physical, chemical, or biologic processes.

Labeled molecule: A molecule containing one or more atoms distinguished by unnatural isotopic composition (with radioactive or stable isotopes).

LD$_{50}$ (lethal dose): The dose of radiation that causes mortality in 50% of a species.

Lead equivalent: The thickness of lead that results in the same reduction in radiation dose rate under specified conditions as the material in question.

Line space: The distance between lines of dots on a dot or photo scan; usually expressed in centimeters.

Linear absorption coefficient: An expression of the fraction of a beam of radiation absorbed in unit thickness of material.

Linear accelerator: A device for accelerating charged particles, using alternate electrodes and gaps arranged in a straight line. These electrodes and gaps are so proportioned that when their potentials are varied in the proper amplitude and frequency, particles passing through them receive successive increments of energy.

Linear amplifier: A pulse amplifier in which the output pulse height has been amplified to a height that is proportional to the input pulse height.

Mass absorption coefficient: The linear absorption coefficient per centimeter divided by the density of the absorber in grams per cubic centimeter.

Mass defect: The difference between the mass of the nucleus as a whole and the sum of the nuclear components weighed separately.

Mass number: Symbol: A. The number of nucleons in the nucleus of an atom.

Maximum permissible dose (MPD): The maximum dose of radiation permitted by persons working with ionizing radiation. MPD for whole body $= 5(N - 18)$ rems; $N =$ age.

Median lethal dose (MLD/30): The dose of radiation required to kill 50% of the individuals in a large group of animals or organisms within 30 days.

Metabolism: The sum of all the physical and chemical processes by which a living substance is produced and maintained and by which energy is made available for the uses of the organism.

Metastable state: An excited state of a nucleus that returns to its ground state by the emission of a gamma ray. Ground state is not achieved immediately, but over a measurable half-life.

mev: 1 million electron volts (10^6 ev).

Microcurie (μCi): 3.7×10^4 disintegrations per second (one millionth of a curie).

Micromicrocurie (Picocurie) ($\mu\mu$Ci): 3.7×10^{-2} disintegrations per second (one millionth of a microcurie).

Millicurie (mCi): 3.7×10^7 disintegrations per second (one thousandth of a curie).

Millimicrocurie (Nanocurie) (mμCi): 37 disintegrations per second (one thousandth of a microcurie).

Milliroentgen (mr): One thousandth of a roentgen.

Molecule: The ultimate unit of a compound that can exist by itself and retain all the properties of the original substance.

Monitoring: The periodic or continuous determination of the amount of ionizing radiation or radioactive contamination present in an occupied region. **Area monitoring:** routine monitoring of the level of radiation or of radioactive contamination of any particular area, building, or room. **Personnel monitoring:** monitoring of any part of an individual such as breath, excretions, or clothing.

Monoenergetic radiation: Radiation of a given type in which all photons or particles have the same energy.

Mutation: A change in the characteristics of any organism as a result of an alteration of the usual hereditary pattern.

Negatron (β^-): A particle having a mass and charge equal to that of an electron, but originating from the nucleus. Its mass is 0.000548 amu. This term is not used in the United States.

Neutrino: A neutral particle of very small mass (approaches zero rest mass) emitted during various processes of decay.

Neutron: An elementary, electrically neutral nuclear particle with a mass approximately the same as that of a proton. Its mass is 1.00898 atomic mass units (amu).

Nuclear reactor: An apparatus in which the nuclear fission reaction may be self-sustaining.

Nucleon: A common term for a constituent particle of the nucleus; usually applies to protons and neutrons.

Nucleus (of an atom): That part of an atom in which most of the mass and the total positive electric charge are concentrated.

Nuclide: A general term referring to any nucleus (stable or radioactive) plus its orbital electrons.

Operating voltage: The voltage across the electrodes in the detecting chamber required for proper detection of an ionizing event.

Pair production: An absorption process for x- and gamma radiation in which the incident photon is annihilated in the vicinity of the nucleus of the absorbing atom, with subsequent release of a positron and a beta particle. This reaction cannot occur for incident radiation energies of less than 1.02 mev.

Parent: A radionuclide that yields another nuclide upon disintegration. The latter (the daughter) may be radioactive or stable.

Photoelectric effect: A process by which a photon ejects an electron from an atom and thereby is totally absorbed.

Photographic dosimetry: The determination of the accumulative radiation dosage by use of photographic film.

Photomultiplier tube: A tube in which small electron currents are amplified by a cascade process employing secondary emission.

Photon: A quantity of electromagnetic energy.

Photo scan: A display, on x-ray film, of variable density dots in a manner that reproduces the spatial distribution of radioactivity in the area desired to be visualized.

Physical half-life (T_p or $T_{1/2}$): The time required for a source of radioactivity to lose 50% of its activity by decay.

Pile; *see* **Nuclear reactor.**

Planck's constant: A natural constant of proportionality *(h)* relating the frequency of a quantum of energy to the total energy of the quantum; equivalent to 6.61×10^{-27} erg-sec.

Plateau: As applied to radiation detector chambers, the level portion of the voltage curve where changes in operating voltage introduce minimum changes in the counting rate.

Positron: A particle having a mass equal to the electron and having an equal, but opposite charge. Its mass is 0.000548 atomic mass units (amu).

Proportional counter: A gas-filled radiation detector in which the pulse produced is proportional to the number of ions formed in the gas by the primary ionizing particle.

Proportional region: The voltage range in which the gas amplification is greater than 1 and in which the charge collected is proportional to the initial ionizing event.

Proton: An elementary nuclear particle with a positive electric charge equal numerically to the charge of the electron and having a mass of 1.00759 atomic mass units (amu).

Pulse height analyzer: Any circuit designed to select and pass voltage pulses in a certain range of amplitudes.

Quantum; *see* **Photon.**

Quenching: The process of inhibiting discharge in a counter tube that uses gas amplification.

Quenching gas: A polyatomic gas used in Geiger-Mueller counters to quench or extinguish avalanche ionization.

Radiation absorbed dose (rad): A measure of the amount of energy imparted to matter by ionizing radiation per unit mass of irradiated material at the place of interest; equivalent to 100 ergs of absorbed energy per gram of irradiated material.

Radioactive half-life; *see* **Physical half-life.**

Radioactivity: The process whereby certain nuclides undergo spontaneous disintegration in which energy is liberated, generally resulting in the formation of new nuclides. The process is accompanied by the emission of one or more types of radiation, such as alpha and beta particles and gamma radiation.

Radioresistance: The relative resistance of cells, tissues, organs, or entire organisms to the injurious action of radiation.

Radiosensitivity: The relative susceptibility of cells, tissues, organs, entire organisms, or any substances to the injurious action of radiation. Radioresistance and radiosusceptibility are at present employed in a qualitative or comparative sense, rather than in a quantitative or absolute one.

Readout: A method of presenting a total count or rate of detected radiation events.

Relative biologic effectiveness: The ratio of x- or gamma ray dose to the dose that is required to produce the same biologic effect by the radiation in question.

Relativistic mass: The increased mass associated with a particle when its velocity is increased. The increase in mass becomes appreciable only at velocities approaching the velocity of light (3×10^{10} cm/sec).

Resolving time, counter: The minimum time interval between two distinct ionization events that will permit both to be counted.

Roentgen: The quantity of x- or gamma radiation such that the associated corpuscular emission per 0.001293 gm of air produces, in air, ions carrying 1 electrostatic unit of electrical charge, either positive or negative.

Roentgen equivalent, man (rem): A unit of human biologic dose as a result of exposure to one or many types of ionizing radiation. It is equal to the absorbed dose in rads times the RBE of the particular type of radiation being absorbed.

Scaler: An electronic device that produces an output voltage pulse whenever a prescribed number of input pulses has been received.

Scanner: A device used to display a two-dimensional portrayal of the variations of concentration of radioactivity in any volume of material.

Scan speed: The rate of travel of the scanner detector as it traverses the area being visualized.

Scattering: The change of direction of particles or photons as a result of a collision or interaction.

Scintillation counter: The combination of phosphor, photomultiplier tube, and associated circuits for counting light emissions produced in the phosphors by ionizing radiation.

Secondary radiation: Radiation originating as the result of interactions of other radiation in matter. It may be either electromagnetic or particulate in nature.

Self-absorption: The absorption of radiation by the matter in which the radioactive atoms are located; in particular, the absorption of radiation within the sample being assayed.

Somatic cells: Body cells, usually having two sets of chromosomes. Germ cells have only one set.

Specific activity: (1) Of a compound: fatal radioactivity per gram of compound; (2) of an element: total radioactivity per gram of element; (3) of an isotope: total radioactivity per gram of radioisotope.

Spectrometer: A device used to count an emission of radiation of a specific energy or range of energies to the exclusion of all other energies.

Spurious count: The count caused by any agency other than the radiation desired to be detected.

Stable isotope: An isotope of an element that is not radioactive.

Stray radiation: Radiation serving no useful purpose.

Synchrotron: A device for accelerating particles, ordinarily electrons, in a circular orbit with frequency modulated electric fields combined with an increasing magnetic field applied in synchronism with the orbital motion.

Tagged compound; *see* **Labeled compound.**

Teledeltos paper: A black paperlike material with a white chalklike overlay. The overlay is burned away by the passage of a current pulse through a stylus to a metal back-plate upon which the Teledeltos paper is mounted. The result is a black dot on a white field.

Tracer, isotopic: The isotope or nonnatural mixture of isotopes of an element that may be incorporated into a sample to make possible observation of the course of that element through a chemical, biologic, or physical process.

Tritium (^3_1H or ^3T)**:** An isotope of hydrogen having a mass number of 3 (1 proton, 2 neutrons).

Wavelength: The distance between the same point on two subsequent electromagnetic waves.

Window: A term that describes the upper and lower limits of energy of radiation accepted for counting by a spectrometer; also termed window width.

X-rays: Penetrating electromagnetic radiations having wavelengths much shorter than those of visible light.

Part II Clinical nuclear medicine

Chapter
11 *Hematology*

CONSTITUENTS OF BLOOD

Blood is a part of the main transport system of the body that delivers oxygen, nutrients, hormones, and antibodies to the tissues. Blood also receives waste products, including carbon dioxide from the cells and transports them to the organs involved in their subsequent elimination from the body. Blood makes up approximately 7 to 8% of the total body weight, and consists of a fluid fraction (plasma) and formed elements that can be differentiated into red cells (erythrocytes), white cells (leukocytes), and platelets (thrombocytes). Since the specific gravity of these formed elements is greater than that of the plasma, the cells tend to settle if allowed to stand, provided clotting has been prevented by the addition of an anticoagulant. The rate of this separation can be augmented by centrifugation.

Because of the abundance of red cells (5,000,000 per cu mm) in relation to the leukocytes (8,000 per cu mm), together with the relatively small size of the platelets, most of the volume of the formed sediment can be attributed to the erythrocytes. The volume of the packed erythrocytes expressed as percentage of the blood sample used is called the *hematocrit*. Normally it averages 45%. Therefore, the supernatant plasma expressed as percent of the blood sample (plasmacrit) would be 55%.

In contrast, if the blood is allowed to clot and the clot is removed, the remaining straw colored fluid is called *serum*. This serum differs from the plasma mainly in that it contains no fibrinogen.

Plasma. The plasma is a complex, watery fluid that contains various ions as well as inorganic and organic molecules. Its main solid constituent is represented by the plasma proteins, which average 7.5 gm/100 ml. These are usually divided into albumin, 4.8%; globulin, 2.3%; and fibrinogen, 0.3%. Because of the impermeability of the capillary walls to the plasma proteins, these latter exert an osmotic force across this membrane of about 25 mm Hg, which tends to pull water into the capillaries. Another function of the plasma proteins is their help in maintaining the constancy of the blood reaction. Furthermore, some of the proteins that have been isolated from the globulin fraction have specific functions, such as the transport of hormones, blood clotting, and the development of resistance to infections.

The albumin fraction, together with the proteins concerned in blood clotting, is manufactured in the liver. The globulins, including the fibrinogen, are formed by the reticuloendothelial system, plasma cells, and lymphoid nodules.

The formation, function, and fate of each of the formed elements of the blood differ.

Red blood cells. The red cells are circular, nonnucleated, biconcave discs that are manufactured by the red bone marrow situated in the vertebrae, sternum, ribs, and bones of the skull and pelvis. Because of their hemoglobin content, the red cells form an efficient oxygen-carrying system. Furthermore, the hemoglobin plays an essential role in carbon dioxide transport and in regulation of the blood pH. The average hemoglobin content of the blood in adults is 15 gm/100 ml. In man, the red cells usually survive for about 120 days. Thereafter, they are destroyed by the reticuloendothelial system, and the hemoglobin is released. The iron and globin are split off, leaving bilirubin. The iron is reused in the synthesis of new hemoglobin.

White blood cells. The white blood cells or leukocytes, are nucleated cells that can be differentiated into three main types: granulocytes (polymorphonuclear leukocytes), lymphocytes, and monocytes. The granulocytes are normally formed in the red bone marrow and survive for less than 2 weeks. They can be further subdivided into neutrophils (50 to 70%), eosinophils (1 to 4%), and basophils (0 to 1%). Their main function is to combat infections, and they are destroyed in the spleen and other parts of the reticuloendothelial system.

The lymphocytes are formed chiefly in the lymphoid tissues of the body and to a lesser extent in the bone marrow. They form from 20 to 40% of the total number of white cells and live from 2 to 200 days. The lymphocytes are essential for the development of immunity.

The monocytes form from 2 to 8% of the leukocytes. Their main site of origin is in the lymphoid tissues; a few originate in the bone marrow. Monocytes are phagocytic and play a major role in the production of antibodies.

Platelets. The blood platelets are small, nonnucleated granulated bodies, formed in the red bone marrow. Their number averages 200,000 per cubic millimeter and they survive for about 10 days in the bloodstream. Their main function is the provision of support for the endothelium of injured vessels and formation of a hemostatic plug; they also participate in the processes of blood coagulation and clot retraction.

BLOOD VOLUME DETERMINATION

Although nonradioactive methods are available for the estimation of the blood volume, these techniques are tedious and require meticulous care in their performance. This is mainly because these methods depend on the determination of the concentration of a dye (such as Evans blue) following its intravenous administration. Since the determinations are performed by colorimetry, the readings are affected by turbidity caused by high blood fat content, by the presence of abnormal pigments in the blood, and/or hemolysis. Also, these tests cannot be repeated at frequent intervals. Most of these drawbacks have been obviated with the introduction of radioisotopic techniques for blood volume determination.

Radioactive tracers used for volume measurements must be nontoxic and completely safe for parenteral administration. Furthermore, they should mix rapidly and uniformly with the diluting fluid and remain for a reasonable time interval. In addition, these tracers must be easily detected and quantitated in high dilutions. These criteria are fulfilled to a great extent by most of the radioactive tracers utilized for determination of the blood volume.

Ideally, accurate measurement of the circulating blood volume should be performed by simultaneous determinations of the volume of both plasma and blood cells. Therefore, two radioactive tracers of different energies (so they can be easily differentiated by means of pulse height analysis with a gamma ray spectrometer), such as ^{125}I-human serum albumin and ^{51}Cr-tagged erythrocytes, must be used. However, this procedure necessitates the use of dual tracers and specific equipment, together with time-consuming and tedious calculations. For the sake of simplicity and expedience, a single tracer is used for the determination of the volume of either the plasma or red cells using the principle of dilution. According to this principle:

$$Q = V \times C$$
$$V = \frac{Q}{C}$$

Q = Total quantity of tracer
V = Diluting volume
C = Tracer concentration in duluting fluid

Since the volume of one of the blood components has been determined, the total blood volume can be calculated with the aid of the hematocrit:

$$\text{Total blood volume} = \frac{\text{Plasma volume}}{\text{Plasmacrit}} + \frac{\text{Red cell volume}}{\text{Hematocrit}}$$

Consequently, the volume of the other blood component is obtained by subtraction.

However, it should be remembered that the average whole body hematocrit is roughly 92% of the venous blood hematocrit. This difference in hematocrit values occurs because the blood has been obtained from different size vessels, as well as from different organs. In addition, during hematocrit determination some of the plasma is tagged with the cells, which introduces an error of 2 to 4% in the obtained value. In order to account for both sources of errors, the hematocrit is multiplied by correction factor equal to 0.90 (0.92×0.98) to give a corrected hematocrit that is to be used in the calculations.

Plasma volume determination

Several radioactive tracers have been used for estimation of the plasma volume. All of them depend on the ability of the radioactive tag to attach itself to the plasma proteins.

Radioiodinated ^{131}I human serum albumin (RISA or ^{131}IHSA). Radioiodinated human serum albumin is the tracer most commonly used for plasma volume determination. A venous blood sample is obtained to estimate the background radioactivity in the plasma. The test dose of RISA (5 to 30 μCi) is then transferred into a volumetric container and diluted up to 1,000 ml to act as a standard. Using the same syringe, the technologist injects an exactly equal amount of tracer into one of the patient's antecubital veins, taking care to inject the full amount intravenously. After 15 minutes, a blood sample is withdrawn from the patient's other arm in a heparinized syringe. The hematocrit is determined and the plasma is separated by centrifugation. Radioactivity in equal volumes of the standard and plasma is measured in a scintillation well counter for an equal time. The background is subtracted to give the net counting rate of the plasma. The plasma volume is calculated according to the following equation:

$$\text{Plasma volume (liters)} = \frac{\text{Counting rate of standard}}{\text{Net counting rate of plasma}}$$

Since the volume of the plasma and plasmacrit is known, the total blood volume can be calculated, and by subtraction the red cell volume is obtained.

In addition to technical factors, the main source of error in this technique is the leakage of the tracer from the vascular compartment. The rate of this loss averages about 10% per hour, which makes it negligible within the 15 minutes of the test. However, for increased accuracy, multiple blood sampling is used with backward extrapolation in order to calculate the plasma counts and, subsequently, the plasma volume at zero time.

Using this method, the plasma volume in normal individuals was found to be 43 ml per kilogram body weight.

^{125}**I-human serum albumin.** ^{125}I-human serum albumin is used for plasma volume determination, particularly when simultaneous estimation of the red cell volume is done with ^{51}Cr-tagged sodium chromate. The ^{125}I is a pure but weak gamma emitter, with a longer half-life (60 days) than ^{131}I (8.1 days). Its main disadvantage is its low counting efficiency with ordinary counting equipment.

^{51}**Cr-tagged chromic chloride.** ^{51}Cr-tagged chromic chloride is a trivalent salt. When injected intravenously, about 98% labels the plasma proteins, and the remainder becomes attached to the red cells. Therefore, this radioactive compound can be used for plasma volume determination if a correction factor is applied for the amount of radionuclide that is attached to the erythrocytes. In calculating the result, only 98% of the standard (administered dose) is taken into consideration.

Serum albumin can be also tagged with other radionuclides, such as technetium 99m. The same general principles are still applicable for plasma volume determination.

Red cell volume determination

Determination of the red cell volume depends on the use of labeled erythrocytes as the tracer. Such labeling can be done either in vitro or in vivo by means of various radioactive agents.

Sodium chromate ^{51}Cr. Radiochromate is the most commonly utilized radioactive tagging agent for the red cells in clinical use. It is a hexavalent compound that can easily penetrate the red cell membrane and establish a firm tag with the hemoglobin. Tagging is done in vitro. For this purpose, an anticoagulated blood sample (10 ml) is obtained from the patient and transferred into a sterile container to mix with 50 μCi of radiochromate. The mixture is left at room temperature for 15 minutes if ACD solution is used, or for 60 minutes if the anticoagulant is heparin. Most of the radiochromate enters the cells, but a small portion (10 to 20%) is left in the plasma. To remove this free radiochromate, the red cells are washed three times and then resuspended in normal saline.

An easier and less time-consuming alternative is to add 100 mg ascorbic acid (vitamin C) to the mixture in order to reduce the radiochromate and thus prevent it from tagging any other erythrocytes when reinjected into the patient. An accurately measured volume (m) of this tagged mixture is kept as a standard, and an exactly equal amount (m) is injected intravenously into the patient. After 15 to 30 minutes, a venous blood sample is withdrawn from the patient's other arm. The hematocrit of this blood sample (Hct_{pt}), as well as that of the standard (Hct_s), is determined. Finally, the radioactive content of 1 ml of the whole blood and plasma of the standard (B_s and Pl_s) and that of the venous blood sample (B_{pt} and Pl_{pt}) is estimated in a scintillation well counter.

According to the principle of dilution, the diluting volume (V)—which in this particular situation is the red cell volume—can be calculated by dividing the amount of radioactivity injected (Q) by the concentration of the radioactivity (C). If washing is used, Q is going to equal $m \times B_s$. However, in case washing is not performed (which is more common), the radioactivity in the plasma has to be calculated and subtracted from the radioactivity in the total volume. Radioactivity in the plasma contained in 1 ml of the tagged blood (standard) equals radioactivity in 1 ml of this plasma (Pl_s) times the plasmacrit. Therefore, the amount of radioactivity injected and contained in the red cells can be calculated from the following equation:

$$Q = m\,[B_s - (Pl_s \times plasmacrit_s)]$$

On the same assumptions, radioactivity in the red cells contained in 1 ml of the withdrawn blood sample equals $B_{pt} - (Pl_{pt} \times plasmacrit_{pt})$. Dividing this last value by the hematocrit gives the radioactivity per unit volume of red cells or, in other words, the concentration of radioactivity (c).

By substituting for the values of Q and C in the original equation of dilution:

$$V = Q/C$$
$$V = \frac{m\,[B_s - (Pl_s \times plasmacrit_s)]}{\dfrac{B_{pt} - (Pl_{pt} \times plasmacrit_{pt})}{Hct_{pt}}}$$
$$V = \frac{m\,[B_s - (Pl_s \times plasmacrit_s)] \times Hct_{pt}}{B_{pt} - (Pl_{pt} \times plasmacrit_{pt})}$$

The red cell volume as estimated by this technique in normal male subjects averages 28 ml per kilogram body weight.

Using radioisotopic techniques, the average values for the red cell, plasma volume, and total blood volume expressed in milliliters per kilogram in normal adults are:

	Male	*Female*
Red cell volume	28	24
Plasma volume	39	38
Total blood volume	67	62

Although chromium is not a normal constituent of the red cells, its binding with the cell components is very firm. Thus, its elution is slow. Any released ^{51}Cr is not reusable for further labeling of other red cells. In addition, the physical characteristics of ^{51}Cr are very suitable for counting and external monitoring. The disadvantages of this method are mainly technical, such as the need for multiple vascular injections, the lack of tagging due to the presence of reducing agents in the blood, formation of clots in the standard, and hemolysis of the tagged cells. Some of these drawbacks can be avoided by using labeled cells from fresh blood bank O (Rh−) filtered blood and avoiding washing.

Other methods of blood volume determination

RISA blood volume utilizing whole blood. The easiest but the least accurate method of determining total blood volume is the use of radioiodinated human serum albumin. The same procedure as that described under the plasma volume determination is followed, except that radioactivity in the whole blood, rather than in the plasma alone, is measured and used in the calculation. Under such circumstances, the main sources of error are the lack of uniform mixing and the difference between the average whole body hematocrit and that determined from a blood sample withdrawn from a relatively large vein such as the antecubital.

Sodium phosphate ^{32}P. ^{32}P-labeled sodium phosphate can be used to tag red cells in vitro in order to estimate the red cell volume. The same technique as with the radiochromate is used. However, only 20 to 30% of the radiophosphorus becomes fixed to the erythrocytes. Therefore, washing is essential. Elution occurs at the rate of about 6% per hour. Furthermore, ^{32}P is a beta emitter, which makes its counting efficiency inferior to that of radiochromate.

^{59}Fe. ^{59}Fe, when injected in vivo, becomes incorporated in the hemoglobin during the process of red cell production. Although it can be used for the determination of red cell volume, it needs a compatible donor for the preparation of the labeled cells.

Clinical indications for blood volume determination

Under certain circumstances, alteration might occur in the total amount of cells and/or plasma without a corresponding change in these blood constituents in a given unit of volume. Therefore, neither blood counts nor hematocrit determination, both of which are expressed per unit volume, can detect or accurately quantitate such changes. However, such changes are easily diagnosed and quantitated by means of blood volume determinations. This is why blood volume determinations are advisable following acute blood loss, whether early or late, and following extensive burns. False results, caused by compensatory mechanisms, can therefore be avoided. Blood volume should be determined preoperatively in patients of the extreme age groups (children and the elderly) before any major surgery. In this way any volume deficit that would adversely affect the result of surgery can be detected and treated. Postoperatively, the best guide for transfusion therapy regarding the type and amount required is estimation of the volume of both cells and plasma. In addition, the most reliable measure for the degree of anemia, especially in the presence of a change in the plasma volume, is red cell volume determination.

RED CELL SURVIVAL

Red cell survival is measured by following a given group of erythrocytes to determine the time required for their elimination from the circulation. In order to make this possible, the specified erythrocytes should be easily identifiable from the remainder of the red cells by a label or tag. The tag may be either incorporated during the process of formation of the red cells (selective or cohort labeling) or introduced into a heterogenous group of erythrocytes that happen by mere chance to be present in the circulation at the time of tagging (random labeling).

Selective labeling

Selective labeling is usually done with glycine ^{14}C, glycine ^{15}N, glycine ^{3}H, ^{59}Fe, or ^{75}Se selenomethionine. The tagged cells are of the same age and are followed for their full life-span until they are eliminated from the circulation. This necessitates a long period of observation that might extend for more than 4 months. Furthermore, these radionuclides are expensive, and special preparation and specific equipment are required for counting the radionuclides used. However, this technique can easily differentiate between finite and random destruction of the red cells. Another advantage is the relative insensitivity of the test to concomitant shifts in the red cell volume during the period of the study.

Random labeling

Random labeling is easier and can be performed using radioactive as well as nonradioactive techniques. Since the tagged cells are of different ages, they are eliminated from the circulating blood at different times, making identification of the end point of elimination difficult. Therefore, the red cell survival time is calculated from the percent of surviving tagged erythrocytes as determined at periodic time intervals. However, because of the inaccuracy of determinations encountered during the latter part of the study, when the percent of surviving tagged erythrocytes is rather low it is preferable to rely on the results of the first 3 weeks and to express the survival in terms of the time required for elimination of 50% of the tagged erythrocytes (survival half-life). Since the survival is computed from the percent of surviving tagged cells as determined per unit volume, wide fluctuations in the blood volume would undoubtedly invalidate this result. Another disadvantage of the random labeling technique is the inability to differentiate a short finite life-span from random destruction of the red cells.

Ashby's differential agglutination technique. Ashby's differential agglutination technique is a method of measuring the survival time of transfused, but immunologically identifiable, erythrocytes that have been obtained from a donor. The surviving donor cells are enumerated following agglutination or hemolysis of the patient's erythrocytes by appropriate antisera. Thus, it is not possible to study the survival of the red cells of a specified subject in his own circulation. Furthermore, this technique suffers from the inherent errors in cell counting, together with the hazards of transfusion.

Sodium chromate. The disadvantages associated with Ashby's method are completely obviated by tagging the erythrocytes with sodium chromate (^{51}Cr).

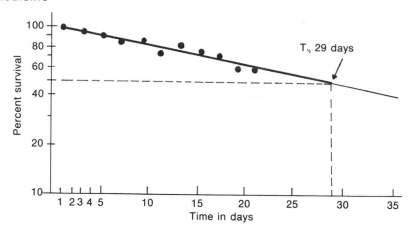

Fig. 11-1. Radiochromate-tagged red cell survival in a normal subject plotted on semilogarithmic scale. Level of radioactivity at 24 hours is considered 100%. The red cell survival half-time ($T_{1/2}$) is 29 days.

The tagged cells are reinjected into the patient and a blood sample is obtained after 30 minutes for blood volume determination. A heparinized blood sample is withdrawn after 24 hours; thereafter one is withdrawn every third day for a period of 3 to 4 weeks. In order to abolish the effect of physical decay, all the samples are counted on the day they are withdrawn in a scintillation well counter. Radioactivity per milliliter of red cells is estimated as previously described under red cell volume determination, and is plotted as a function of time on semilogarithmic paper, starting with the 24-hour sample to avoid errors caused by loss of radioactivity (5 to 10%) during the first 24 hours. The data is made to fit a straight line from which the red cell survival half-time is calculated (Fig. 11-1).

This half-life averages 25 to 35 days, which is shorter than the expected normal half-life of 55 to 60 days. A major part of this difference is attributed to elution of the ^{51}Cr from the intact surviving cells (roughly 1% per day). To apply a fixed correction factor to account for such an error is impossible, because of the unpredictable variability in the rate of ^{51}Cr elution.

Therefore, the estimated or apparent red cell survival half-time is used. At the end of the study, the red cell volume is determined again to exclude any gross change in the blood volume that might invalidate the obtained result.

If the red cell survival half-time is found to be shorter than normal, the test may be repeated by injecting the patient's cells into a normal recipient or by injecting normal erythrocytes into the patient. This is done in order to determine whether the cause of this decreased survival is corpuscular and/or extracorpuscular in nature. Further helpful information is obtained by periodic measurement of the radioactivity over the precordium, sacrum, liver, and spleen at the same time the blood samples are withdrawn. External monitoring is performed by a collimated scintillation detector in a trial to determine the site of red cell sequestration.

Diisopropyl (^{32}P) fluorophosphate. Diisopropyl fluorophosphate is less effective than sodium chromate in labeling the red cells, whether used in vitro (5 to 10%) or in vivo (25 to 40%), but it is much easier to use. Furthermore, there is no elution of the radionuclide after the first few days, which makes the determination of red cell survival more accurate. However, ^{32}P, which acts as the radioactive label, is a beta emitter, and diisopropyl fluorophosphate labels the leukocytes and platelets, together with the red cells. Consequently, the preparation for counting the radioactivity is not easy. In addition, external monitoring of the radioactivity accumulating in the different organs cannot be performed.

Clinical applications

Measurement of red cell survival is invaluable in the study of cases of unexplained anemia, especially the hemolytic type. Further help can be obtained from determination of the nature of the defect causing the shortened red cell survival, whether the cause is intrinsic in the cells and/or extracorpuscular in origin. Also, investigation of the site of red cell sequestration helps in the choice of the proper line of treatment. For example, with exaggerated splenic sequestration of the tagged erythrocytes, splenectomy usually proves beneficial.

IRON METABOLISM AND FERROKINETICS

Although radionuclide techniques have provided valuable information concerning the proper understanding of iron metabolism, such techniques are still far from being routine laboratory clinical tests. This is generally because of the complexity of the factors involved in the regulation of iron metabolism.

The total body iron content, which averages 4.5 gm (2 to 6 gm), tends to remain fixed within narrow limits. Therefore, the amount lost must be matched by absorption. Apart from blood loss, iron is lost through desquamation of cells from the skin and intestinal mucosa, cells discharged in body secretions, falling hair, and cut nails. Traces are excreted through the urine and bile. Normally this loss ranges from 0.5 to 1.5 mg of iron per day. Since only about 10% of food iron is absorbed, the daily dietary iron intake should be from 10 to 15 mg in order to maintain a steady state. Foods known to be rich in iron are liver, meat, eggs, peas, lentils, and leafy vegetables. Favored by the acid medium in the stomach, the dietary iron complexes are broken down and ultimately reduced to the absorbable ferrous form. Absorption takes place mainly in the duodenum. The rate and degree of absorption depend on the state of iron stores, the degree of hemopoietic activity, and the dietary iron intake. The absorbed iron is transported through the plasma by a beta globulin called transferrin. Normally, only about one-third of transferrin is saturated with iron. The plasma iron concentration, which averages 100 mg/100 ml, represents the result of iron delivery to the circulating blood by absorption, hemoglobin breakdown, and release from the iron stores against iron removal by hemoglobin synthesis, cell metabolism, excretion, and deposition in the iron stores.

The available radionuclide techniques provide information about measurement of iron absorption as well as determination of the rate of disappearance of radioiron from the plasma and its subsequent distribution in the body.

Measurement of iron absorption. After a night's fast, 10 μCi of ferrous (^{59}Fe) citrate in a ferrous sulfate carrier are administered orally to the patient. The total fecal radioactivity during the next 5 days is computed as percentage of the oral dose. Care must be taken to use identical geometry during each counting.

The main sources of error in this technique are encountered during the collection and counting of the stool samples. These drawbacks are easily overcome by the use of whole body counting. The percentage of radioiron retention is calculated by comparing whole body radioactivity recorded at 4 hours and at 14 days after the oral administration of the tracer dose. Normally, the amount of radioiron absorbed ranges between 5 and 15% of the orally administered dose.

Plasma iron disappearance. For this test about 10 μCi of ferrous (^{59}Fe) citrate are injected intravenously into the patient. The ferrous citrate is used as is or bound to transferrin by incubation with fresh plasma for 30 minutes. Serial blood samples are collected for a period of 2 hours. Radioactivity per unit volume of plasma is estimated and plotted on semilogarithmic paper against time in order to calculate the time required for half of the radioactivity to disappear from the plasma. Normally, the plasma radioiron disappearance half-time ($T_{1/2}$) averages 90 minutes.

From the plasma radioiron disappearance half-time, together with the plasma volume and the level of serum iron as determined by the available chemical methods, the plasma iron turnover rate (PITR) can be calculated as follows:

$$PITR = \frac{0.693}{T_{1/2}}(hours) \times serum\ iron \times plasma\ volume \times 24$$

The normal plasma iron turnover rate ranges between 20 to 42 mg per day (average 37 mg per day) and can be used as an index of total erythropoietic activity.

Red cell iron turnover rate and utilization. For this test a blood sample is obtained 15 minutes after the intravenous injection of the plasma bound iron complex. Thereafter, blood samples are collected every third day for 2 weeks. Radioactivity per unit volume of the hemolyzed blood is determined and expressed as a percentage of the radioactivity present in the first sample (obtained 15 minutes after the dose was given) in order to determine the maximum red cell uptake of radioiron.

Normally, more than 80% of the injected radioiron is incoporated in the newly formed erythrocytes and appears in the circulating blood within 10 days.

From the maximum red cell uptake of radioiron (MC) and the plasma iron turnover rate (PITR), the red cell iron turnover rate (RCITR) can be calculated:

$$RCITR = PITR \times \frac{MC}{100}$$

In normal subjects, the RCITR averages 29 mg per day, with a range from 20 to 40 mg per day, and indicates the effectiveness of red cell production.

From the red cell iron turnover rate, the fraction of red cell iron renewal per day, as well as the mean red cell life-span, can be calculated.

In vivo distribution and movement of radioiron. Following the intravenous injection of the radioiron complex, external counting is performed periodically and simultaneously over the precordium, sacrum, spleen, and liver over a period of 2 weeks.

Normally, within the first few hours after the injection of the tracer dose, the counting rate over the precordium, which represents the blood radioactivity, diminishes. Consequently, the counting rates over the spleen and liver decrease. In contrast, radioactivity over the sacrum, which represents the bone marrow radioactivity, increases and remains at a peak for about 2 days before it rapidly diminishes. In the meantime, precordial radioactivity increases to reach a maximum within 7 to 10 days, which denotes the appearance of radioactivity within the newly formed erythrocytes in the circulating blood. A similar, but much less pronounced, increase in the counting rate is noticed over the liver and spleen.

A significant increase in the splenic counting rate, which exceeds the original level of radioactivity as measured after radioiron injection, denotes splenic sequestration of red cells. If radioactivity over the liver or spleen behaves in a similar way to that over the sacrum, extramedullary erythropoiesis is suggested.

The main indication for ferrokinetic studies is the investigation of obscure hematologic disorders. In this respect, simultaneous studies with ^{51}Cr (for red cell survival) and ^{59}Fe (for ferrokinetics) using pulse height analysis would be of great help.

VITAMIN B$_{12}$ ABSORPTION

Vitamin B$_{12}$ is a very potent, cobalt-containing, dietary factor available in many foods of animal origin, such as liver, kidney, muscle, milk, and eggs. It plays a major role in the synthesis of nucleic acid, and therefore is particularly important in the process of cell maturation. Consequently, the first cells to suffer from its deficiency are the rapidly dividing cells, such as those of the bone marrow and gastrointestinal tract. The proper absorption of the small amounts of vitamin B$_{12}$ available in the daily food intake depends on the adequate secretion of intrinsic factor by the glands of the body of the stomach. The vitamin B$_{12}$-intrinsic factor complex thus formed is mainly absorbed in the terminal ileum. After absorption, vitamin B$_{12}$ is carried by the blood, bound to the plasma proteins. It goes to the liver, which serves as its main storage depot. It stays in the liver for months or even years, and is slowly released to carry out its normal cellular metabolic functions. Vitamin B$_{12}$ is generally excreted through the urine, but any that is not absorbed in the ileum is excreted in the stool.

The presence of a cobalt atom in each molecule of vitamin B$_{12}$ made it possible to synthesize a radioactive cobalt-labeled vitamin B$_{12}$. The radionuclides used are ^{57}Co, ^{58}Co, and ^{60}Co. The long half-life of ^{60}Co (5.26 years) has made its use limited. Although ^{57}Co has a longer half-life (270 days) than ^{58}Co (71.3 days), ^{57}Co is preferred because of its better counting efficiency and the absence of beta radiation.

Absorption of vitamin B$_{12}$ can be studied by one or more of the following tests: fecal excretion, plasma radioactivity, hepatic uptake, or urine radioactivity. Since many of the patients to be tested have already received other radionuclides for diagnostic purposes, it is advisable to obtain control samples of stools, plasma, or urine before giving the test dose of radioactive vitamin B$_{12}$ in every case. The usual dose of radioactive vitamin B$_{12}$ is 0.5 μCi, which is given orally with half a glass of water on an empty stomach. A light breakfast is given after approximately

2 hours. The remainder of the procedure depends on the type of test to be performed.

Fecal excretion method. All stools of the patient are collected for at least 72 hours. The net amount of radioactivity in all the stools is counted and expressed as percentage of the administered dose. This represents the amount of radioactive vitamin B_{12} that was not absorbed. Therefore, the remainder should be the amount absorbed.

Normally, the stools contain from 30 to 70% of the administered dose. With defective absorption, the amount of radioactivity recovered in the stools is higher than these normal values.

Using this technique, erroneous results might be obtained because of contamination of the stools during their collection with urine and/or incomplete stool collection. This, together with the unpleasant task of dealing with fecal matter, has limited the use of this method.

Level of plasma radioactivity. Approximately 8 to 10 hours after the oral administration of the tagged vitamin, plasma radioactivity reaches its peak level. Accordingly, a blood sample of about 20 ml is obtained at that time. Radioactivity in 10 ml of the plasma is estimated in a scintillation well counter, and the background count is subtracted to give the net counting rate. The obtained figure is multiplied by 100 to give the net radioactivity per liter of plasma. Similarly, the net counting rate of 1% of the test dose dissolved into 10 ml of water is estimated and designated as the standard. Dividing the net plasma radioactivity by the counting rate of the standard gives the percentage of dose per liter plasma.

Normally, the level of plasma radioactivity ranges between 0.25 and 2.54% of the administered dose per liter plasma. However, because of some overlap between the low normal and abnormal results, values between 0.25 and 0.50% should be considered suspicious.

The main advantages of this method are that it requires minimum cooperation from the patient and nurses, and errors caused by loss of samples are avoided. The test is completed on the same day it is given and there is no need to inject nonradioactive vitamin B_{12}, which might affect any subsequent studies. However, because of the low counting rate, extreme caution must be given to the preparation and counting of the plasma. In addition, the counting time should be reasonably long, and the use of pulse height analysis is advisable.

Hepatic uptake test. Five days after the oral ingestion of the tracer dose of radioactive vitamin B_{12}, the subject is given a laxative to clear his alimentary tract of any remaining radioactive material. Two days later, radioactivity accumulating in four different areas over the liver, left iliac fossa, and thighs is measured by means of a collimated scintillation detector. The mean of the counts over the thighs is considered as body background. This is subtracted from the average counting rates over both the liver and left iliac fossa. The ratio between the net hepatic counting rate and that over the iliac fossa is then calculated.

In normal subjects, the ratio between the counts over the liver and those over the left iliac fossa should be at least 2.5:1.

The time required for completion of the test and the fact that it is a qualitative rather than a quantitative test are the main disadvantages.

Urine radioactivity (Schilling test). This method is the most commonly applied one. For this test the patient is given nonradioactive vitamin B_{12} which will reach and block the specific binding sites before the absorbed radioactive vitamin B_{12} can arrive at them. Consequently, the absorbed unbound radioactive vitamin is excreted with the urine. In order to achieve this purpose, 1,000 μg of stable vitamin B_{12} are injected within 2 hours after the oral administration of the tracer dose. The urine is collected for the next 24 hours, and its radioactivity is estimated and expressed as percentage of the administered oral dose. Urine should have been collected from the patient the day before the test. This urine is diluted with water up to 1 or 2 liters in a volumetric container. The radioactivity in this urine is measured on top of a well counter, and is considered as background. Exactly the same is done to the urine collected after the test dose is given and to the test dose itself. The background is subtracted to give the net counting rate. Finally, the result is obtained by dividing the urine radioactivity by that of the tracer dose and multiplying times 100 to express it as a percent.

The percent of dose that is absorbed and, consequently, recovered in the urine by flushing with stable vitamin B_{12} is normally 7% or more.

The main sources of error in this test lie in the collection of urine and measurement of its radioactivity. Furthermore, the result can be affected by renal diseases. The possible effects of the injected stable vitamin B_{12} on subsequent studies, as well as on the course of the disease, should be considered.

Although most workers use one of the above procedures to test vitamin B_{12} absorption, a combination of two of these methods using the same oral tracer dose would definitely give more accurate information.

If the obtained result indicates impaired absorption of vitamin B_{12}, the test should be repeated after about 1 week, using 30 mg of intrinsic factor together with the radioactive tracer dose. Normalization of the result after the addition of intrinsic factor denotes that the impaired absorption of vitamin B_{12} is caused by lack of adequate secretion of intrinsic factor. This is seen following gastrectomy and in cases of pernicious anemia and gastric carcinoma.

If the result of the absorption test remains within the abnormal range, the cause should be looked for in the intestine. In some cases the basic defect is competition for vitamin B_{12} by intestinal parasites or by microorganisms, as in the blind loop syndrome, intestinal strictures, and diverticulosis. Defective absorption in the remaining cases can be explained on the basis of a quantitative and/or qualitative diminution in the intestinal absorptive surface as seen after extensive intestinal resections, regional enteritis, tropical sprue, celiac disease, and idiopathic steatorrhea.

Clinical indications

The main clinical indication for vitamin B_{12} absorption studies is the differential diagnosis of pernicious anemia. Pernicious anemia is directly related to a lack of vitamin B_{12} and the signs and symptoms are those of anemia. Laboratory signs

217

are directly related to a maturation of the rapidly developing cells of the body. Associated symptomatology is related to a specific neural disorder caused by degradation of specific areas of the spinal cord. Utilized intelligently in conjunction with other laboratory studies, the radioactive vitamin B_{12} absorption test can be a very useful diagnostic test in patients with the early signs and symptoms of pernicious anemia.

Chapter
12   *Surface anatomy*

There is no doubt that an accurate description of the site and size of the various internal organs would be much easier with the use of known and fixed reference points or landmarks. Although soft tissue landmarks (such as the nipple and umbilicus) have been commonly used, their positions are affected by various factors as age, sex, pregnancy, and intraabdominal and pelvic tumors. In contrast, bony landmarks are fixed; they can be easily recognized on x-ray films and enable accurate superimposition of a radioisotope photoscan on the corresponding roentgenogram (Fig. 12-1).

Some of the main bony landmarks in the head are the nasion, inion, mastoid process, and mandible. The nasion is the depression at the root of the nose; the inion, or external occipital protuberance, is the midline bony prominence situated on the back of the skull at the junction of the head and neck. The mastoid process is the bony projection behind the ear which points downward and forward.

Passing the finger along the midline from the mandible downward, one encounters the hyoid bone, thyroid cartilage, cricoid cartilage, and trachea in that order (see Fig. 13-1).

Two of the major landmarks in the neck are muscles, the sternocleidomastoid and trapezius. The sternocleidomastoid, as its name implies, extends from the mastoid process to the upper part of the sternum and clavicle. The trapezius forms the upper border of the shoulder and slopes upward from the point of the shoulder toward the back of the head and medially toward the midline of the back. The neck can therefore be divided into two main triangles—the anterior and the posterior. The anterior triangle is bounded anteriorly by the midline, by the anterior border of the sternocleidomastoid posteriorly, and by the lower border of the body of the mandible upward. The boundaries of the posterior triangle are the posterior margin of the sternocleidomastoid, by the anterior margin of the trapezius, and by the middle third of the clavicle downward.

The clavicles, the sternum, and the ribs (with the intercostal spaces) form the main landmarks over the front of the chest. The suprasternal or jugular notch lies at the upper border of the manubrium sterni, between the sternal attachments of both sternocleidomastoid muscles. About 2 inches along the midsternal line there is a transverse ridge at the junction of the manubrium with the body of the sternum (Fig. 12-2). This ridge is called the sternal angle (angle of Louis or Ludwig's angle) and lies opposite the sternochondral junction of the second rib. Therefore the second rib is the most easily and accurately identifiable one, and the one from which other ribs can be recognized. The second intercostal space is the one immediately below this rib. The lowest part of the sternum is called the xiphoid

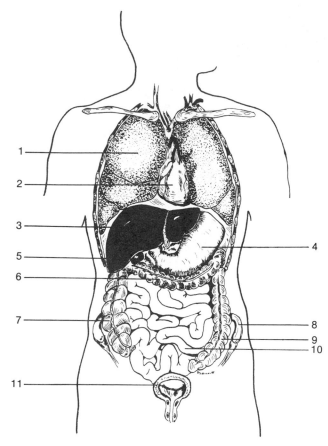

Fig. 12-1. Soft tissue organs of the body: *1,* lung; *2,* heart; *3,* liver; *4,* stomach; *5,* gallbladder; *6,* transverse colon; *7,* ascending colon; *8,* iliac crest; *9,* descending colon; *10,* small bowel; *11,* bladder.

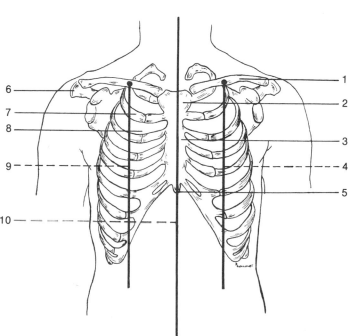

Fig. 12-2. Anatomic landmarks of the thorax: *1,* clavicle; *2,* manubrium sterni; *3,* sternum; *4,* midclavicular line; *5,* xiphoid; *6,* acromion; *7,* second rib; *8,* second intercostal space; *9,* midclavicular line; *10,* midline.

process. It varies in shape and is usually cartilaginous. Parallel to the midsternal line and passing through the middle of the clavicle is the midclavicular line, which forms an important line of orientation over the front of the chest.

On each side of the chest, the hollow of the armpit, or axilla, is limited by two muscular folds, the anterior and posterior axillary folds. Halfway between these folds, the midaxillary line is drawn to serve as a landmark.

On the back, the furrow down the midline corresponds to the tips of the spinous processes of the vertebrae.

For descriptive purposes, the abdomen is divided into nine regions by two horizontal and two sagittal planes. The transpyloric plane lies half way between the suprasternal notch and the upper margin of the pubic symphysis, which is situated at the lowest part of the front of the abdomen. This plane cuts through the pylorus, the tip of the ninth costal cartilage, and the lower border of the first lumbar vertebra. The transtubercular plane joins the highest points on the iliac crests as identified on both sides of the body, and passes through the body of the fifth

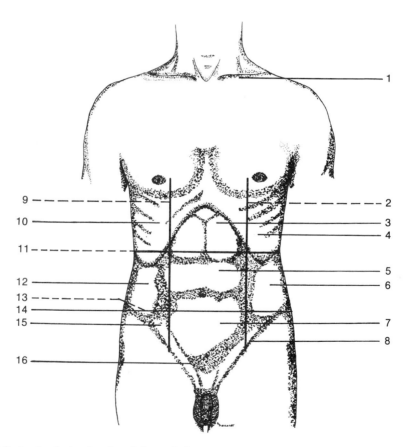

Fig. 12-3. Anatomic landmarks of the anterior thorax and abdomen: *1*, clavicle; *2*, left lateral line; *3*, epigasterium; *4*, left hypochondrium; *5*, umbilical region; *6*, left lumbar; *7*, hypogasterium or suprapubic region; *8*, left iliac; *9*, right lateral line; *10*, right hypochondrium; *11*, transpyloric plane; *12*, right lumbar; *13*, transtubercular plane; *14*, anterior superior iliac spine; *15*, right iliac; *16*, inguinal ligament.

221

lumbar vertebra. The two sagittal planes are drawn parallel to the midline from the midinguinal point. This point lies half way between the symphysis pubis and the anterior superior iliac spine, which is the anterior end of the iliac crest. These regions, from top to bottom, are the epigastric, the umbilical, and the hypogastric (suprapubic) regions in the middle. On both sides of these areas, the hypochondriac, lumbar, and iliac (inguinal) regions are situated. The abdomen may be also sub-divided by means of two planes drawn at right angles giving four quadrants. These planes are a midsagittal and a transverse plane passing through the umbilicus. However, the position of the umbilicus is affected by so many factors, that this subdivision is inaccurate.

Chapter

13 *Thyroid*

The thyroid is an endocrine organ, and thyroid hormones have a direct effect on the body's metabolism. The thyroid's function is under the direct control of the anterior pituitary gland, which secretes thyroid stimulating hormone. The output of thyroid stimulating hormone is directly related to the secretion of a thyroid factor (thyrotropin releasing factor) by the hypothalamus. The relationship between thyroid factor, TSH, and thyroxine is called the hypothalamic pituitary thyroid axis.

ANATOMY AND PHYSIOLOGY OF THE THYROID GLAND

During embryonic development, the thyroid is derived from the ventral wall of the primitive pharynx (Figs. 13-1 and 13-2). This median outgrowth migrates downward and at its lower end it bifurcates to form the isthmus and lateral lobes of the thyroid. In some cases the thyroid does not progress down into the neck,

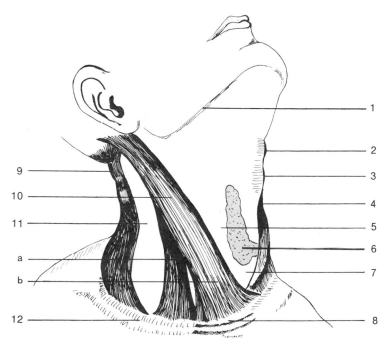

Fig. 13-1. Anatomy of the neck region: *1*, mandible; *2*, hyoid bone; *3*, thyroid cartilage; *4*, cricoid cartilage; *5*, anterior triangle; *6*, thyroid gland—right lobe; *7*, suprasternal notch; *8*, sternum; *9*, trapezius; *10*, sternocleidomastoid muscle (*a*, sternal head; *b*, clavicular head); *11*, posterior triangle; *12*, clavicle.

223

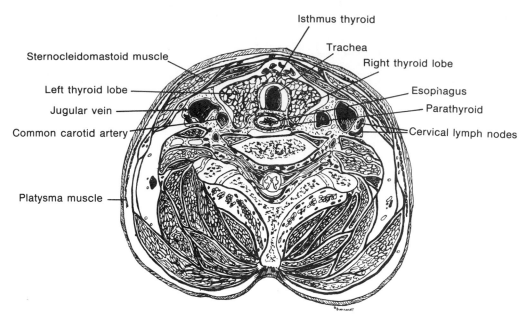

Fig. 13-2. Transverse section through the seventh cervical vertebra.

but remains at the base of the tongue. Thyroid tissue may also continue down into the mediastinum and thus become substernal. However, the thyroid is usually found between the thyroid cartilage and the suprasternal notch. The isthmus is astride the trachea with one lobe on either side of the trachea. In many cases there is a slight extension of thyroid tissue from the lobes and/or from the isthmus. This is normal thyroid tissue which lines the tract the thyroid follows down into the neck. This tissue is called the pyramidal lobe.

Thyroid tissue is composed of cuboidal epithelial cells arranged in single layers around spherical spaces called follicles. In the human fetus, the thyroid becomes functional during the third month of gestation.

The thyroid's blood supply arises from the superior and inferior thyroid arteries; the blood flow to the thyroid, as well as its capillary bed, is quite profuse.

Normally, control of thyroid activity is exerted by the thyroid thyrotropic hormone (TSH), which is secreted by the anterior pituitary. The normal weight of the human thyroid is from 20 to 35 gm, and the usual normal adult thyroid gland is barely palpable if at all. The thyroid gland's primary function is to synthesize, store, and secrete the thyroid hormones.

The thyroid extracts iodide from the blood supply (I^-) and converts iodide to iodine (I^2), which is utilized in the synthesis of thyroid hormone.

Iodine and thyroid hormone metabolism

The hypothalamus regulates the pituitary secretion of thyrotropic hormone (TSH) by secreting a thyroid factor (thyrotropin releasing factor) into the portal vessels of the pituitary stalk (Fig. 13-3). Cells of the anterior pituitary secrete TSH, which has four distinct effects on the thyroid gland. There is a reciprocal relation-

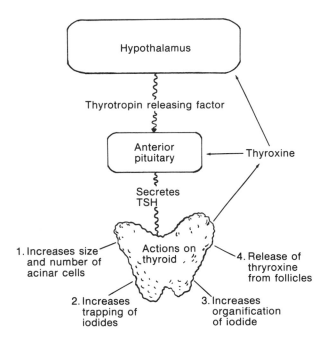

Fig. 13-3. Interrelationships of thyroid stimulating hormone and the thyroid.

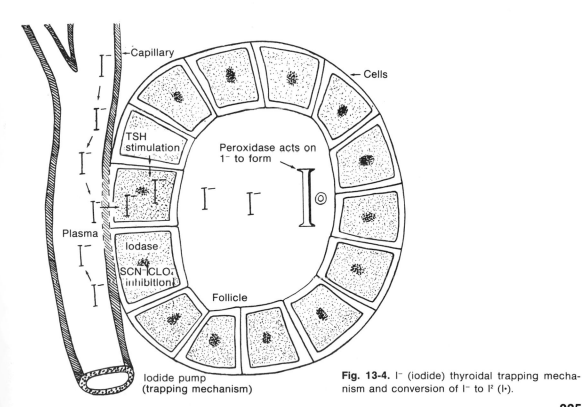

Fig. 13-4. I⁻ (iodide) thyroidal trapping mechanism and conversion of I⁻ to I² (I·).

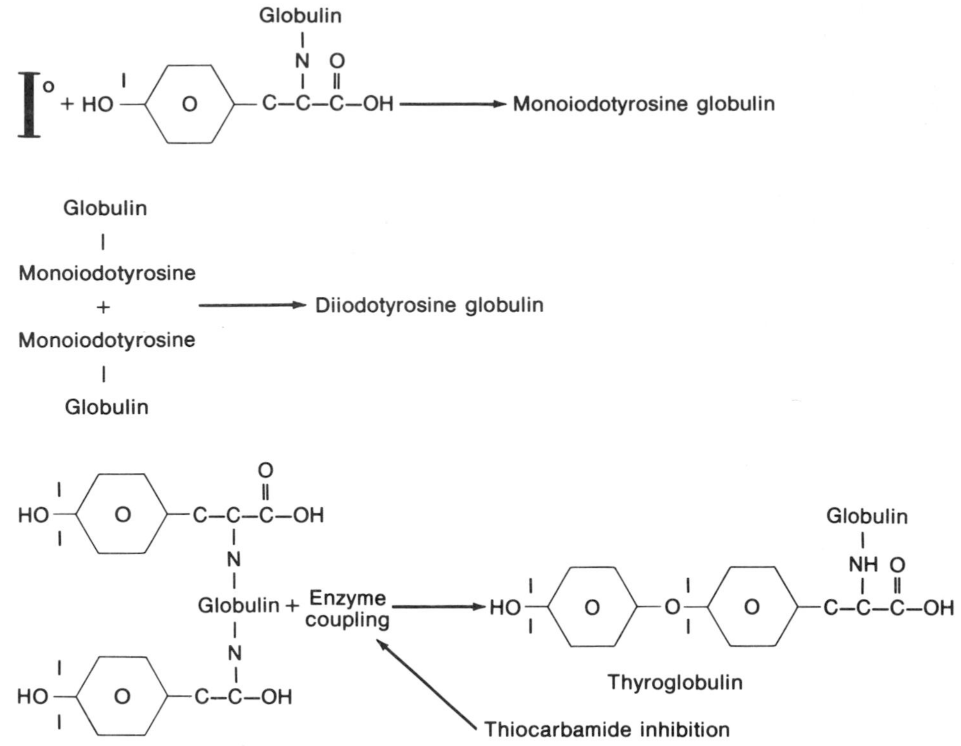

Fig. 13-5. Thyroid hormonal synthesis.

ship between TSH output and the serum and/or tissue levels of the thyroid hormone. It is not known whether the level of thyroid hormone acts primarily through its effect on the hypothalamus or on the pituitary. It is possible that the feed-back mechanism of the thyroid pituitary axis operates at both levels.

The ability of the thyroid gland to concentrate iodine is found in the thyroid epithelial cells (Fig. 13-4). The iodide concentrating mechanism of the thyroid gland is referred to as the iodide trap or iodide pump. This mechanism may concentrate iodide to 25 times that of the plasma level or, in some abnormal instances, may increase this concentration to 500 times that of the plasma concentration. The iodide pump is so efficient that tagged iodine has been found in the colloid (which is on the other side of the epithelial cell), as early as 2 minutes after iodide was injected intravenously. The next step that iodide takes in the course of biosynthesis of thyroid hormone is the formation of iodinated amino acids. This is also an extremely rapid process and takes place in the colloid at the surface of the thyroid epithelial cells (at the cell colloid interface). At this stage it is thought that the iodide is oxidized to iodine, which in turn reacts with the tyrosyl residues of the protein chain of tyroglobulin to form monoiodotyrosine globulin (Fig. 13-5).

Further iodination leads to the formation of diiodotyrosine globulin, and subsequent coupling of the two iodinated tyrosyl groups will form the tetraiodinated compound, thyroxine, still attached to the globulin moiety. If one monoiodotyrosyl molecule couples with a diiodotyrosyl molecule, triiodothyronine globulin is formed.

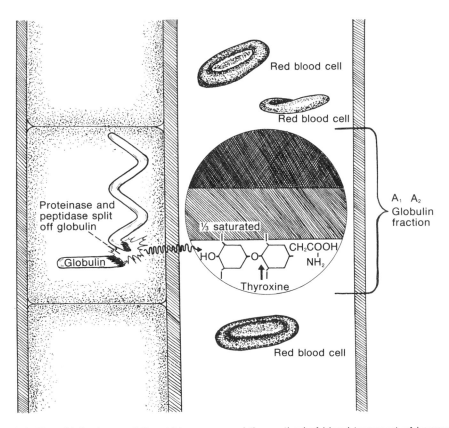

Fig. 13-6. Thyroidal release of thyroid hormone and the method of blood transport of hormone.

These compounds are then stored in the thyroid follicle in the form of thyroglobulins. Active proteolytic enzymes release thyroxine and triiodothyronine from thyroglobulin. This process is probably intracellular, as small fragments of colloid appear as droplets in thyroid epithelial cells. Free thyroxine (T 4) and triiodothyronine (T 3) are then released into the venous drainage of the thyroid gland (Fig. 13-6).

The thyroid gland has a remarkable affinity for iodide; although the gland constitutes only 0.05% of the total body weight, the normal gland contains half the body's entire iodine content.

Iodine turnover in the human

The most commonly used radioactive form of iodine is ^{131}I, which will act exactly as stable iodine [127]I in the body. Therefore, very small amounts of ^{131}I may be introduced into the body in order to trace the role of stable iodine in metabolic pathways.

Since iodine is distributed in all areas of the body there are several iodine "compartments"; these include the intracellular, extracellular, thyroid, and extrathyroidal compartments. There are also extrathyroidal iodide spaces and intra- and extrathyroidal organic iodine compartments. The terminology in this section

227

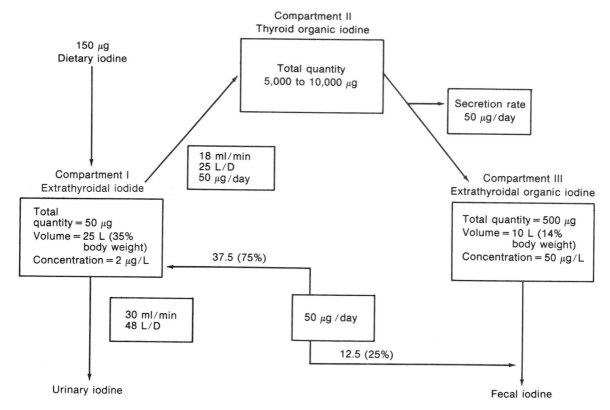

Fig. 13-7. Iodine and iodide body compartments.

should not be too difficult and this portion of the chapter should be studied in detail. With the understanding of the iodide and iodine compartments, the student will be able to predict the results of almost all of the radioactive iodine studies, as well as the chemical iodine studies which will be discussed later in this chapter.

Iodine metabolism in the body has been roughly divided into a three compartment model. Compartment I is the extrathyroidal iodide pool which receives its iodide from both the diet and the extrathyroidal deiodinization or removal of iodine from secreted thyroid hormone. Iodide is removed from this pool by thyroid accumulation and renal excretion. Compartment II is the thyroidal organic iodine pool from which hormonal iodine is secreted into Compartment III, the extrathyroidal organic iodine pool. Iodine is transported from Compartment III by removal of iodide from the organic thyroid hormone (which reenters Compartment I) and by fecal excretion in an organic form (Fig. 13-7).

Compartment I—extrathyroidal iodide pool. Approximately 150 to 300 μg of dietary iodide are normally ingested by the human daily. For purposes of this discussion, an ingested amount of 150 μg will be used.

Iodine is absorbed by the gastrointestinal tract, largely by the stomach mucosa, in the first 15 to 30 minutes after ingestion, and thus enters the extrathyroidal pool. This pool is approximately 25 liters in volume, (35% of the total body weight). Therefore, at any period in time approximately 50 μg (or 2 μg/liter) of iodide should be found in this pool. As mentioned previously, iodide leaves this pool by two routes: (1) by entering the thyroid organic iodine pool and (2) by renal excretion. The kidneys have a rather fixed rate of excretion of iodide and will clear approximately 40 ml plasma of iodide per minute; in a 24-hour period, approximately 48 liters of the extrathyroidal iodide pool is cleared of iodide.

Compartment II—thyroid organic iodine pool. The thyroid actively extracts iodide from the extrathyroidal iodide pool converting the iodide into thyroid organic iodine. The thyroid normally contains 5,000 to 10,000 μg of thyroid organic iodine. The thyroid normally extracts iodide from 18 ml of plasma per minute (50 μg of iodide are extracted from the plasma per 24-hour period). The thyroid then clears approximately 25 liters of the extrathyroidal iodide pool of iodide per 24 hours. The thyroid organic iodine pool, as can be seen by the quantity of iodine extracted, contains a rather static quantity as compared to compartment I. The majority of the thyroid organic iodine compartment is composed of the central follicular storage of thyroid hormone, which is the static moiety of this compartment. The dynamic portion of the compartment is the external follicular areas, which are close to the thyroidal cells. These are the areas where most of the synthesis and release of thyroid hormone takes place. The thyroid organic iodine pool actively secretes thyroid hormone into the extrathyroidal organic iodine compartment (compartment III). The secretion rate of thyroid hormones is approximately 50 μg per 24-hour period.

Compartment III—extrathyroidal organic iodine pool. The extrathyroidal organic iodine pool contains approximately 500 μg of iodine, which is distributed in a 10 liter space (about 14% of the body weight). By measurement the organic iodine in this pool is approximately 50 μg per liter; the extrathyroidal organic iodine pool is known as the protein-bound iodine pool. The extrathyroidal organic iodine pool is decreased in a 24-hour period by approximately 50 μg, primarily due to thyroxine degradation. Approximately 25% of the iodine freed by thyroxine degradation is excreted in the feces. The remainder returns to the extrathyroidal iodide space.

Special clinical note

Now that the student has an introductory understanding as to the quantities of iodine in the various spaces he will be able to recognize that if Lugol's solution, which contains 130,000 μg of iodine per milliliter (a 1,000 day supply of the iodine requirements), is introduced into the body, any study utilizing an infinitesimal tracer dose of ^{131}I will be invalidated. Another commonly used pharmaceutical, potassium iodide, contains 800,000 μg of iodine (a 20 year supply of the iodine requirements) in 1 ml. Obviously, the iodide pool would be greatly increased and its specific activity would be reduced to exceedingly low levels. If the stable iodine uptake of the thyroid remains unchanged, the tracer ^{131}I would be taken up in reduced amounts, since ^{131}I is being used to measure the percentage of the iodine pool that is being trapped by the thyroid. If the total amount of iodide trapped in compartment I is to be measured, it must be of normal size for these measurements to be of any value. If substances in which iodine is bound to an organic nucleus

229

(such as compounds employed for urography, cholecystography, and opacification studies) are introduced into the bloodstream or intracavitary spaces, the tracer iodine studies will be influenced. In their original state these compounds would not influence thyroid function, as the iodine is not ionized. However, these compounds undergo degradation when introduced into the body and the iodine that is freed enters the iodide pool. The compounds can then disturb tracer studies for months or even years.

TESTS FOR ASSESSING TURNOVER OR RELEASE OF THYROIDAL IODINE
Thyroid accumulation of iodine (thyroid uptake of iodine)

The radioactive estimation of iodine accumulation by the thyroid is a dynamic study, which is directly related to the flow of iodide from compartment I to compartment II and the flow of organic iodine from compartment II to compartment III. Iodide leaves the extrathyroidal pool and enters the thyroid cell through an active metabolic process (the thyroid trapping mechanism) and thus enters the thyroid organic iodine pool and is involved in thyroxine synthesis. The thyroid clearance of iodide from the extrathyroidal pool is usually measured soon after ^{131}I administration, and appropriate corrections for the extrathyroidal neck radioactivity are essential. Under normal circumstances the clearance of circulating thyroid is unidirectional, with iodide being actively transported into the gland so rapidly that the efflux of trapped iodide from the gland into the circulation is not appreciable. As mentioned previously, iodide is almost instantaneously organified and, therefore, the accumulation of iodide is almost always the same as the thyroid rate of binding iodide.

The thyroid uptake of radioiodine should be done at varying time periods—from 2 to 24 hours after administration of the tracer dose. Normal values for euthyroid, hypothyroid, and hyperthyroid subjects should be indivdually established and correlated with the results obtained by other workers in the same geographic area.

Table 13-1 shows uptake figures obtained in various sections of this country at given time periods. It should be understood by the student that even if the figures are statistically sound, there will be overlapping of patient populations; that is, hypothyroid in the euthyroid range, euthyroid in the hypothyroid range and so on. In this case a value is measured at one period of time and any par-

Table 13-1. Normal values of radioactive iodine uptake after oral administration of [131]I

	Number of hours after dose	Normal value (% of dose as a range or mean ±SD)
Ann Arbor, Mich.	2	1.4 to 13.4
	6	2.0 to 25.9
	24	10.5 to 38.9
New England	24	20.0 to 50.0
Cleveland	24	15.0 to 45.0

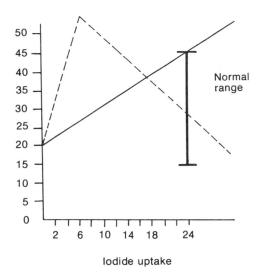

Fig. 13-8. Comparison of normal thyroid up-take values and those of differing forms of hyperthyroidism.

ticular physiologic happening in the thyroid gland (such as true accumulation gradient or secretion gradient) is not being measured. Any gross increase or decrease in the iodine pool will invalidate the thyroid uptake measurement as a diagnostic entity. It must also be understood that in approximately 20% of the hyperthyroid patients, the secretion rate of organically bound iodine (thyroid hormones) is greatly increased. Therefore, the iodide uptake, if it is done later than 6 hours after ingestion of iodine, will be falsely low (Fig. 13-8). Likewise, earlier uptakes are more likely to be abnormal in hypothyroid patients, because slow trapping of ^{131}I in hypothyroidism will make the uptake closer to normal at 24 hours than at the shorter time period. Therefore, it is strongly recommended that 2-hour and 24-hour uptakes be completed on every patient, in questionable cases, a 6-hour uptake should be obtained.

Direct measurement of ^{131}I release

If serial counts are taken after the accumulation of ^{131}I by the thyroid gland, a direct measurement of organically bound ^{131}I release may be obtained. In order that the study not be obscured by reaccumulation of ^{131}I, the function of the patient's thyroid is blocked utilizing an antithyroid agent. After this is done, the curve of thyroid counts will indicate the release of a constant fraction of thyroidal ^{131}I per unit time. When corrected for physical decay of the isotope, the observations indicate a rate of turnover of accumulated ^{131}I, which is accelerated in thyroid hyperfunction.

Measurement of the protein-bound ^{131}I in serum

As will be more fully described, the radioiodinated thyroid hormones secreted by the gland are bound to thyroid hormone binding proteins in serum and, therefore, are measurable. This moiety is separated from radioiodine by trichloroacetic acid precipitation of the serum or passage of the serum through an ion exchange column or by chromotography. The concentration of protein-bound ^{131}I in serum

231

is then related to the administered dose of ^{131}I in samples obtained at 24, 48, and 72 hours. This test has been used primarily to indicate thyroidal hyperfunction.

The conversion ratio. The conversion ratio relates the quantity of protein-bound ^{131}I in the serum after administration of radioiodine to the quantity of the dose remaining in the serum of iodine. The conversion ratio is determined at a fixed time interval (usually at 24 hours) after administration of [131]I. Approximately values in excess of 50% at this time indicate hyperfunction, and values below 20% indicate hypofunction. This test is not useful.

In vitro studies of thyroid function

Thyroxine is bound primarily in the globulin portion of plasma. However, three proteins that carry thyroxine have been identified: (1) thyroxine-binding pre-albumin, which on electrophoresis has a mobility greater than that of serum albumin, (2) serum albumin, and (3) thyroxine-binding globulin, which on electrophoresis has a mobility intermediate between alpha 1 and alpha 2 globulin. Approximately 10% of thyroxine is associated with thyroxine-binding prealbumin, 60% with thyroxine-binding globulin, and the remaining 30% with serum albumin. T 3 (triiodothyronine) is bound primarily to thyroid-binding globulin and secondarily to serum albumin. However, it has been shown that the association is much looser than the corresponding thyroxine-protein complex. T 3 is not bound to thyroxine-binding prealbumin.

Thyroxine-binding globulin, which is the most important of the binding site for thyroxine, has a normal binding capacity ranging from 16 to 24 μg/100 ml. Thyroxine-binding globulin has a molecular weight of 59,000 and is probably a glycoprotein. Thyroxine-binding globulin is normally one-third saturated with thyroid hormone. The concentration of free thyroxine in normal human plasma is less than 0.01 to 0.04% of the total plasma thyroxine concentration, and, therefore, is extremely difficult to measure by conventional chemical measurement.

SPECIAL PROCEDURES IN THE STUDY OF THYROID FUNCTION
In vitro tests of thyroid function

In clinical medicine many nonradioactive tests of thyroid function are used routinely. Therefore, the student must have a general understanding of these tests and what the specific tests measure.

Protein-bound iodine. The protein-bound iodine (see Table 13-2) is simply a measure of the protein precipitable iodine or the organified iodine in the serum. This test measures the amount of T 4, T 3, iodinated dyes, thyroglobulin, and iodoprotein in the blood. It, therefore, is an indirect study of organified iodide in the form of thyroid hormone. However, any iodine contamination will invalidate this particular study. The protein-bound iodine can be improved on slightly by a butanol extraction, which will remove the thyroglobulin, iodoprotein, and free iodide. However, even with the use of butanol extraction, contrast media such as iodinated dyes cannot be removed and the studies will be invalidated.

Measurement of T 4 iodine. There have been chemical techniques designed specifically to separate T 4 from contaminated iodinated materials. These methods

Table 13-2. Factors that may increase or decrease T 3 uptake and protein bound iodine values

Factor	Protein bound iodine	T 3 uptake
Hyperthyroidism	Increased	Increased
Hypothyroidism	Decreased	Decreased
Inorganic iodides	Increased	No change
Contrast media containing iodine	Increased	No change
Estrogens (including oral contraceptives and pregnancy)	Increased	Decreased
Acidosis	No change	Increased
Cancer	No change	Increased
Subacute thyroiditis	Increased	Increased

depend upon ion exchange or thin layer chromography separation of T 4, the iodine content of which is then measured. At this time the methods appear successful and are becoming available to the clinician.

Radioactive in vitro tests of thyroid function. Many procedures have been developed to assess the state of the thyroid hormone plasma protein interaction. The in vitro uptakes generally reflect a portion of hormone in serum that is free. Because of the intense binding of T 4 by plasma proteins, in vitro uptake values for labeled T 4 are usually quite low. Greater ease in counting is obtained when labeled T 3 is employed. The weaker binding of T 3 results in higher uptake values and almost all of the clinical in vitro radioactive tests employ radioactive triiodothyronine.

Hamolsky and Freedberg developed the first (and still one of the most popular) in vitro tests of thyroid function. It was shown that if triiodothyronine labeled with ^{131}I was incubated with whole blood and the erythrocytes were then separated and washed, diagnosis could be drawn from the percent of the original labeled T 3 that remained fixed to the red blood cells. That is, the more saturated the binding protein is with thyroxine the greater the quantity of the added radioactive T 3 available for absorption on the red cell. The T 3 in vitro test has been changed by many investigators with replacement of the red cell by anion exchange resins, however, the basic principles are relatively the same. In hyperthyroidism, the binding sites are more filled and, therefore, a greater proportion of the added radioactive T 3 will be found unbound to the serum protein. In hypothyroidism the binding sites are not saturated and, therefore, the added radioactive T 3 will be bound to the available binding sites. Therefore, the results of the in vitro uptake studies will be relatively diagnostic. A large amount of unbound T 3 will occur in patients with hyperthyroidism, and decreased amounts will be found in patients with hypothyroidism. Values are greatly influenced by changes in the activity in the binding proteins as well as by changes in hormonal concentrations. For instance, estrogens increase the amount of binding sites available, therefore, a greater amount of the added radioactive T 3 will be found on the binding sites, which will invalidate the test. It has also been found that this particular in vitro test is relatively accurate in the diagnosis of hyperthyroidism and relatively inaccurate for diagnosing hypothyroidism.

Measurement of T 4 by binding displacement. A method for the measurement of T 4 in serum has been recently introduced. The method depends on the ability of increments of stable T 4 to progressively displace ^{125}I-labeled T 4 from thyroid-binding globulin. Ethanol, which denatures thyroxine-binding globulin (TBG), is added, releasing thyroxine into the serum. Following centrifugation a sample of the supernatant that contains free T 4 is obtained, the ethanol is evaporated, and a known quantity of TBG with ^{125}I-labeled T 4 is added. The combination is incubated with a resin sponge. Since the stable T 4 will displace the labeled T 4 on TBG, it is then possible to calculate the amount of T 4 in the patient's serum utilizing a standard curve of known concentrations of T 4. By knowing the total amount of thyroxine in the patient's blood, we have a better estimation of the patient's metabolic status. However, this test has the fallacy that the patient's binding globulins may be abnormal and indirectly cause peripheral effects of a thyroid disorder that is related to the amount of free T 4 in the patient's blood.

Free thyroxine measurements. Recently, it has been shown that the measurement of the concentration of free thyroxine in serum is possible. Serum is enriched with a very low concentration of ^{131}I-labeled T 4, to determine the proportion of endogenous hormone that is free to cross a semipermeable membrane. Normally, the proportion of free thyroxine in serum is no more than approximately 0.01 to 0.04% of the total amount of thyroxine. Obviously, increased concentration of thyroxine in serum is found in hyperthyroidism, but high values may also be obtained if there is decreased binding by the binding proteins.

DISEASES OF THE THYROID

To understand why the physician should want so many tests to study a small 20 to 35 gm organ, the student will have to understand both the importance of the thyroid gland to the body's metabolism and how diseases that affect the thyroid can have far-reaching metabolic effects in the human body. It is obvious that since there are so many tests to study the thyroid that no single test will give the clinician a definitive answer as to the thyroid status of his patient. The thyroid uptake test is used only to study how much radioiodine is found in the thyroid gland at given time intervals. The in vitro T 3 test is an indirect study of the thyroid hormone–binding proteins, and even the direct assessment of free thyroxine may lead to an erroneous diagnosis if the patient's thyroid hormone–binding proteins are abnormal in quantity or quality. Therefore, a discussion of all the ramifications of the results of these tests, as well as a discussion of thyroid diseases is necessary.

Hyperthyroidism

An excess of free thyroid hormone has a direct effect on the metabolic rate of the patient. Therefore, with an excess of free thyroid hormone, the patient becomes hypermetabolic. Hyperthyroidism is a relatively common disease and may be roughly broken down into two distinct entities: (1) Graves' disease and (2) Plummer's disease. The following outline gives the symptoms and the pathophysiology for each.

Graves' disease
  Signs and symptoms
    Diffuse thyroid enlargement (goiter)
    Hypermetabolism
    Exopthalmalopathy
    Dermopathy (pretibial myxedema)
  Pathophysiology
    Autonomous thyroid tissue
    Long-acting thyroid substance (LATS)
    Normal plasma levels of thyroid stimulating hormone (TSH)
    Increased serum levels of thyroxine
  Etiology—unknown

Plummer's disease
  Signs and symptoms
    Nodular thyroid enlargement
    Hypermetabolism
  Pathophysiology
    Autonomous nodularity
    Normal levels of TSH
    Increased serum levels of thyroxine
  Etiology—unknown

Graves' disease. Graves' disease is usually characterized by diffuse, smooth thyroid enlargement and the patient is hypermetabolic. The majority of patients with Graves' disease will have exophthalmopathy and dermopathy. The exophthalmopathy may be either minor or severe and may lead to subsequent blindness. The dermopathy usually takes the form of pretibial myxedema which is a pale, nonpitting swelling in the tibial areas.

The thyroid of the patient with Graves' disease is always autonomous (no longer under pituitary control). Formation and release of hormone are entirely under thyroid control. Generally, the patient will have increased serum levels of thyroxine and will always have normal plasma levels of thyroid stimulating hormone. In the majority of cases, long-acting thyroid stimulator substance (LATS) may be found. Long-acting thyroid stimulator substance has been found recently to be a 7 S gamma globulin, therefore, it is probably an antibody; this form of hyperthyroidism may have an immunologic basis. It has been shown that LATS does stimulate the human thyroid. However, LATS probably has no relationship to the ophthalmopathy of Graves' disease.

Graves' disease is of uncertain etiology and is known to remit spontaneously. It is difficult to treat. Approximately 50% of the patients with this disease will have spontaneous remissions; therefore, there is always a therapeutic dilemma. (This dilemma will be discussed in Chapter 23.) This disease occurs in persons of all age groups. Although classically patients have obvious signs of hypermetabolism, there are many in the younger as well as in the elderly groups who have few, if any, signs of hypermetabolism. Graves' disease is extremely protean. Classically, the patient with Graves' disease will have extreme nervousness, fatigue, weight loss, proximal muscle wasting, protrusion of the eyes, heat intolerance, and a wasting-away of the nail beds. A great many of the patients will have pretibial myxedema. Therefore the radioactive studies of the thyroid have been popular because of ease of both administration of the tests and interpretation of results.

Plummer's disease. Patients with Plummer's disease are hypermetabolic and have solitary or multiple nodules in the thyroid. These nodules are autonomous and are not under pituitary control. Normal serum levels of thyroid stimulating hormone and increased serum levels of circulating free thyroxine are found.

The etiology of Plummer's disease is unknown. Since Plummer's disease is a nodular autonomous disease, the therapy of this particular form of hyperthyroidism is much different from that for Graves' disease (see p. 348). It will be noted in the outline on p. 235 that patients with Plummer's disease do not have circulating LATS and, therefore, this form of hyperthyroidism is different from that of Graves' disease.

Hypothyroidism

The signs and symptoms of hypothyroidism are all related to hypometabolism, which is secondary to decreased tissue levels of thyroid hormone. In all patients except those with pituitary failure, increased serum levels of thyroid stimulating hormone and decreased serum levels of thyroxine are found. The following is an outline of the symptoms, pathophysiology, and etiologies of hypothyroidism.

Signs and symptoms
    Hypometabolism
Pathophysiology
    Increased serum TSH level in all except pituitary failure
    Decreased serum levels of thyroxine
Etiology
    Iodine deficiency
    Iatrogenic
        Iodine 131 therapy
        Antithyroid therapy
        Surgery
    Inborn error of metabolism (trapping iodine through secretion of thyroxine)
    Inflammatory (thyroiditis)
        Bacterial
        Viral
        Autoimmune

The etiologies of hypothyroidism are quite varied. Many cases of hypothyroidism in children are of the inherited enzyme defect type. In the baby and child hypothyroidism is quite severe. The baby born hypothyroid is called a cretin and has a very definite lethargic appearance, pot belly, and enlargement of the tongue. Physical and mental growth and development are severely retarded.

Hypothyroidism in the adult may be secondary to iodine deficiency. However, since iodized salt is used throughout the world, iodine deficiency is much less common than it was formerly. There is a large group of patients that have inborn errors of metabolism. These adults have a very slow onset of hypothyroidism and the defect may be found anywhere from the trapping of iodine through the secretion of thyroid hormone. The patient with an inborn error of metabolism of thyroid hormone production usually has an enlarged thyroid (a goiter), and the patient with pituitary failure or thyroid failure will have no palpable thyroid.

Another major cause of hypothyroidism is inflammatory diseases of the thyroid (thyroiditis). The inflammatory process may be bacterial, viral, or autoimmune.

Autoimmune disease is being recognized more frequently. In patients with autoimmune thyroiditis, there is a process of immunization against the body's own protein (in this case protein derived from the thyroid) and the body's reaction causes the thyroiditis.

Hypothyroidism may also occur secondary to ^{131}I therapy or to medical therapy of hyperthyroidism. It may also be caused by surgical ablation of the thyroid. A rare cause of hypothyroidism is pituitary failure or insufficient secretion of thyroid stimulating hormone by the pituitary.

True myxedema, which is the end stage of hypothyroidism, is fairly easy for the physician to recognize. However, the lesser forms of hypothyroidism are much more difficult to recognize. The classic myxedematous patient is extremely pale, has puffy facies, obvious fluid retention, and is lethargic. Few studies are necessary to make a diagnosis. However, other signs of hypometabolism, such as excessive tiredness, fatigability, and irritability, are common signs and symptoms of anxiety. Therefore, there is always a large group of patients under study for possible hypometabolism. If the administration of exogenous thyroid hormone completely corrects the hypometabolic state, thyroid therapy is indicated, regardless of the cause of the hypometabolism.

THYROID SCANNING WITH RADIONUCLIDES

Imaging and/or scanning of the thyroid is performed in order to (1) estimate the site, size, and shape of the thyroid gland and/or (2) define visually whether all or part of the thyroid is functional and/or nonfunctional. A combination of both purposes is usually involved when the physician sends the patient for a thyroid scan, after he has palpated an abnormality in the thyroid gland. The various disease states associated with an enlargement of the thyroid gland are listed below.

1. Decreased iodine intake
2. Goiterogenic agents
3. Familial goiter
4. Hashimoto's struma; chronic thyroiditis; lymphadenoid goiter; autoimmune thyroiditis
5. Subacute thyroiditis
6. Graves' disease
7. Autonomous nodular thyroid disease
8. Carcinoma

The relationships involved in the pituitary thyroid axis explain why many of the disease states listed would increase the size of the thyroid by interfering with the usual thyroid pituitary relationships. For example, if there was a decreased intake of iodine by the patient, there would be an increased output by the pituitary of thyroid stimulating hormone, and this would cause physical enlargement of the thyroid gland. In familial goiter a similar process takes place because of various biochemical defects in the thyroid; there is decreased output of thyroxine and an increased stimulation of thyroid stimulating hormone. In chronic thyroiditis the gland enlarges partially because of its decreased output of thyroxine, but also because of growth of replacement tissue caused by the destruction of the thyroid gland. It is obvious that the cancer would cause disruption of the thyroid gland and enlargement of all or part of the area palpated as thyroid tissue. It is also true that various thyroid carcinomas will metabolize iodine when they metastasize. Therefore, metastatic disease of the thyroid can sometimes be evaluated by radioiodine scanning.

In Graves' disease and Plummer's disease, enlargement of the thyroid gland is not under thyroid stimulating hormone control, and the cause for the enlargement is still unknown.

Radionuclides utilized in thyroid scanning and imaging

The most common radiopharmaceutical utilized in thyroid scanning is ^{131}I because of its relatively short effective half-life and ease of handling. ^{125}I has also been used for scanning because it is easier to collimate and it has a longer half-life and therefore a longer shelf-life than ^{131}I. Also the use of ^{125}I may possibly decrease the radiation dose received by the thyroid. Technetium 99m (in the form of pertechnetate) has also been utilized to image thyroid tissue. This radiopharmaceutical is becoming more popular, since the thyroid can be scanned a few minutes after the administration of pertechnetate and the image obtained is similar to that obtained with radioiodine.

Normal thyroid scan

The normal thyroid scans (Fig. 13-9) have an even distribution of the radioisotope throughout the area of the thyroid gland. The isthmus is so thin that it is

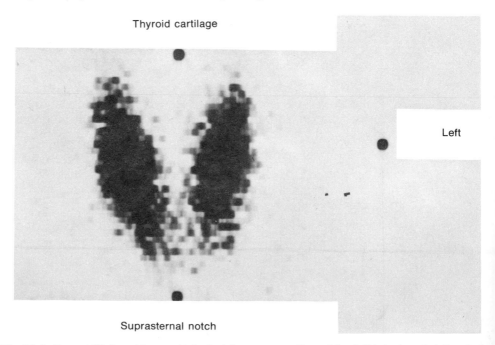

Thyroid cartilage

Left

Suprasternal notch

Fig. 13-9. Normal ^{131}I thyroid scan. Note that the upper portion of the left lobe is not delineated well. This is not uncommon as the upper poles of the thyroid go posteriorly around the trachea. This again emphasizes that palpation is necessary when interpreting the thyroid scan.

poorly delineated on most thyroid images; however, the lobes can be visualized quite well. With today's instrumentation the pyramidal lobe is seen frequently and since the embryologic as well as the adult anatomy of the thyroid is understood, tissue that could be found at the base of the tongue will be picked up on a thyroid scan, as would a thyroid in the mediastinum, where it is occasionally found. Aberrant thyroid tissue is found infrequently, however, aberrant thyroid tissue can be found both in the neck and in the abdomen. The thyroid tissue in the abdomen is usually found in female patients where it is associated with the ovaries.

Scanning of the abnormal thyroid

All thyroids that are scanned should be palpated before, during, and after the scanning procedure so that the radionuclide localization on the scan can be correlated with what is palpated by the referring and consulting physician.

Nonfunctioning areas of the thyroid are called "cold" areas; functioning areas are called "hot" areas. Since the student now understands collimation he can

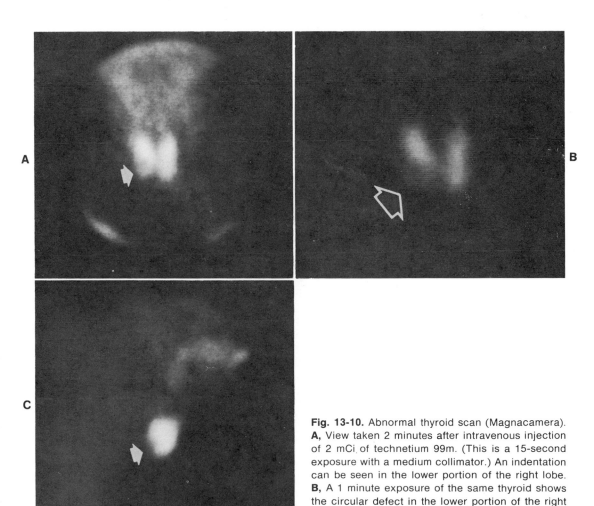

Fig. 13-10. Abnormal thyroid scan (Magnacamera). **A,** View taken 2 minutes after intravenous injection of 2 mCi of technetium 99m. (This is a 15-second exposure with a medium collimator.) An indentation can be seen in the lower portion of the right lobe. **B,** A 1 minute exposure of the same thyroid shows the circular defect in the lower portion of the right lobe. **C,** A 15 second lateral exposure revealing the lesion to be a posterior lesion.

readily see that the same problems encountered in scanning other organs are present in thyroid scanning. If an area is either hot or cold there is little difficulty in performing the study. However, if there is functioning tissue between a cold area and the detector or in the field of resolution of the detector, there are no longer black and white guide lines. Therefore, the thyroid, as well as other organs, should be scanned in various positions to clearly delineate whether a palpable mass is nonfunctioning or has some functional tissue residing in the area.

Cold nodule. It has been found through long experience that 25% of the cold nodules (Fig. 13-10) are malignant. Therefore, physicians place much emphasis on the patient who is found to have a solitary nodule by palpation. It is also known that when there are multiple cold nodules in the thyroid, as well as multiple areas of nodularity, the incidence of malignancy decreases quite sharply. The cold nodules may be thyroid adenomas, cysts, degenerated areas, areas of hemorrhage, or areas of lymphoid infiltration. A cold nodule in the thyroid may also be caused by metastatic disease from another primary site.

Hot nodule. Hot nodules (Fig. 13-11) are almost always benign. The hot nodule has significance when it leads to the diagnosis of autonomous nodular thyroid disease, as in Plummer's disease.

Thyroid scanning of a hot nodule is interesting, as the patient usually has a solitary palpable nodule which is found on scan to be hyperfunctional, and the remainder of the gland nonfunctional. In these patients, the thyroid hormone put out by the autonomous nodule is enough to shut off the normal pituitary thyroid relationship. The amount of thyroid hormone put out by the autonomous

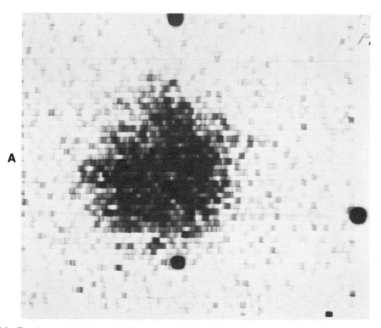

Fig. 13-11. For legend see opposite page.

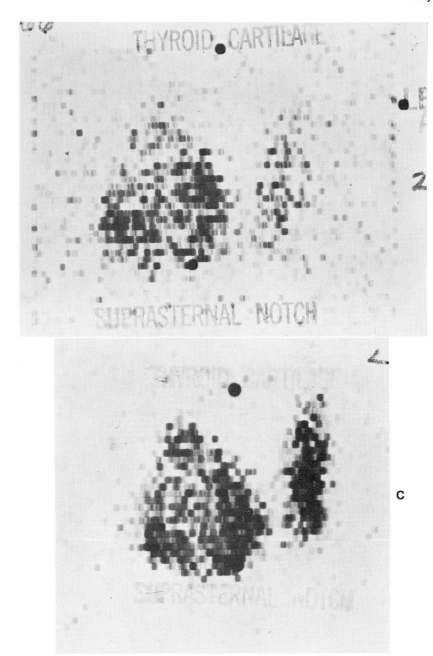

Fig. 13-11. Abnormal ^{131}I thyroid scan. **A,** A large autonomous nodule in the area of the right lobe is suppressing the left lobe. (This area was proved with Cytomel suppression and TSH studies.) **B,** This scan was done approximately 6 months later following a therapeutic dose of radioiodine. Enough radioiodine was given to destroy the nodule and the patient was placed on thyroid therapy to protect the remaining thyroid tissue. The patient had been off thyroid therapy for approximately 1 month at the time this scan was taken. The normal portion of the gland is just recovering. **C,** Scan performed 4 months after the patient had been taken off thyroid therapy. The patient has returned to a euthyroid state. Note the area of the right lobe which had contained the autonomous nodule that was destroyed by the ^{131}I therapy.

241

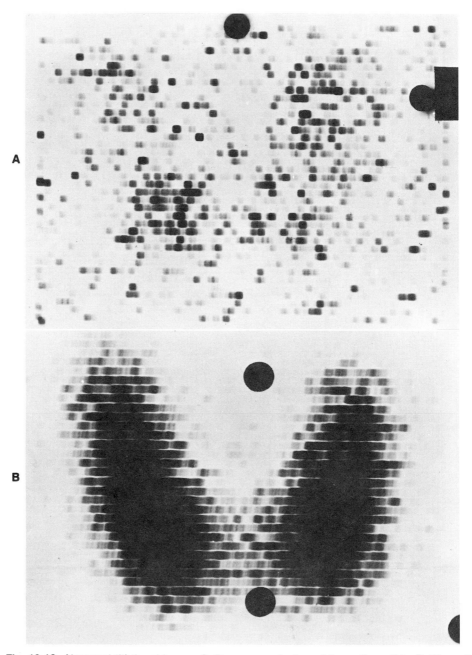

Fig. 13-12. Abnormal ¹³¹I thyroid scan. **A,** Poor concentration of the radionuclide. **B,** The patient was placed on therapy and restudied. Note the marked improvement in the scan picture. This study is compatible with subacute thyroiditis.

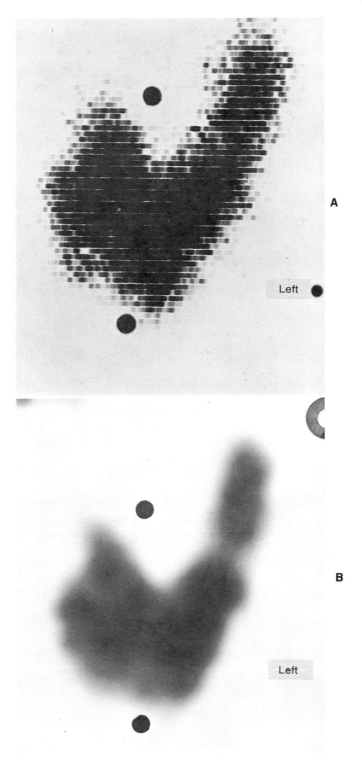

Fig. 13-13. Abnormal ¹³¹I thyroid scan. **A,** Enlarged multinodular thyroid gland. **B.** A light diffused ¹³¹I scan, which clearly shows the multinodularity of the gland.

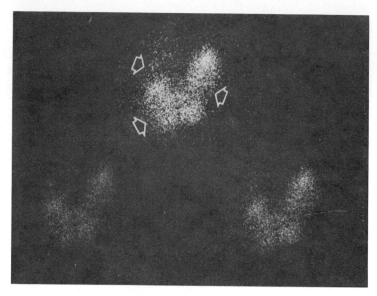

Fig. 13-14. Abnormal ^{131}I thyroid image of a multinodular, enlarged gland with multiple warm and cold nodules.

nodule may be enough to make the patient hyperthyroid. However, the patient may be found to be euthyroid or hypothyroid.

Mixed lesions in the thyroid (Figs. 13-12 and 13-13). It is obvious that there can be all gradations of abnormality in the thyroid, which will cause varying degrees in concentration of the radionuclide (Fig. 13-14). When the diagnostician has gained experience, he may be able to infer certain diagnoses by his palpatory findings in relation to the differing concentrations of the radionuclide on the thyroid scan. However, a definitive diagnosis is usually made only by biopsy and by pathologic examination.

SPECIAL STUDIES OF THYROID FUNCTION AND SCANNING

Thyroid stimulation tests and suppression tests have been developed to help the diagnostician come to a definitive diagnosis. The methodology of the best known tests is listed below.

I. Suppression tests
    A. Werner's suppression test
    B. Modified suppression test
        1. A baseline 24 hour RAIU is given
        2. Triiodothyronine, 75 μg, q.i.d. is given for 2 days, followed by 25 μg q.i.d. on days 3 and 4
        3. Residual activity is measured; repeat 24 hour RAIU between days 3 and 4
        4. If inadequate suppression is induced, T 3 is continued through day 8
        5. Residual activity is measured, and a third 24 hour RAIU is given between days 8 and 9
II. Stimulation tests (TSH)
    A. Use
        1. Differentiation of primary thyroid failure from hypothyroidism associated with pituitary hyposecretion
        2. Diagnosis of type of myxedema (primary or pituitary)
    B. Procedure
        1. A baseline 24 hour RAIU and a PBI are given

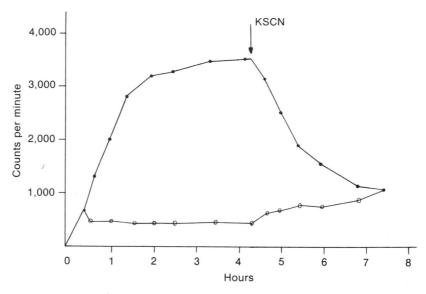

Fig. 13-15. Potassium thiocyanate (KSCN) release test which reveals a defect in organification of iodine.

2. Thyrotropin, 5 units, is given intramuscularly
3. Twenty-four hours after the thyrotropin injection, and following a count of residual activity in the gland, a second tracer of ^{131}I is administered, and a 24 hour RAIU is completed the following day (48 hours after injection of TSH)
4. A second PBI is obtained 48 hours after the TSH injection

Both the stimulating and the suppression tests will give physiologic information, and may also give anatomic information to the physician. In the case of thyroid stimulating hormone stimulation, the physician may want to see whether there is tissue in the neck that cannot be palpated or whether nonfunctional tissue as seen on an initial scan is still nonfunctional tissue after administration of thyroid stimulating hormone. The suppression study is usually used by a physician to identify autonomous thyroid tissue, which is found in both Graves' disease and Plummer's disease. It is used particularly for scanning a patient with a nodular thyroid, where the physician would like to know whether a nodule can be suppressed or not.

The physician may have a basic interest in intrathyroidal biochemical disturbances, such as may be found in congenital goiters. One test that is used to define one aspect of this disease process is the potassium thiocyanate discharge study, which is illustrated in Fig. 13-15. Since potassium thiocynate blocks the iodide trapping mechanism, if the patient has any defect in organification, nonorganified iodide will return through the cell wall back into the patient's vascular system.

A study under investigation at the present time is the technetium 99m pertechnetate accumulation study. Since pertechnetate lodges in the iodide trapping mechanism, it has been found that patients with hyperthyroidism will accumulate more pertechnetate per unit time than normal persons. It has also been shown grossly that in the majority of the hypothyroid patients, there is a decreased ability to lodge pertechentate in the trapping mechanism.

Chapter

14 *Brain*

ANATOMY AND PHYSIOLOGY

The nervous system together with the endocrine system, controls the functions of the body. The nervous system controls the rapid activities of the body, which include muscular contraction, perception of changing visual events, and the secretion rates of endocrine glands. The nervous system is the computer of the body; it receives thousands of bits of information from the internal and external environments and integrates all of these to determine the response to be made by the body. The nervous system is usually described as having a sensory division and a motor division. The cerebral cortex integrates the body's higher functions; most of the cerebral cortex is located in the cerebral hemispheres.

Cerebral hemispheres

The twin cerebral hemispheres, which make up a large portion of the brain, are separated by the longitudinal cerebral fissure (Fig. 14-1). The falx cerebri, an

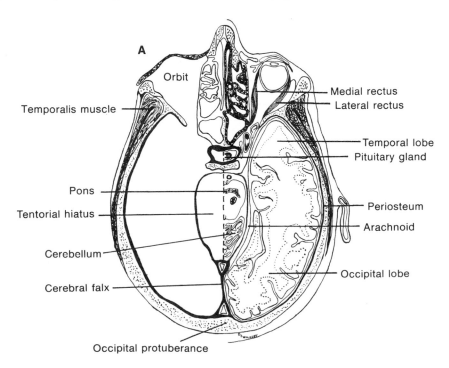

Fig. 14-1. The cerebral hemispheres. **A,** Horizontal section; **B,** sagittal section; **C,** posterior section.

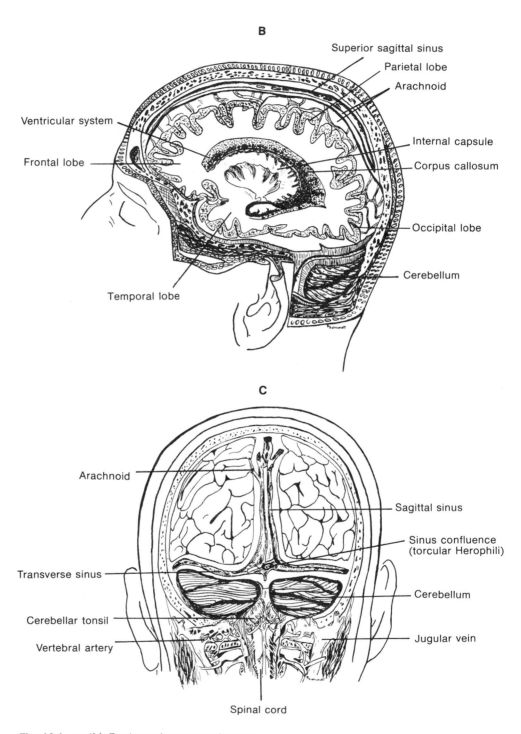

Fig. 14-1, cont'd. For legend see opposite page.

extension of the dura mater, projects into the longitudinal cerebral fissure. The cerebral hemispheres have dorsolateral, medial, and basal surfaces, which contain many grooves or furrows known as fissures and sulci. The part of the brain that lies between the grooves is known as convolutions or gyri. The cerebral hemispheres are divided into four lobes—the frontal, parietal, occipital, and temporal lobes. The lateral cerebral fissure (the fissure of Sylvius) separates the temporal from the frontal lobe. The central sulcus (fissure Rolando) separates the frontal lobe from the parietal lobe; the parietal occipital fissure passes along the medial surface of the posterior portion of the cerebral hemisphere dividing the parietal from the occipital lobe. The cerebral cortex has an area of approximately 2,200 square millimeters, and not more than one-third of this area lies upon the free surface or crown of the convolutions. The total number of the nerve cells in the human cerebral cortex has been estimated at between 7×10^9 and 14×10^9. There are approximately 200 million nerve fibers that are received from and projected to the lower levels of the nervous system. Many times this number of fibers associates the cells within the cortex.

Function of cerebral hemispheres. The functions of the four lobes can be grossly subdivided as follows. The posterior portion of the frontal lobe, the so-called prefrontal cortex of man, affects the motor system. This posterior portion is called the motor cortex, and it controls discrete voluntary movements of skeletal muscles. (The right side of the motor cortex controls the left side of the body and vice versa.) The parietal lobe receives the somatic sensory messages, and separate parts of the body are represented in a pattern closely resembling that of the adjacent motor cortex. The parietal lobe is also the part of the brain that receives sensations of stereoperception and can discriminate between differences in weight, texture, and position. The temporal lobe contains the cortical representation for hearing and is necessary to recognize and organize language. The occipital lobe's function is entirely related to vision. The nerve fibers that emanate or end in the cerebral cortex, cross in the brain stem; therefore, lesions of the left cerebral cortex are recognized peripherally in the opposite extremities.

Basal ganglia

The basal ganglia are masses of gray matter situated deep within the cerebral hemispheres. These ganglia exert important regulating and controlling influences on motor integration, in addition to relaying messages to the cerebral cortex. This area of the brain may also inhibit somatic reactions initiated by the cerebral cortex.

Thalamus and hypothalamus

The thalamus is a large ovoid gray mass located on either side of the third ventricle. It is crucial for the perception of some types of sensations. The hypothalamus lies below or ventral to the thalamus and forms a floor and part of the inferior and lateral walls of the third ventricle. This small area of the brain has diversified activities. The hypothalamus has a stimulatory control over many of the hormonal activities of the pituitary gland.

Cerebellum

The cerebellum is located in the posterior fossa of the skull behind the pons and medulla and is separated from the overlying cerebrum by an extension of the dura mater, the tentorium cerebri. The surface of the cerebellum, as does the surface of the cerebrum, has many sulci in furrows. The cerebellum is composed of a small, unpaired medium portion of the vermis and two large lateral masses, the cerebellar hemispheres.

Cerebellar functions. The cerebellum controls individual orientation in space and the antigravity muscles of the body. The nerve fibers that emanate from and end on one side of the cerebellum control that same side of the body (ipsilateral control).

Medulla oblongata

The medulla oblongata is a pyramid-shaped portion of the brain stem located between the spinal cord and the pons. The dorsal portion of the upper half forms the floor of the body of the fourth ventricle. The majority of the so-called cranial nerves have their primary nuclei in this portion of the brain. The cranial nerves are listed in Table 14-1. Since most of them have very specific functions, they can be easily learned and remembered and are quite useful in the localization of neurologic lesions in patients.

Spinal cord

The spinal cord, which traverses the vertebral column, consists of thirty-one symmetrically arranged pairs of spinal nerves, each derived from the spinal cord by two roots, a sensory root and a motor root. The nerves can be divided topographically, into eight cervical pairs, twelve thoracic pairs, five lumbar pairs, five sacral pairs, and one coccygeal pair. Each nerve contains several kinds of fibers. The motor fibers originate in large cells in the anterior gray column of the spinal cord. These form the ventral root and pass to the skeletal muscles. Sensory fibers originate in unipolar cells in the spinal ganglia within the ventricles.

Ventricle system

The ventricular system is a communicating system of four cavities or ventricles.

Lateral ventricles. Each of the two lateral ventricles has an anterior horn and a posterior horn. The anterior horn is imbedded in the frontal lobe and the posterior horn extends into the occipital lobe. The inferior horn traverses the temporal lobe. Cerebral spinal fluid, which bathes the brain, is manufactured in the choroid plexus, which is found on the interior of the lateral ventricles as a vascular fringe-like process of cellular material projecting into the ventricular cavity. It is covered by an epithelial layer of cells.

Third ventricle. The third ventricle is a vertical cleft between the two lateral ventricles.

Fourth ventricle. The fourth ventricle is a cavity which transverses the pons and medulla oblongata and is bordered dorsally by the cerebellum. The cerebral

Clinical nuclear medicine

Table 14-1. Cranial nerves

Nerve	Component	Course	Peripheral termination
Abducens	Somatic motor	Under pons, into orbit	Rectus lateralis
Accessory	Branchial motor	Side of neck	Sternomastoid
Facial	Branchial motor	Temporal bone, side of face	Muscles of expression, hyoid elevators
	Visceral motor	1. Greater superficial petrosal to sphenopalatine ganglion	Glands of nose, palate; lacrimal gland
		2. Chorda tympani to submaxillary ganglion	Submaxillary and sublingual glands
Glossopharyngeal	Branchial motor	Jugular foramen side of pharynx	Superior constrictor, stylopharyngeus muscles
	Visceral motor	Lesser superficial petrosal, to optic ganglion, to auriculotemporal nerve	Parotid gland
Hypoglossal	Somatic motor	Side of tongue	Muscles of tongue
Oculomotor	Somatic motor	Orbit	Rectus superior, inferior, medial; obliquus inferior; levator palpebrae muscles
Olfactory		Through roof of nasal cavity	Olfactory epithelium
Optic	Special somatic sensory	Orbit, to optic chiasm, to optic tracts	Bipolar cells of retina; rods and cones
Trigeminal	Branchial motor	With mandibular	Muscles of mastication
	General somatic sensory	Ophthalmic, maxillary, mandibular branches	Face, nose, mouth
Trochlear	Somatic motor	Orbit	Obliquus superior muscle
Vagus	Branchial motor	Recurrent and external branch of superior laryngeal nerve	Pharyngeal and laryngeal muscles
	Visceral motor	Along carotid artery, esophagus, stomach	Viscera of thorax and abdomen
	Visceral sensory	With motor	Viscera of thorax and abdomen
	General somatic sensory	Auricular branch	Pinna of ear
Vestibular	Special somatic sensory	Internal acoustic meatus	Cristae of semicircular canals, maculae of utricle and saccule
Cochlear	Special somatic sensory	Internal acoustic meatus	Organ of Corti

spinal fluid bathes the entire brain and the spinal cord. It is reabsorbed by the arachnoid—a tissue that covers the surface of the brain.

BRAIN CIRCULATION

Studies of the extent and quantity of arterial flow to the brain are important, since the brain is very sensitive to oxygen deprivation.

Arterial circulation

Arterial blood is delivered to the brain through the twined internal carotid arteries and the vertebral artery. The internal carotid artery primarily branches into the anterior cerebral artery, the middle cerebral artery, and the posterior cerebral artery. There is communication between the blood delivered by the internal carotid artery and that delivered by the vertebral arteries in the communicating circle of Willis at the base of the brain.

Venous circulation

The venous drainage of the brain is primarily through the dural sinuses, which are vascular channels lying within the dura. The superficial cortical veins drain largely into the medial superior longitudinal sinus. The two major cortical veins are the great veins of Trolard and the smaller anastomotic vein of Labbe, which drains caudally into the transverse sinus. Other important internal venous drainage veins are the internal cerebral vein, the great vein of Galen, and the inferior sagittal sinus, all of which flow into the straight sinus. The straight sinus drains caudally into the junction (torcular Herophili) of the superior sagittal sinus and the lateral sinuses. The lateral sinuses drain primarily into the internal jugular vein.

Pathophysiology of the cerebral circulation

The brain has great need of oxygen. It has been shown that brain metabolism accounts for approximately 8% of the total oxygen consumption of the body. Oxygen is used primarily for the oxidation of glucose; in the brain, carbohydrate metabolism is a chief source of energy. In man, the brain contains approximately 7 ml total oxygen, which, at normal rates of use, would last approximately 10 seconds. Therefore, the central nervous system tissues cannot withstand an oxygen deficit for longer than a few minutes.

The oxygen supply of the brain is maintained primarily by controls upon cerebral circulation. The most important of these are systemic blood pressure, certain vasomotor receptors (such as the carotid sinus receptor), and the aortic receptor. Vasomotor centers in the reflex regulation of blood flow depend upon cortical senstivity to both blood pressure and metabolic changes.

Each internal carotid artery supplies the cerebral hemisphere on its respective side of the body, and the basilar artery carries blood to the posterior fossa. The circle of Willis functions as an anastomotic pathway whereby, if an internal carotid artery is occluded, a pressure of about half of normal blood flow can be maintained through collateral blood vessels.

The blood-brain barrier

In the central nervous system of an adult, all cellular processes and vascular elements are closely packed; there is little or no extracellular space. The capillaries are completely invested by glial or neural processes, so there is no perivascular space. In the immature cerebral spinal central nervous system, there is incomplete glial development; neurons may contact capillary surfaces and there is direct neuron-to-neuron contact. There may also be space between cells and around capillaries.

In the immature central nervous system there is permeability to certain dyes, such as ferricyanide or blood bilirubin. Radioactive phosphorus enters more readily and in greater amounts in the brains of the newborn, since the central nervous system is incompletely developed. With complete glial investment, there develops a blood-brain barrier that hinders the free passage of many metabolites into the brain, thus protecting the brain from variations of blood composition and from entry of any toxic compound.

Simple expansion of the intracellular volume of water of the brain cells will cause the breakdown in this blood-brain barrier. Other disease states that influence the brain will also influence the breakdown of this protective blood-brain barrier. Inflammations involving the brain, brain tumors, or simple anoxia can also cause a breakdown of this protective barrier. Whether this barrier is intact or broken is most important in diagnosis of disease states.

NONRADIOACTIVE STUDIES OF BRAIN PATHOPHYSIOLOGY
Cerebrospinal fluid tests

Examination of the cerebrospinal fluid for pressure, protein, sugar, cell count, cultures, serologic tests, and cytologic analysis is usually helpful in the diagnosis of intracranial tumor. The incidence of abnormalities varies with the stage of the disease and the site and nature of the neoplasm. With slowly growing neoplasms, the intracranial pressure will remain normal until late in the illness. Many tumors cause a significant elevation of the protein level in the cerebrospinal fluid. With slowly growing tumors the protein may be normal, despite the presence of a huge mass. The lumbar puncture is contraindicated for critically ill patients with clinical signs of increased intracerebral pressure. However, the hazard is minimal if the patients do not have clinical signs of incipient herniation of the temporal lobe or of the cerebellar tonsils through the foramen magnum.

Electroencephalography

The electroencephalograph (EEG) is a method of studying the electrical brain wave pattern. Persons with epilepsy or seizures will have an abnormal EEG. The electrical discharges will be essentially synchronous discharges, interspersed with nonspecific patterns of high amplitude spikes and flow waves. Flow wave discharges localized in one region may suggest a focal cerebral lesion. In other types of epilepsy, such as petit mal (absence attack) which usually consists of a loss of consciousness for a short time, the electroencephalographic record reveals a slow rhythmic spike and wave discharge. The electroencephalograph has been used in screening for possible brain tumors. Focal changes, particularly a slowing in frequency of the record, are indications of neoplasm in the cerebral hemispheres. Rapidly growing tumors are more likely to evoke focal changes than are slowly progressive tumors; with the latter the record may be entirely normal. The EEG is often normal with posterior fossa neoplasms.

Roentgenographic contrast studies

Pneumoencephalography by the lumbar route (the introduction of air into the cerebrospinal fluid), ventriculography, and arteriography are of importance in the diagnosis and localization of brain tumors. Pneumoencephalography delineates the ventricular system and the subarachnoid space. It may reveal the presence of a mass lesion by displacement of the ventricles or invasion of the ventricular system. In ventriculography, air is injected through burr holes in the skull directly into the lateral cerebral ventricles. Cerebral angiography, via the carotid, vertebral, or brachial arteries may reveal the vascular patterns of the tumor, since the main arterial tree of the cerebrum may be displaced by the tumor or contrast media may stain the tumor. All of the roentgenographic contrast studies are special procedures and merit special handling techniques of the patient by specialized personnel.

The pneumoencephalography studies are best suited for small midline lesions and the arteriography techniques are limited if a space occupying lesion has not disrupted the normal arterial tree.

Echoencephalography

Ultrasonic energy transmitted from one side of the head to the other may indicate differences in the density of the intervening structures. Therefore, a shift of the intracranial context may be determined. For tumors or other lesions that will cause a shift of the intracerebral structures, this test is a useful screening device.

RADIONUCLIDE LOCALIZATION OF BRAIN PATHOLOGY

Brain imaging utilizing radionuclides was introduced in the late 1940's and early 1950's. Since that time this technique has become a well-established technique for the screening of suspected neuropathology. The popularity of brain scanning or brain imaging as a screening technique is based on the fact that localization of neuropathology on the basis of altered function is quite difficult. Such localization is difficult because localization of function is not fully understood and localizing clinical signs may be produced by involvement of structures remote from the original lesion. Based on the previously discussed neurology, it can be readily understood that signs and symptoms of cerebral vascular disease may be quite diffuse. The medical procedures mentioned previously to localize neuropathology have serious limitations when compared to radionuclide localization. Electroencephalography and echoencephalography are innocuous procedures, but many lesions may be missed utilizing these two screening modalities. Radiographic contrast studies as performed today are not harmless, since they necessitate the intraarterial injection of contrast media. All of these procedures have known morbidity. Therefore, because brain scanning and imaging are safe procedures, they have earned a place in the medical armamentarium.

Radionuclides utilized in brain scanning and imaging

A major reason for the passage of radionuclides into abnormal areas of the brain is the breakdown of the so-called blood-brain barrier. Obviously, there are many disease states that will influence the blood-brain barrier and will increase permeability to substances not normally found in the cerebral cells. True proof of this localization has awaited the increasing use of the electron microscope and microautoradiography techniques. These improved qualitative and quantitative techniques will open the way for further improvements in this field.

Radioiodinated human serum albumin (RISA). Radioactive albumin injected intravenously diffuses slowly into brain tumors, but not into normal brain cells. The blood level remains high since labeled albumin is not excreted and is catabolized at a slow rate. Persistence of a high level of radioactivity in the blood enhances diffusion of the albumin into tumors and/or abnormal tissue; however, it decreases the so-called target (tumor) to nontarget (normal brain) ratio. It has been shown that radioiodinated albumin is transferred into the capillary endothelium of tumors by pinocytosis and that the degree of pinocytotic activity is increased in neoplastic cells. (Pinocytosis is the process by which particles, molecules, or ions are engaged by the cytoplasmic membrane of the cell, which creates a vesicle including them. The vesicle is then pinched off from the cell surface and it travels into the intracytoplasmic compartment. Here the vesicles may release their contents or remain as cell components, or they may extrude the contents from the cell. Therefore, the uptake of RISA is explained by high pinocytotic activity of the tumor cells.) Twenty-four hours after the injection of radioactive albumin, 59% of the radioactivity of the tumor is found in the tumor cell, 25% is intravascular, and 16% is interstitial. All of the radioactivity in the tumor is protein bound. Radioactive albumin has been utilized for brain work since 1953. However, because of the initial concentration of labeled albumin in the vasculature, scanning or imaging has to be delayed at least for 24 hours. Also, because ^{131}I is used, some of the high energies of iodine penetrate commercial collimators, which impairs spacial imaging.

Although it has been reported that albumin-bound substances have a greater tumor to normal brain ratio than other substances, investigators have been able to quantitatively demonstrate in vitro that the radioactive mercurial nuclides have twice the uptake in abnormal tissue as compared to radioactive albumin.

^{131}I albumin has also been utilized intrathecally. It has been introduced into the ventricular system to aid in the diagnosis of brain tumor, internal hydrocephalis, and cerebrospinal fluid rhinorrhea. The leaking site may be found with apparent ease utilizing this technique.

Radioactive mercury chlormerodrin. Chlormerodrin is a mercurial diuretic that is rapidly excreted by the kidneys following intravenous injection. It, therefore, decreases the blood level much more rapidly than RISA. ^{203}Hg chlormerodrin was first used for brain scanning; however, ^{197}Hg chlormerodrin is now preferred, since ^{203}Hg causes irradiation of the kidneys. ^{197}Hg chlormerodrin has a blood clearance half-life from 1 to 3 hours. It has been shown through microautoradiography of tumors that radioactive mercury is deposited on or in abnormal tumor cells. By the use of quantitative counting, it has been shown that the majority of the radioactive mercury ions are concentrated in tumor cells. It has also been shown that radioactive mercury localizes in nearly all areas of cerebral pathology.

Obviously, if the radionuclide is injected intra-arterially, arteriovenous fistulas or other arteriovenous anomalies may be demonstrated also.

[197]Hg chlormerodrin has been found to be a most useful radiopharmaceutical as a brain screening agent because of the retention of the mercury by abnormal tissue. Thus, a lesion may be rescanned or reimaged at a later time to validate previous results.

Technetium 99m pertechnetate. Technetium 99m pertechnetate has an ionic extracellular distribution pattern; however, it remains mainly in blood pools for 5 to 15 minutes after intravenous injection. Technetium 99m has gained popularity because it has a half-life of 6 hours, it emits monoenergetic gamma rays at 140

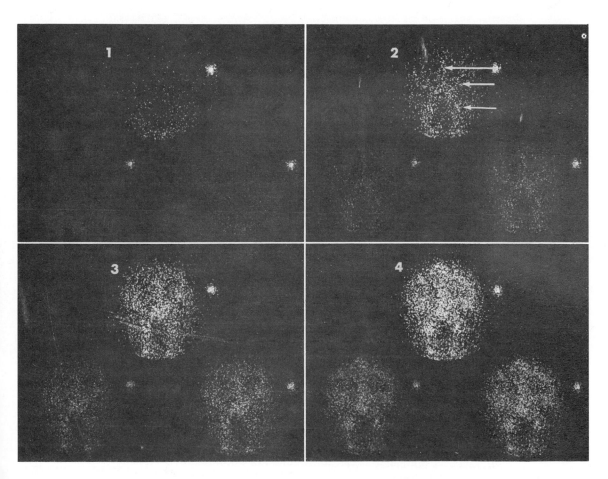

Continued.

Fig. 14-2. Normal technetium 99m brain flow study and static imaging study. Views *1* through *3* cover the 6 seconds after the bolus of 10 mCi of ^{99m}Tc has reached the level of the common carotid artery. Note that the carotids, the anterior cerebrals, and the middle cerebrals can be delineated as can the areas that they perfuse. The series of images from *5* through *8* cover the static imaging studies that were done between 30 minutes and 1 hour after injection of pertechnetate. These images are the four routine views done: anterior, posterior, and the laterals. These images delineate the large vascular sinuses.

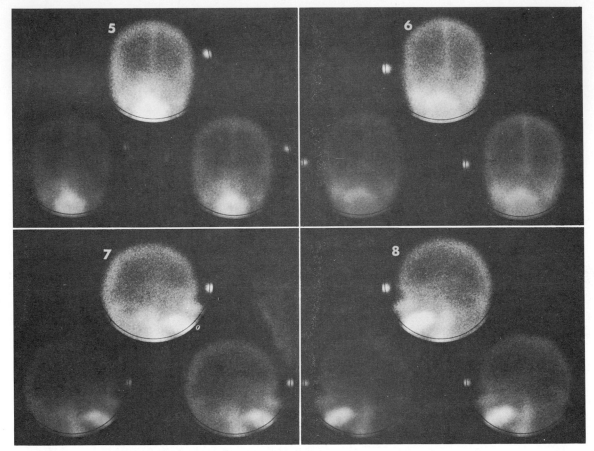

Fig. 14-2, cont'd. For legend see page 255.

kev, and it is easily collimated. One of the main screening defects of the pertechnetate is the fact that it localizes in the choroid plexus. The choroid accumulation at times makes the interpretation of this area difficult.

Positron emitters and other generator-produced radionuclides. The positron emitters such as arsenic 74 and rubidium 84 are primarily found in the intracellular spaces and are characterized by a rapid rate of diffusion into brain tumor. However, cyclotron facilities are needed for their production. Indium, a generator-produced radionuclide, appears to have the same potential as ^{99m}Tc pertechnetate; however, it is still under research investigation.

BRAIN SCANNING AND IMAGING

The routine positions that are used in brain scanning or imaging are illustrated in Fig. 14-4.

Accurate positioning is more important in nuclear medicine than in roentgenology. In nuclear medicine the physician does not have the bony landmarks

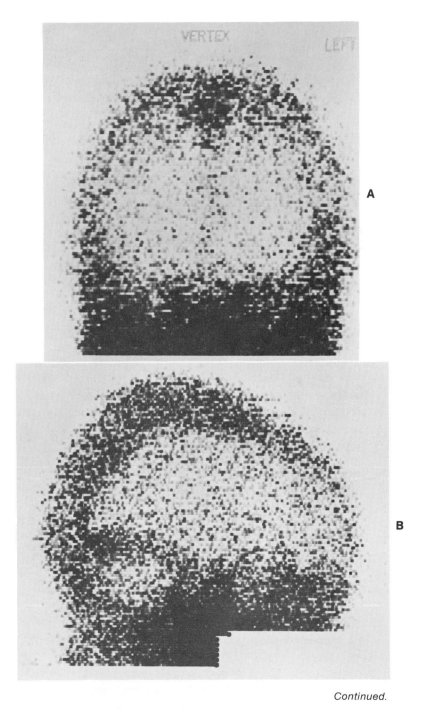

Continued.

Fig. 14-3. Normal brain scan series: anterior **(A)**, right lateral **(B)**, and posterior **(C)** views.

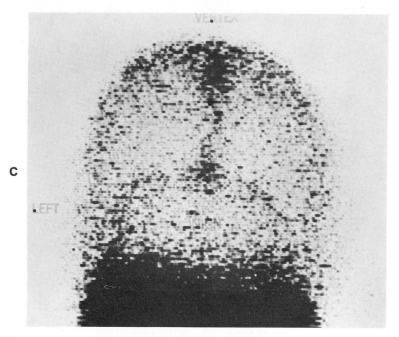

C

Fig. 14-3, cont'd. For legend see page 257.

portrayed on his scan, therefore, the technician must place markers on the scan that accurately denote the landmarks.

There is little reason to spend much time on the portrayal of the normal brain image. If the technician utilizes the proper radionuclides and uses acceptable data presentation, the dynamic camera studies which image the flow of the radionuclide through the brain will give a representation of the arterial flow of the brain in the first 8 seconds. If the imaging of the gross arterial tree of the brain is done immediately after the injection of the radionuclide the physician may be able to infer whether there is decreased flow to an area of the brain or absent flow to an area of the brain. In this way there is a rather gross presentation of the early portion of arteriography. Rectilinear brain scanning and a longer imaging time will primarily portray the venous mixing phase of the radionuclide and will also portray abnormal accumulation of the radionuclide in brain tissue. Thus, normal and abnormal architecture of the brain can be inferred from a brain image or scan.

Clinical indications for brain scanning

Brain tumors and other neuropathology. One of the fundamental reasons for employing brain scanning as a screening study is to localize a brain tumor (Figs. 14-5 and 14-6). Brain tumors account for approximately 3% of all neoplasms and occur in all age groups. Metastatic brain tumors, however, are now recognized with increasing frequency since brain scanning is more widely used. In metastatic disease there are usually multiple sites, whereas primary tumors usually occur singly.

Positive brain scans are related to the amount of neovascularity in the abnormal

Text continued on p. 265.

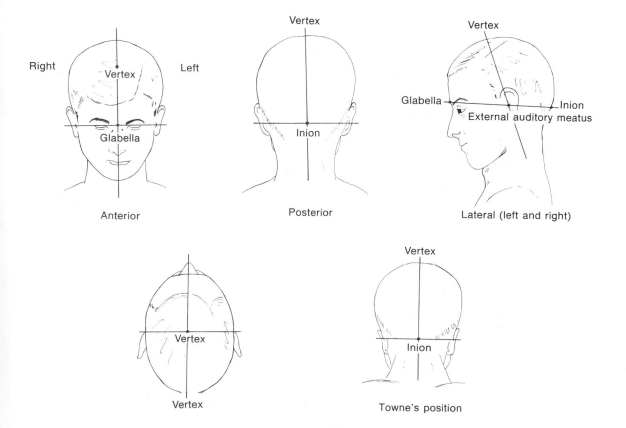

Fig. 14-4. Nuclear medicine brain scanning positions. *Anterior position.* The patient is in a supine position; his head is elevated and his chin is tucked down until a horizontal line passes through the external auditory meatus and the outer canthus of the eye; the midsagittal line is perpendicular to this line. *Posterior position.* The patient is in a prone position. The chest is elevated and the chin is tucked down as in anterior view. The chin is tucked toward the chest so that a horizontal line will pass through the external auditory meatus and the outer canthus of the eye and the midsagittal line forms a perpendicular with the horizontal line. *Lateral position.* With patient on his side, his head is positioned so that a line drawn from vertex to external auditory meatus superimposes an identical line on the other side of the head. The chin should be brought toward the chest until a horizontal line can be drawn from the glabella to the inion. *Vertex position.* The patient is sitting; midsagittal and coronal lines are drawn crossing at the vertex. Of all positions, this is the least useful. *Towne's position.* The patient is positioned as for a posterior view, however greater angulation of approximately 10 to 30 degrees is obtained by pulling the chin toward the chest to allow the straight sinus to be tipped out of view so that the cerebellum (posterior fossa) can be observed without background interference.

259

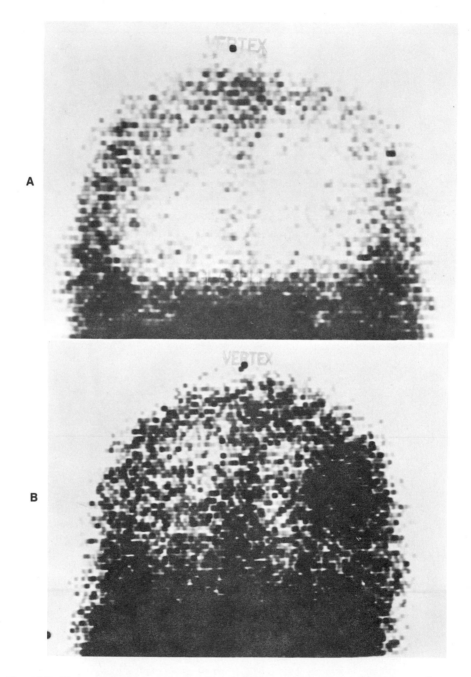

Fig. 14-5. Abnormal brain scan series demonstrating a right parietal astrocytoma. **A** through **D,** Scans obtained after administration of ^{99m}Tc. **E,** Right lateral view done 10 days later using the same dosage and technique. There is no change in the lesion.

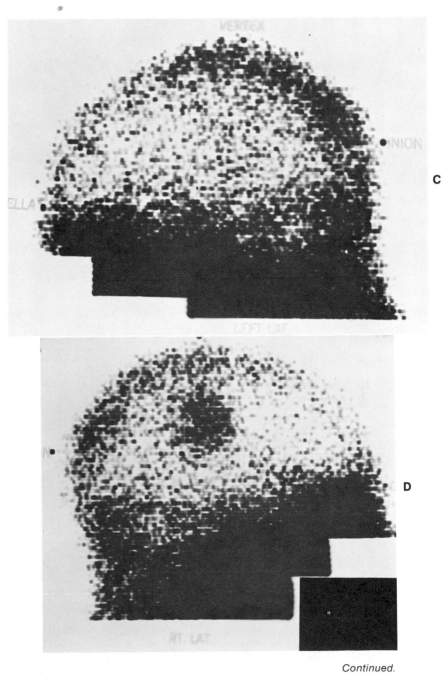

C

D

Continued.

Fig. 14-5, cont'd. For legend see opposite page.

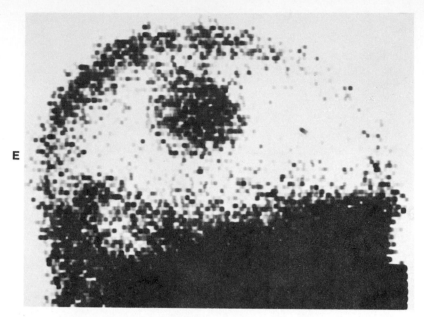

E

Fig. 14-5, cont'd. For legend see page 260.

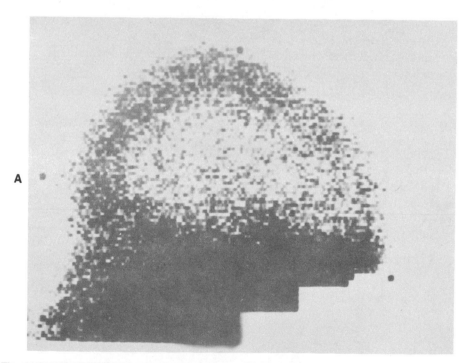

A

Fig. 14-6. Abnormal brain scan series demonstrating metastatic disease. **A,** A 1 hour ^{99m}Tc right lateral brain scan reveals no evidence of a space-occupying lesion. **B,** A 6 hour ^{197}Hg right lateral brain scan reveals no conclusive evidence of a space-occupying lesion. **C,** ^{197}Hg right lateral scan done 24 hours after administration of ^{197}Hg reveals two separate metastatic sites, one in the prefrontal region and one in the occipital lobe. **D,** The test was repeated 12 days later after cortisone therapy. This scan, taken 24 hours after ^{197}Hg injection, reveals slightly decreased count rate in the previously noted lesions, and the possibility of a third metastatic site. **E,** A 24 hour post-injection scan was performed 2 months later and revealed an apparent increase in the number of lesions.

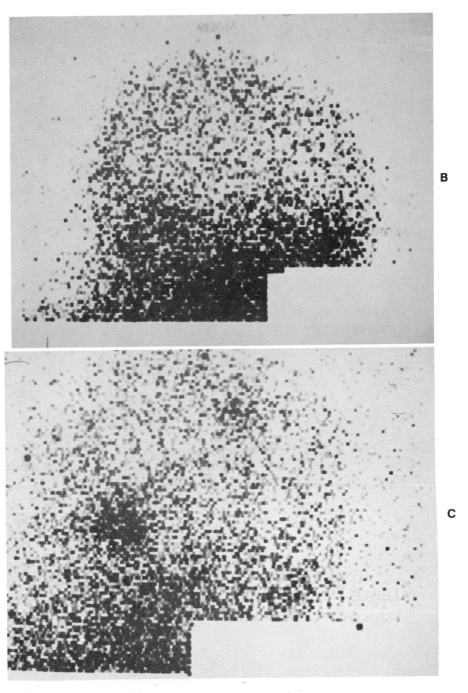

B

C

Continued.

Fig. 14-6, cont'd. For legend see opposite page.

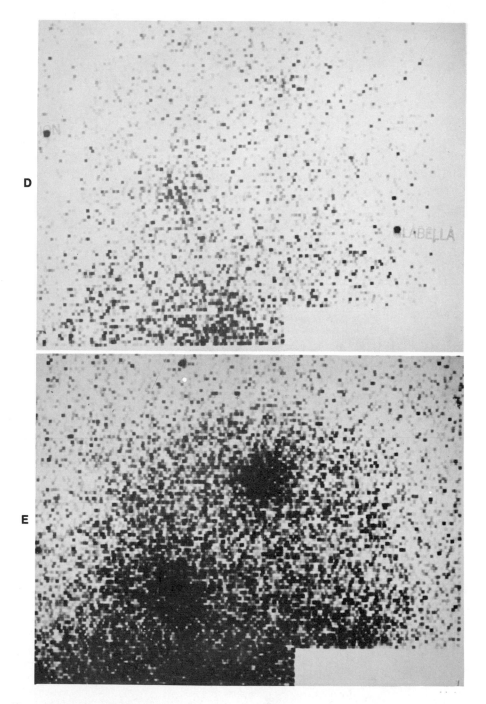

Fig. 14-6, cont'd. For legend see page 262.

brain tissue. Therefore, in certain cases scans obtained with a short-lived radio-pharmaceutical, such as ^{99m}Tc pertechnetate, are negative, while delayed scans (6 to 48 hours) with a longer-lived radiopharmaceutical, such as ^{197}Hg chlormerodrin, are positive. In such disease states, because of the decreased vascularity of the lesion, it takes longer to obtain sufficient concentration of radioactivity in the area to visualize the abnormality. Metastatic brain disease, infarcts, inflammatory disease, and intracerebral hemorrhage have decreased vascularity. Therefore, both early and delayed imaging or scanning using several radiopharmaceuticals are indicated.

Cerebrovascular diseases. Abnormalities of the circulation of the brain (Fig. 14-7) may result from decreased oxygen content in the brain, emboli to the brain, hemorrhage from one of the cerebral vessels, and cerebral contusion. Positive brain scans may be obtained when there is hemorrhage into surrounding brain tissue, infarction (death of tissue), and possibly severe anoxia. All three of the above etiologies would cause a defect in the normally intact blood-brain barrier.

Obviously, small cerebral thromboses or small areas of embolization may not cause gross defects in the blood-brain barrier, because of the collateral circulation of the brain. However, for reasons that are difficult to define, approximately one-half of the patients with clinical vascular occlusions will develop a positive brain scan over a period of as long as 3 weeks following the insult. These lesions, cannot be differentiated from brain tumors without special techniques.

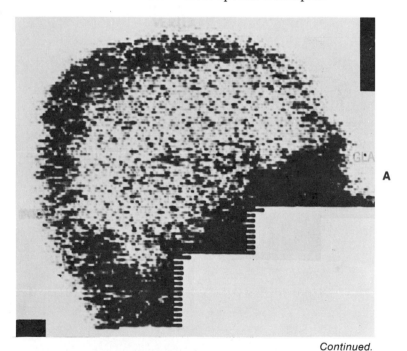

Continued.

Fig. 14-7. Abnormal brain scan series demonstrating a middle cerebral artery thrombosis. **A,** The scan taken 1 to 2 hours after administration of ^{99m}Tc. This scan could be read as being within normal limits. **B** and **C,** Right residual lateral scans taken 24 and 48 hours after administration of ^{197}Hg show gross abnormalities.

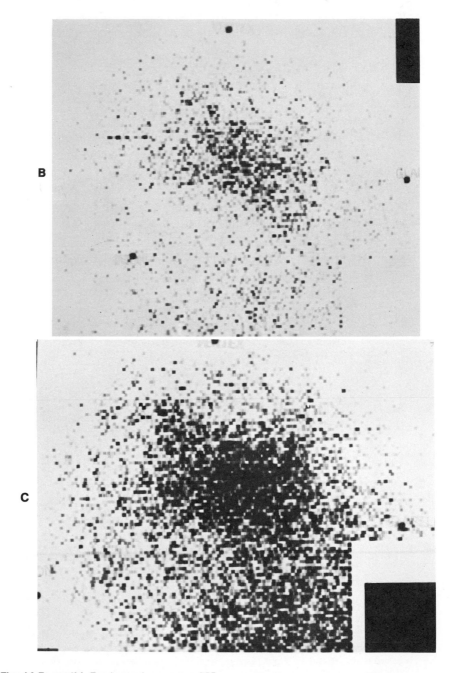

Fig. 14-7, cont'd. For legend see page 265.

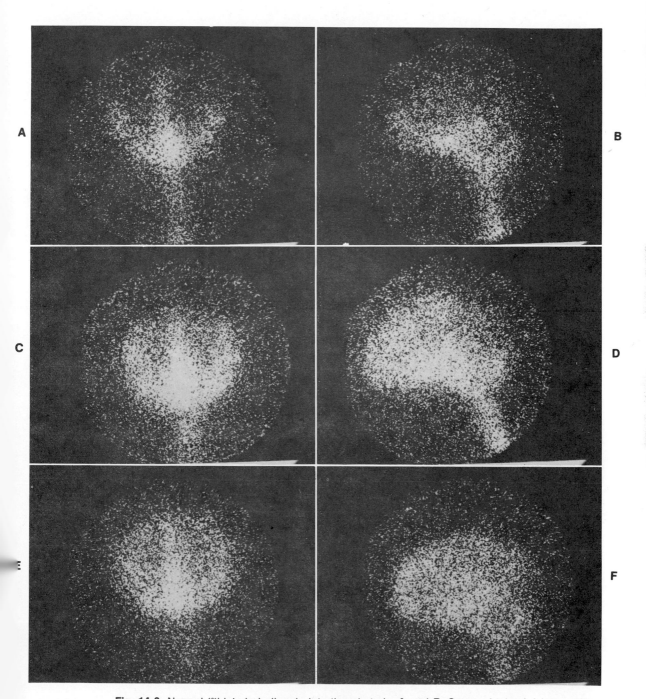

Fig. 14-8. Normal ¹³¹I-labeled albumin intrathecal study. **A** and **B,** Scans obtained 4 hours after injection of ¹³¹I-labeled albumin. **A,** Anterior view; **B,** left lateral view. **C** and **D,** Scans obtained 8 hours after injection. **C,** Anterior view; **D,** left lateral view. **E** and **F,** Scans obtained 24 hours after injection. **E,** Anterior view; **F,** left lateral view.

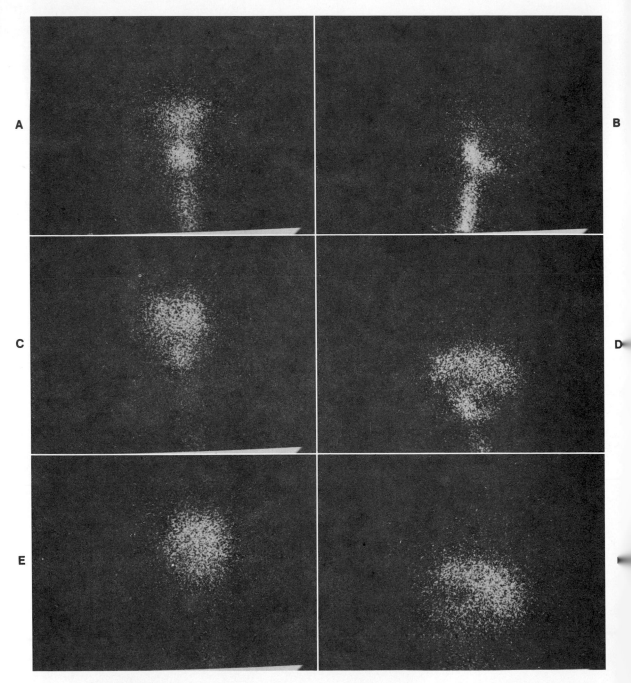

Fig. 14-9. Abnormal ^{131}I-labeled albumin intrathecal study in a 3-month-old infant with hydro-
cephalus. **A** and **B,** Scans obtained 30 minutes after injection of ^{131}I-labeled albumin. **A,** Anterior
view; **B,** left lateral view. **C** and **D,** Scans obtained 1 hour after injection. **C,** Anterior view;
D, left lateral view. **E** and **F,** Scans obtained 4 hours after injection. **E,** Anterior view; **F,** left
lateral view. (Courtesy, August Miale, Jr., M.D. and Glen A. Landis, M.D.; Radioisotope Unit,
Georgetown University Hospital, Washington, D.C.)

With knowledge of the arterial tree of the brain it is sometimes possible to tell whether or not the abnormality on the brain scan has been caused by a specific vessel that is occluded. Nearly half of the large vascular occlusions occur in the middle cerebral artery. It has also been found that in most of the patients who have vascular accidents which produce abnormal brain scans, there is gradual clearing of part or all of the abnormality over a period of weeks. In brain tumors, this change is not seen; the count rate in the area of the brain tumor over a period of weeks will increase as the size of the lesion increases.

STUDIES OF THE CEREBROSPINAL FLUID

There are certain conditions that may be studied with injection of radionuclides into the spinal fluid (Figs. 14-8 and 14-9). Certain tumors involve the cerebrospinal space and cause total or subtotal blocks that can be easily studied. The intrathecal injection of ^{131}I albumin has been used to study the ventricular system, brain tumor, internal hydrocephalis, and cerebral rhinorrhea. The latter diagnosis is interesting and is a sequel to skull fracture. With a basilar skull fracture cerebrospinal fluid will leak through the bony tables into the nasal region. This may be visualized on multiple postinjection views of the radionuclide into the cerebrospinal fluid as a leak of radioactivity into the nasal region.

Cerebral circulation time and cerebral blood flow

Cerebral circulation time and blood flow are not unlike the dynamic function and flow studies of other organs of the body. In studying the cerebral circulation time, a nondiffusable radionuclide, such as ^{131}I albumin, is injected intravenously and its course through the brain is measured with appropriate instrumentation. Diffusable tracers are utilized for the measurement of total cerebral blood flow. The most common diffusable tracers are the inert gases, such as krypton 79 and xenon 133. These agents may be injected interarterially or may be administered by inhalation.

The above techniques are applicable in very few medical centers. However, there is much interest in the possible screening reliability of these procedures in cerebral vascular disease.

SUMMARY

Radionuclide brain imaging or scanning is an accepted screening procedure which is now widely utilized by all medical specialties. The procedure as performed today has no patient morbidity and patients with the earliest of neurologic symptoms or behavior disorders may be studied. Therefore, correctable neurosurgical lesions may be inferred at a stage in their development for which greater cure rates are possible. Because there are accurate imaging and scanning techniques and an increasing number of interpreters who have the necessary training and clinical experience, the referring physician can be reassured that if a normal report is given, the patient, in all probability, does not have a neurosurgical lesion.

The cerebral blood flow studies are now under investigation and will probably have great clinical applicability in the study of cerebral vascular disease.

15 *Lung*

ANATOMY AND PHYSIOLOGY

The main function of the lung is gaseous exchange. This exchange consists of the extraction of oxygen from atmospheric air and the disposal of gaseous waste products of the body. The diseases that affect the lung can be understood in terms of the anatomy of the airway system in which atmospheric air flow takes place and of the histology of the large membrane system through which the exchange of oxygen and gaseous products takes place.

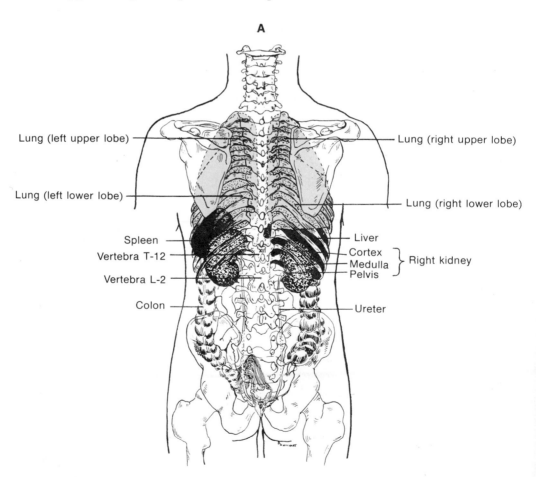

Fig. 15-1. A, Posterior anatomic relationships of large organs; **B,** right lateral relationships; **C,** left lateral relationships; **D,** posterior view of tracheobronchial tree.

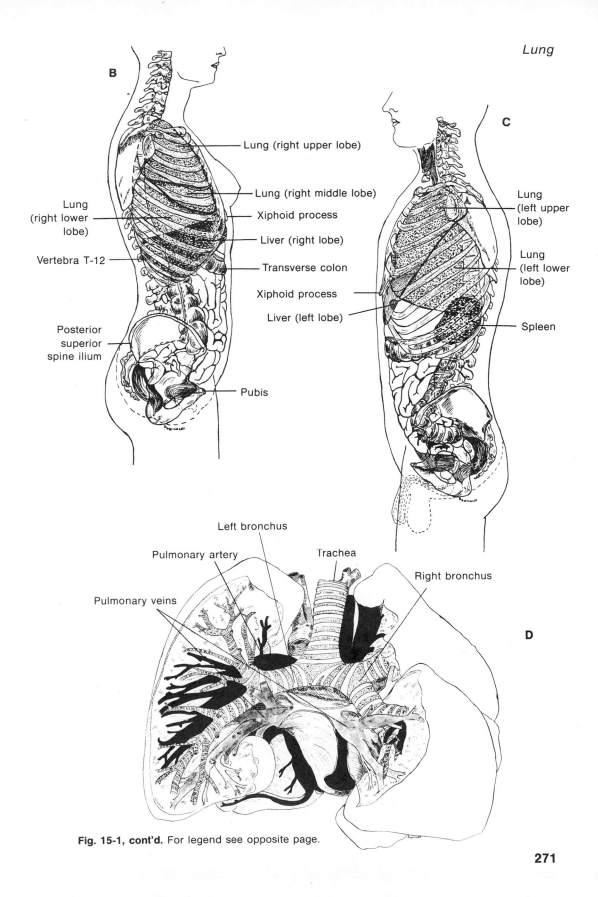

B

Lung (right upper lobe)

Lung (right middle lobe)

Xiphoid process

Lung
(right lower
lobe)

Liver (right lobe)

Vertebra T-12

Transverse colon

Posterior
superior
spine ilium

Pubis

C

Lung
(left upper
lobe)

Lung
(left lower
lobe)

Xiphoid process

Liver (left lobe)

Spleen

Left bronchus

Pulmonary artery

Trachea

Right bronchus

Pulmonary veins

D

Fig. 15-1, cont'd. For legend see opposite page.

The airway

Air is carried to the lung through a system of airways that begins at the trachea and extends into alveolar units. The trachea divides into the two bronchi, which in turn divide into progressively smaller units, and end at the terminal bronchials. These bronchials deliver air to the alveoli, the final air sacs where the exchange is made between the inspired air and the bloodstream. The airways are lined with two different types of cells, the ciliated and the goblet cells. The goblet cells produce mucus, and the ciliated cells have cilia which protect the airways. The unidirectional action of the cilia propels substances toward the mouth (Fig. 15-1).

The lung has two separate and vital functions—a ventilatory function and a respiratory function. The ventilatory function is the process of moving gas in and out of the lungs from the external environment to the alveolar wall.

The respiratory function is more complex than the ventilatory function as the transfer of gas between the alveoli and blood is an active metabolic process and is also dependent on the delivery of blood to the alveolus.

Pulmonary circulation

Approximately 90% of the blood supply of the lung is carried through the right and left pulmonary arteries, and 10% of the blood supply comes from the systemic circulation through the bronchial arteries, which come off the aorta. The pulmonary arterial system branches to the right upper lobe, to the right middle lobe and right lower lobe, and to the two major portions of the left lung (the left upper and lower lobes). The arteries then subdivide segmentally, finally to end in an arteriolar capillary unit which surrounds the alveolus.

METHODS OF STUDYING LUNG FUNCTION

The ventilatory function of the lung is studied by pulmonary function studies. Volumes of air in the lung are usually studied by means of an instrument called a *spirometer.* The *residual volume,* approximately 1,200 ml of air, is the air found within the chest after a maximal expiration. A *functional residual capacity* is the resting lung volume at the end of a quiet expiration. *Tidal volume,* approximately 500 ml, is the volume of one normal breath. *Vital capacity,* approximately 4,800 ml of air, is the total volume that can be delivered after a full inspiration. *Total lung capacity,* approximately 6,000 ml, is the volume within the chest at full inspiration. *Maximal voluntary ventilation* is the greatest rate that the patient can sustain for 15 seconds and is usually expressed as amount of air exchanged per minute. With the above nonradioactive studies, physicians can judge whether ventilatory impairment is obstructive or just restrictive.

Utilizing special equipment, the physician can also measure gas concentrations if the patient is rebreathing in a closed system.

Tests of respiratory function usually need technical equipment and are more difficult for the physician to interpret. These studies include evaluation of the arterial and venous blood gases, both oxygen and carbon dioxide. Finally, using radiographic techniques, the radiologist may instill contrast media into the tracheobronchial system to demonstrate patency of the airway; contrast media can also be injected to visualize the major arterial system of the lung.

Nuclear medical tests of pulmonary function

Radioactive tracers have made estimation of regional pulmonary function as well as a simple estimation of pulmonary arteriolar perfusion possible.

Radioactive tests of ventilation

Recently, several investigators have utilized radioactive aerosol in the evaluation of the function of the tracheobronchial tree. Aerosol particles have varied in size from 5 to 100 μ and various radiopharmaceuticals have been utilized including macroaggregates of albumin labeled with iodine 131 and technetium 99m. The studies are said to have accuracy in the evaluation of the patency of the tracheobronchial tree by scanning.

Respiratory ventilation has also been studied by having the patient breathe radioactive gas through a closed system. Multiple detectors or scanners, qualitatively and quantitatively measure the amount of radioactivity found over areas of the lung. Oxygen 13, carbon 11, and nitrogen 13 have been used for these lung function studies. These radionuclides are primarily produced by a cyclotron. More recently, xenon 133 has been utilized to estimate both respiration and ventilation of the lung. Using a closed breathing system the patient inspires radioactive xenon and the radioactive gas enters various regions of the lung at a rate directly related to ventilation. This method also may be extended until the radioactivity reaches equilibrium. This particular equilibrium time method gives an indication of alveolar ventilation.

A measure of both perfusion and respiration can also be tested with radioactive xenon by placing it in solution and injecting it intravenously into the patient. The patient holds his breath during injection so the xenon will reach the pulmonary capillary bed and diffuse into the air within the alveoli. As the patient holds his breath for 10 seconds, intrapulmonary distribution of radioactivity is determined primarily by regional pulmonary blood flow, which can be measured with external radiation detectors.

Radioactive study of lung perfusion

In recent years it has been shown that injected radioactive macroparticles lodge in the capillary bed of the lung. This has been demonstrated with the use of such materials as macroaggregated albumin [131]I. A direct estimation of regional perfusion can be made utilizing external detectors. In this case, quantitative and qualitative information of perfusion can be obtained rapidly with scanners or cameras.

Macroaggregated albumin ^{131}I can be safely administered to man. There are no hemodynamic effects from the use of the macroaggregates, which range from 10 to 50 μ in size. It has been stated that the lung contains approximately 280 billion capillary segments and in the dose of 250 to 300 μCi of macroaggregated albumin ^{131}I utilized in lung scanning fewer than 1 million particles are injected. Therefore, this is a relatively safe clinical procedure.

Pulmonary arterial blood flow

The major contribution of nuclear medicine to the study of lung physiology has been the evaluation of arterial blood flow. To better understand the application of this procedure the student must first know something of the normal pulmonary blood flow.

It has been shown that the regional distribution of blood flow in the lung is affected by gravity. The interalveolar structure is the same throughout the lung; however, the standing blood pressure decreases 1 cm of water per centimeter distance from the base to the apex of the lung. Therefore, the interalveolar pressure exceeds the blood pressure at the apex, and the alveolar blood vessels are compressed and the apical flow is minimal. When the patient is in a supine position, blood pressures become equal in the apical and basal lung regions, and the distribution of pulmonary blood flow becomes uniform. Different phases of the respiratory cycle may also influence distribution of pulmonary arterial blood flow. Therefore, the injection of the radioactive particles should take several seconds and the patient should be in a supine position. Either a scanner or a camera is

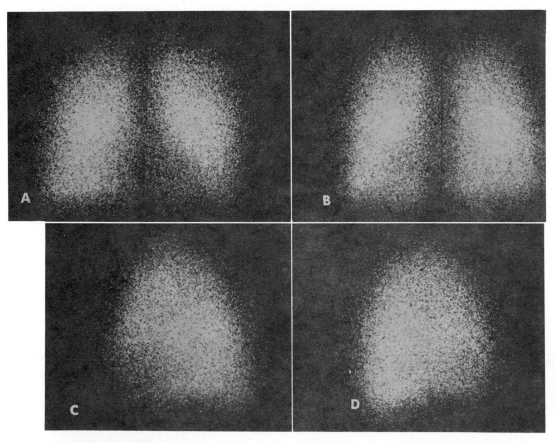

Fig. 15-2. Normal ^{131}I MAA lung image. **A,** Anterior view; **B,** posterior view; **C,** left lateral view; **D,** right lateral view. (Courtesy, August Miale, Jr., M.D. and Glen A. Landis, M.D.; Radioisotope Unit, Georgetown University Hospital, Washington, D.C.)

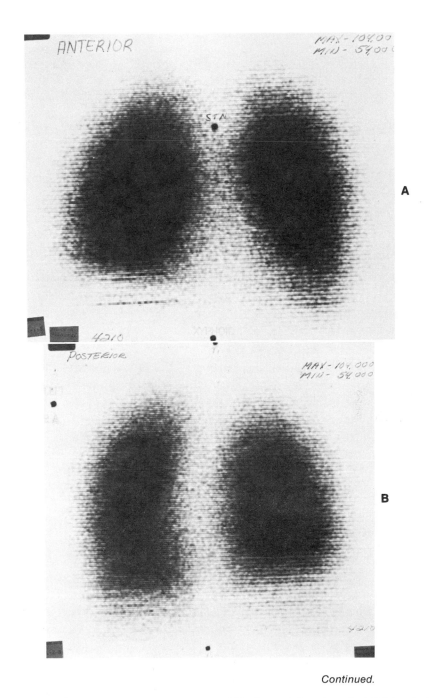

Continued.

Fig. 15-3. Normal ^{131}I MAA lung scan. **A,** Anterior view; **B,** posterior view; **C,** left lateral view; **D,** right lateral view.

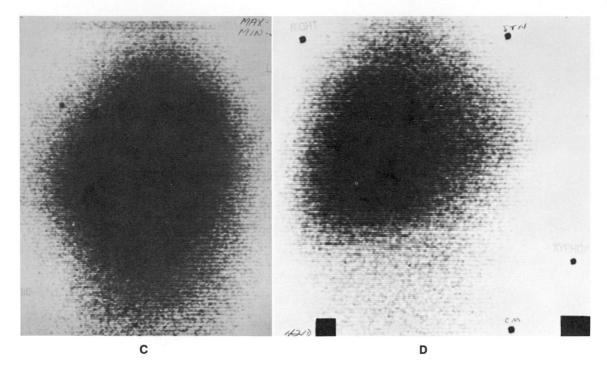

C   D

Fig. 15-3, cont'd. For legend see page 275.

used for imaging distribution of the radioactivity, and several views are usually obtained (Figs. 15-2 and 15-3). A note of caution should be given concerning this type of injection. The macroaggregated matter must be evenly distributed in the syringe and blood should not be drawn back into the syringe. If a nonuniform mixture is administered or small blood clots are injected with this particular material, small areas of microembolization may be visualized.

The majority of lung tissue is posterior, therefore the best view is obtained posteriorly. Because of the focusing collimation used with rectilinear scanners, the anterior view usually does not depict the bases of the lobes, and the cardiac space will be prominent. Because the counting rate is best at the surface of the camera, it is still true that the posterior view is the best single view. Generally, however, the anterior, posterior, and both lateral views are obtained.

The student will recognize that emphasis is placed on complete absence or patchy absence of radioactivity in areas of the lung. Therefore, in rectilinear scanning, contrast enhancement should be minimal; otherwise areas of poor distribution will be made absent by enhancement. As long as there is a measure of background activity on the image, minor variations in perfusion will be ascertained.

DISEASE STATES INFERRED FROM PERFUSION LUNG IMAGING
Pulmonary embolism

The search for pulmonary emboli has been one of the major uses of perfusion lung imaging. The major cause of pulmonary embolization is usually deep venous

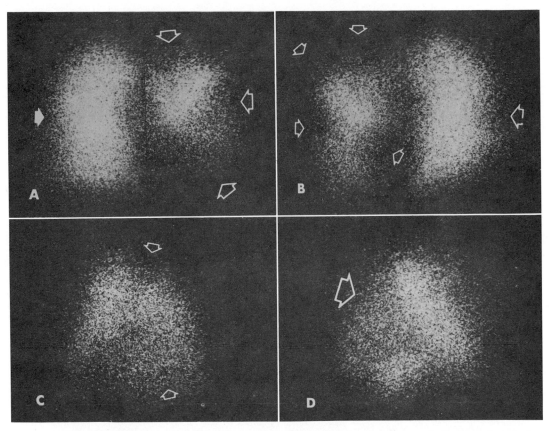

Fig. 15-4. Abnormal ¹³¹I MAA lung image compatible with pulmonary embolization. **A,** Anterior view; **B,** posterior view; **C,** left lateral view; **D,** right lateral view. (Courtesy, August Miale, Jr., M.D. and Glen A. Landis, M.D.; Radioisotope Unit, Georgetown University Hospital, Washington, D.C.)

thrombophlebitis. Small fragments of the clot break loose, pass through the inferior vena cava through the right side of the heart, and lodge in the pulmonary arteriolar system. Obviously, pulmonary embolization can be caused by tumor emboli, foreign bodies, or thrombi located anywhere along the vena cava or in the right side of the heart. Pulmonary embolization may be life threatening, however, now that the diagnosis is being made with frequency, it is known that many patients who have pulmonary embolization recover without incident. The student must recognize that the signs and symptoms of this particular disease were not as well understood in the past, since the physician had no easy, direct way of estimating pulmonary perfusion. Lung scanning has given the physician a simple, nontraumatic, indirect study of pulmonary perfusion.

The signs and symptoms of pulmonary embolization listed in the medical textbooks are quite dramatic, but many patients with pulmonary emboli have very vague symptomatology. Frequently patients will have a fast respiratory rate and a rapid heart rate, and may also have a slight fever. The patients complain of being uncomfortable and at times have slight dyspnea. However, the cardinal signs of disease, such as pain, are usually lacking in this particular disease.

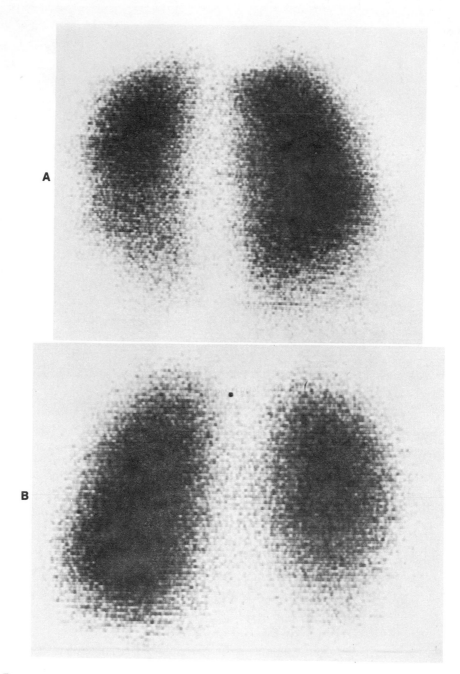

Fig. 15-5. Abnormal ¹³¹I MAA pulmonary scans. **A** and **B,** The anterior scan reveals decreased perfusion of the left lower lobe area and a probable decrease in perfusion in the right lobe area. Posterior view reveals a medial defect of the right midlung field, as well as a decrease in perfusion of the lower portion of the right lower lobe. On the left side there is decreased to absent perfusion of the left lower lobe. **C** and **D,** The study was repeated 1 week later. This series reveals almost complete reperfusion of the abnormalities noted on the previous series of scans with the exception of a small area of the left lower lobe. These studies are compatible with pulmonary embolization with subsequent reperfusion.

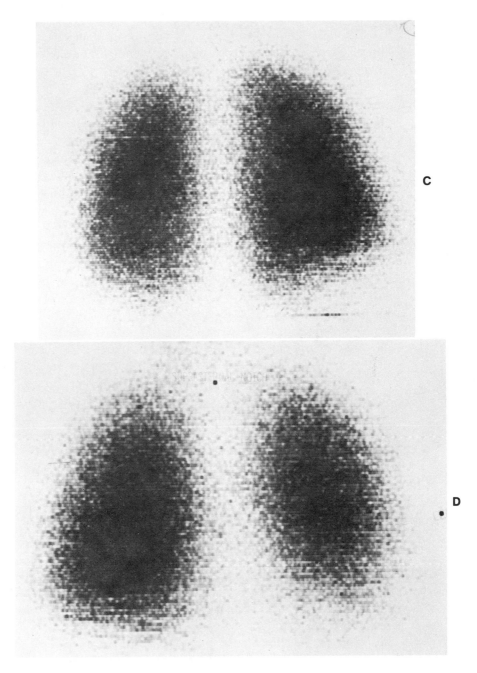

Fig. 15-5, cont'd. For legend see opposite page.

A chest roentgenogram in the diagnosis of pulmonary embolism is only positive in 10 to 15% of the patients. Usually hemorrhagic infarction is necessary before the roentgenogram is positive. Minor changes may be visualized which are indicative of pulmonary embolism, but these are also indicative of other disease processes. The electrocardiogram is frequently used to aid in the diagnosis of pulmonary emboli, but it is usually positive only when patients have had massive pulmonary emboli.

Chemical serum enzyme studies may be of value in the diagnosis; however, only 20% of the patients with pulmonary embolization have changes in the serum enzymes associated with this diagnosis.

Finally, the radiologist may inject contrast media into the patient to visualize the pulmonary artery and its ramifications. Pulmonary arteriography, however, cannot be classed as a screening study and is usually done only when surgery of a massive pulmonary embolic insult is being considered.

Lung scan of pulmonary embolism. The most frequent lesion visualized on a lung scan in pulmonary embolization is a concave defect in the periphery of the lung (Figs. 15-4 and 15-5). A second type of defect is a diffuse decrease in perfusion of one or several segments of the lung. Occasionally, there will be complete absence of perfusion of a segment or segments. By planemetry it has been shown that the majority of patients with pulmonary embolization will have a decrease in or absence of perfusion of less than 20% of the total lung area.

Serial scans done on patients who have had proved pulmonary embolization have been an aid in the evaluation of the recanalization of the vessels involved in the lung. Infrequently, the lung scan will revert to normal within a very short time (within the first few days of insult). Usually, reperfusion will take place over a period of months. In older patients or those with cardiovascular conditions longer periods of time are necessary for pulmonary reperfusion. The repeated lung scans have been very helpful in following patients that reembolize, even though they are under corrective therapy. These are the patients that are selected for surgical therapy. The primary site of the emboli is usually the deep iliac veins or the vena cava, and the surgical therapy is usually vena cava plication and/or ligation.

Pulmonary emphysema

The etiology of pulmonary emphysema is usually closely related to heavy smoking. In this disease the normal architecture of the tracheobronchial tree is disrupted, and bronchiolar and alveolar walls break down resulting in large air sacs called blebs or bullae. These sacs do not exchange air and, therefore, become dead air spaces. In this group of patients pulmonary function studies are usually abnormal. Regional vascular defects are observed by scanning in approximately 90% of the cases. The perfusion defect is usually a diffuse diminution of perfusion involving one or more areas. This perfusion defect is usually a direct effect of the distended alveoli pressing on pulmonary capillaries.

This disease could also be studied by having the patient breathe a radiocolloid aerosol and imaging the normal and abnormal tracheobronchial tree.

Lung carcinoma

Lung scanning can delineate a perfusion defect caused primarily by broncho-genic carcinoma of the lung before it can be seen by standard roentgenogram studies (Fig. 15-6). These particular tumors start deep in the mediastinum and usually by reflex action cause a decrease in pulmonary perfusion. Since broncho-genic carcinoma begins in the lumen of the bronchus, it has been found that with just a small amount of obstruction, there is a 50% decrease in perfusion in that segment of the lung. Complete absence of perfusion is the most common sign of lung carcinoma.

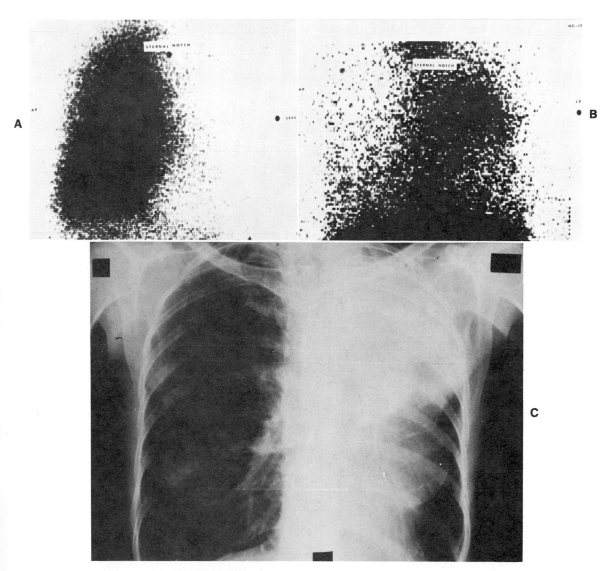

Fig. 15-6. A, Abnormal ^{131}I MAA lung scan, with complete absence of vascularity in the left lobe. **B,** ^{197}Hg scan revealed retention throughout the region of the left upper lobe and mediastinum. Study compatible with bronchogenic carcinoma.

281

Inflammatory disease of the lung

In bacterial, viral, or tuberculous inflammations of the lung, the lung scan is usually abnormal. The defects described are primarily of the diffuse variety; however, concave defects, as well as complete absences, have been observed. Blunting of the costophrenic angle has also been seen on scans in patients with pneumonia.

Congenital and acquired heart disease

Congenital disorders of the heart will affect pulmonary circulation and the lung scan can be informative. For example, if a single pulmonary artery has not formed, the scan will have the appearance of aplasia of the lung. When right to left side cardiac shunting is pronounced, a portion of the injected dose will often appear in other organs, such as the kidney. All of the rare congenital heart diseases have a bearing on pulmonary perfusion and may be studied by lung scanning. The lung scan may be of value in the diagnosis of congenital heart disease, as well as in the estimation of the amount of lung perfusion. Serial lung scans are very effective in evaluating corrective surgery.

Acquired heart diseases may be typified by mitral stenosis, which is usually a direct result of rheumatic heart disease. Patients with mitral stenosis have been found to have reversal of the gravitational perfusion of the lung. The advancing mitral stenosis will occur in the upright as well as in the supine position, there will be increased blood perfusion of the apices of the lung, and decreased perfusion at the bases of the lung.

Other types of heart disease, such as arteriosclerotic and hypertensive heart disease, may also change this perfusion relationship so that apical and basilar flow are almost equal.

SUMMARY

The study of pulmonary physiology with radionuclides is a relatively new addition to nuclear medicine. The study of air exchange (radioactive pulmonary function studies) are still in the research development phase. However, the study of the bronchopulmonary tree with radioactive particles and the study of pulmonary circulation with large radioactive particles have been accepted and are now used routinely for pulmonary diagnostic problems. Of particular usefulness is the lung perfusion scan that utilizes large particles which lodge in the pulmonary arteriocapillary bed after injection. Intelligent use of the perfusion lung scan, in conjunction with routine procedures such as the chest roentgenograms, now gives a simple indirect method of distinguishing pulmonary embolism from other common lung diseases.

Chapter

16 *Liver*

ANATOMY AND PHYSIOLOGY

The liver is the largest solid organ in the body, weighing almost 3 pounds (1.5 kg) in the adult. It occupies the right hypochondrium and part of the epigastric area, extending into the left hypochondrium and downward into the right lumbar region. It lies directly under the diaphragm and is sheltered in its greater part by the ribs (See Figs. 12-1; 15-1, *B*; and 16-1).

The liver consists of two main lobes, the right much larger than the left. On the medial portion of the right lobe are two lesser segments (called the caudate and quadrate lobes). They are separated on the inferior or visceral surface of the liver by a deep, short fissure called the porta hepatis. Through the porta most of the blood vessels, nerves, and lymphatics as well as the hepatic bile ducts enter and leave the organ.

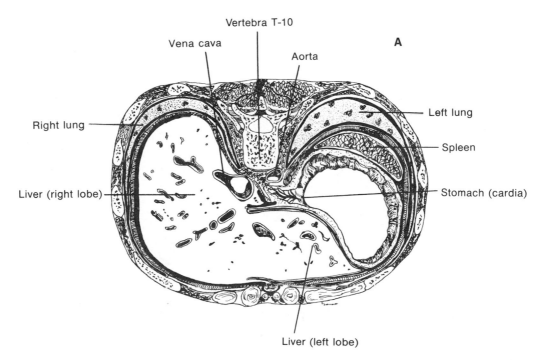

Fig. 16-1. Transverse sections through the abdomen to demonstrate the relative positions of the internal organs. **A,** At the level of the tenth thoracic vertebra; **B,** at the level of the twelfth thoracic vertebra; **C,** at the level of the third lumbar vertebra.

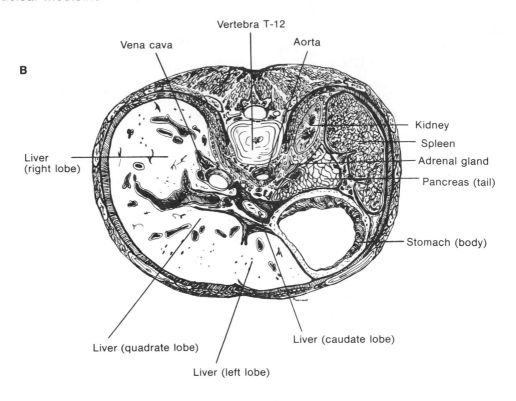

Vertebra T-12

Vena cava

Aorta

B

Kidney

Spleen

Adrenal gland

Pancreas (tail)

Liver
(right lobe)

Stomach (body)

Liver (caudate lobe)

Liver (quadrate lobe)

Liver (left lobe)

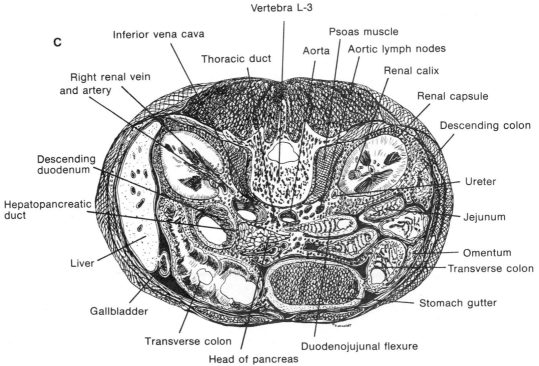

Vertebra L-3

Inferior vena cava

Psoas muscle

C

Aortic lymph nodes

Thoracic duct

Aorta

Renal calix

Right renal vein
and artery

Renal capsule

Descending colon

Descending
duodenum

Ureter

Hepatopancreatic
duct

Jejunum

Omentum

Liver

Transverse colon

Stomach gutter

Gallbladder

Transverse colon

Duodenojujunal flexure

Head of pancreas

Fig. 16-1, cont'd. For legend see page 283.

The liver has a dual blood supply. The portal vein brings venous blood from the intestine and spleen, and normally accounts for 65 to 75% of the total flow. The remainder is delivered by the hepatic artery, which supplies the liver with arterial blood. Both vessels enter the liver through the porta hepatis. In the liver, the portal venous and hepatic arterial bloods mix at different levels in the hepatic sinusoids. Blood is then drained by way of the central hepatic veins into the hepatic veins, which emerge from the back of the liver and enter into the inferior vena cava.

Most of the lymphatic vessels of the liver terminate in a small group of glands around the porta hepatis. Others pierce the diaphragm to end in the mediastinal glands, and the remainder accompany the inferior vena cava to terminate in glands around it in the thorax.

On the surface of the body, the outline of the liver can be simulated by a triangle. The upper border of the liver corresponds to a line drawn from a point slightly medial to the left midclavicular line at the upper border of the sixth rib, crossing the midline at the junction of the body of the sternum and the xiphoid process and ending at the level of the fifth rib in the right midclavicular line. The lateral border extends from this point downward and outward to meet the seventh rib at the side of the chest and continues downward to about one-half inch below the costal margin. The lower border can be indicated by a line drawn one-half inch below the costal margin to the right ninth costal cartilage, then obliquely upward to cross the midline at the transpyloric plane and meet the left eighth costal cartilage. From there it extends with a slight downward convexity to end at the beginning of the first line.

Structure and function

The liver is covered by a connective tissue capsule that dips at the porta hepatis, where it grows deep and branches into the substance of the organ, providing it with internal support.

For descriptive purposes, the liver can be compared to a sponge. Its main substance suggests anastomosing plates one cell thick or sheets of polyhedral parenchymal hepatic cells. Between the adjacent rows of hepatic cells of the same plate, there are tiny passageways called bile canaliculi or capillaries. The irregularly disposed cavities between the cell plates represent the sinusoids. These sinusoids are lined by a very thin layer of endothelial cells. Some of these are flat, whereas the others bulge with raylike extensions that gave them the name stellate cells (also called Kupffer cells). Pervading the liver and running in variable directions are two separate systems of pipelines: the portal tracts or canals and the hepatic central canals. The portal tracts contain a portal vein radicle, hepatic arteriole, and bile duct. The central hepatic canals contain radicles of the hepatic veins.

The liver receives absorbed products of digestion from the intestine through the portal vein, with the exception of some fats. In the liver these absorbed materials are metabolized by the polygonal parenchymal cells and are prepared either for storage or for use by the various tissues of the body. These parenchymal cells also function in the formation and secretion of bile and the excretion of exogenous substances, particularly dyes such as rose bengal, sulfobromophthalein (BSP) and fluorescein. As a storage organ the liver deals with glycogen, fats, proteins, vitamins, and other substances needed for blood formation and regeneration. In synthesis the liver is active in the anabolic formation of glycogen, serum lipids, ketone bodies, plasma proteins and some of the enzymes. In addition, the liver has a detoxicating action by which endogenous or exogenous harmful substances are made innocuous. Furthermore, the liver plays a major role in the metabolism of blood pigments.

As part of the reticuloendothelial system, Kupffer cells participate in production of antibodies, blood pigment breakdown, and phagocytosis (engulfing of microorganisms, cell fragments, foreign particles, and colloidal suspensions).

The excretory system of the liver begins with the biliary canaliculi, which lie between the hepatic parenchymal cells and communicate with the ducts in the portal canals. In the porta hepatis, the ducts from the different lobes of the liver fuse to form the common hepatic duct. The common hepatic duct, after receiving the cystic duct from the gallbladder, continues as the common bile duct; it opens into the duodenum either by a common orifice with the pancreatic duct or separately.

The gallbladder's main functions are concentration and storage of the biliary secretion during the intervals between meals. Expulsion of the bile from the gallbladder into the duodenum occurs through gallbladder contractions, accompanied by relaxation of the sphincter of Oddi surrounding the end of the common bile duct. The chief components of bile are the bile salts, bile pigments, cholesterol, lecithin, fats, and various inorganic salts. With the exception of bile salts, biliary constituents are excretory products. Bile salts are needed for the proper digestion and absorption of fats and related substances such as fat-soluble vitamins.

RADIONUCLIDE EVALUATION OF LIVER

The introduction of improved radiopharmaceuticals and the availability of sensitive equipment have made it possible to use radionuclide techniques for the study of the hemodynamic pattern, function, and morphology of the liver.

According to their nature, radioactive nuclides used for hepatic evaluation can be classified into two main groups. The first group is represented by radionulcides that are picked up by the phagocytic Kupffer cells. These radiopharmaceuticals are usually colloidal suspensions such as chromic phosphate ^{32}P, colloidal gold ^{198}Au, denatured or microaggregated serum albumin ^{131}I and ^{99m}Tc-labeled sulfur colloid. The second group consists of soluble dyes that are removed from the circulation mainly by the hepatic parenchymal polygonal cells, such as rose bengal ^{131}I and sulfobromophthalein ^{35}S.

Determination of hepatic blood flow and liver function

If a substance that is removable solely by a single organ is injected intravenously, its disappearance from the circulating blood will depend upon the blood flow carrying this substance to the particular organ, together with the state of function of the cells responsible for its removal. Thus with diminution in the blood flow to the organ, the disappearance of the substance is less rapid, which also means that the time taken for removal is longer. The same result can be caused by a decrease in the functional ability of the cells responsible for removal of the test substance.

In the liver, the situation is complicated by the presence of two types of cells, each of which is responsible for the removal of materials of specific nature. The parenchymal cells remove dyes and the Kupffer cells remove colloids. Therefore, each case must be considered separately.

When colloid particles of certain size are injected intravenously, their removal from the circulation should depend upon the amount of blood filtered by the liver, together with the phagocytic activity of Kupffer cells. However, if the number of particles entering the liver is kept low in relation to the number of receptor sites, these particles should be totally phagocytized in a single passage through the liver. Consequently, the rate of removal of the colloid from the blood is no longer affected by the phagocytic activity of Kupffer cells—which is more than enough—but is dependent only on the amount of liver blood flow. Such limitation is easily achieved in clinical practice if the concentration of particles is kept below a certain critical level. This is helped to a great extent by the fact that with inflammation, damage, or exhaustive use of Kupffer cells, the disabled cells are rapidly discharged and replaced by a new generation of phagocytic cells; the phagocytic receptor sites are thus kept in abundance at all times. Therefore, if the rate of disappearance of colloid particles from the circulating blood could be determined, it would represent an index of the liver blood flow.

These assumptions do not hold true in the case of dyes that are removed from the circulation by the hepatic parenchymal cells, presumably through a process of active transport. Their removal is followed by a brief phase of intracellular storage of the dye before its ultimate secretion into the bile. Therefore, the rate of removal of these dyes from the circulating blood depends on both the liver blood flow and the functional capacity of the hepatic parenchymal cells.

Determination of blood flow. Determining the rate of disappearance of colloid particles from the circulation reveals the state of blood flow in the liver. However, the size of these particles is critical if they are to be extracted in a single passage through the liver. If they are too large, they are caught in the pulmonary bed, the first vascular bed encountered by substances injected intravenously. If the particles are too small, they pass through the liver without being picked up by the Kupffer cells.

Various radiocolloids have been tried, but none of them has proved to be completely satisfactory. Chromic phosphate ^{32}P, apart from being difficult to prepare in uniformly sized particles, is a beta emitter and therefore cannot be monitored externally. Similarly, the preparation of denatured albumin tagged with ^{131}I is complicated and rather uncertain. The most commonly used radiopharmaceutical for determination of the hepatic blood flow is colloidal gold particles tagged with the gamma-emitting radionuclide ^{198}Au. This radiocolloid is easy to prepare and widely available. However, because its particles vary in size, some of the particles pass through the liver without being extracted by the Kupffer cells.

In order to determine the disappearance rate of radiogold from the circulation,

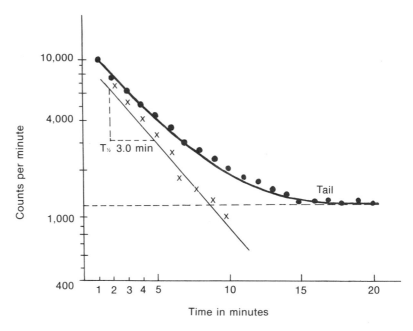

Fig. 16-2. Determination of the disappearance half-time of radiogold from the circulation by means of a detector placed over the temple. The tail of the curve is extrapolated and subtracted from the original readings.

20 to 40 μCi of colloidal gold ([198]Au) is injected intravenously. The level of radioactivity in the circulating blood is followed either by serial blood sampling or, more easily, by external monitoring.

For external monitoring a collimated scintillation detector is either centered over the temple or placed over the thigh. The information collected is counted by a rate meter with a time constant of 3 seconds and drawn on a stripchart recorder moving at a rate of ¾ inch per minute. When the information thus obtained is drawn on semilogarithmic scale, the disappearance of radiogold from the circulation appears to be a complex exponential function of time, being made of an early rapid phase and a later slow phase. This time variation is a result of the varied sizes of the colloid particles, which result in different disappearance rates. In order to correct for the effect of the smaller particles, which are not removed by the liver and which cause the slower phase, the tail of the curve is extrapolated back to zero time and subtracted from the original readings (Fig. 16-2). The resulting values are plotted on a semilogarithmic scale, and the time taken for the disappearance of half of the radioactivity is determined. This is called the disappearance or clearance half-time ($T_{1/2}$). The disappearance rate constant (K) is obtained by dividing 0.693 (natural log of 2) by the disappearance half-time. The disappearance rate constant represents the fraction of total blood volume that is cleared of the colloid by the liver per unit time, that is, the liver blood flow as a fraction of the total blood volume. Therefore, the hepatic blood flow can be calculated by multiplying K times the blood volume.

The disappearance half-time of radiogold can be also determined from the

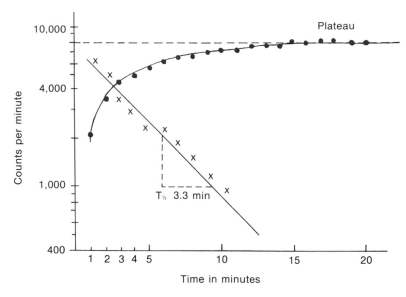

Fig. 16-3. Determination of the disappearance half-time of radiogold by the hepatic uptake technique. The recorded values are subtracted from the level of plateau activity.

hepatic uptake curve as obtained by a collimated scintillation detector placed over the right eighth intercostal space in the midaxillary plane. The obtained readings are subtracted from the level of plateau activity, and the resultant values are plotted on a semilogarithmic scale against time to enable calculation of the disappearance half-time (Fig. 16-3). From this value the disappearance rate constant is calculated and liver blood flow is determined.

Theoretically the hepatic counting rate represents a complex combination of hepatic accumulation of radioactivity versus blood disappearance occurring simultaneously in the field of the detector; however, in reality the level of the decreasing blood radioactivity in relation to the hepatic uptake (especially at the later time intervals) is too low to exert any significant effect. Therefore, it can be ignored during the calculations.

The main advantage of the hepatic uptake technique is that it offers a direct measurement of the hepatic uptake of radioactivity without being affected by the extrahepatic removal of the radiocolloid particles. In addition, the increasing counting rate recorded with time makes it possible to use rather small tracer doses of the radiocolloid, with minimal statistical fluctuations in the obtained values.

Assessment of parenchymal cell function. Because rose bengal ^{131}I is representative of the group of dyes, the rate of its disappearance from the circulation should depend on both the liver blood flow and the functional capacity of the hepatic parenchymal polygonal cells. Therefore, slower removal of the dye from the circulation, as evidenced by prolongation in the disappearance half-time, can be caused by either diminished liver blood flow or impaired parenchymal cell function or both.

Radiogold method. The source of the prolonged removal time can easily be

Clinical nuclear medicine

Table 16-1. Combinations of results of test for parenchymal cell function

Test	Condition	T½ Gold	T½ Rose bengal	T½ Gold/T½ rose bengal
Liver blood flow	Normal	3	6	0.50
Parenchymal cell	Normal	(2.0 to 4.3)	(4.0 to 8.0)	(0.40 to 0.70)
Liver blood flow	Normal	3	9	0.33
Parenchymal cell	Impaired			
Liver blood flow	Diminished	6	12	0.50
Parenchymal cell	Normal			
Liver blood flow	Diminished	8	30	0.27
Parenchymal cell	Impaired			

identified by the subsequent determination of the liver blood flow by the radiogold method. If the liver blood flow is normal, then the fault is in the parenchymal cells. However, if the hepatic blood flow is diminished, the answer depends on the degree of abnormality, whether it can totally explain the prolongation in the disappearance half-time of rose bengal or not.

The test itself is performed by the consecutive determination of the disappearance half-times of rose bengal and of radioactive colloidal gold. This can be done by external monitoring of either tracer disappearance from the blood or, better, of accumulation of tracers in the liver. The dosage used is 20 to 30 μCi of each, beginning with rose bengal ^{131}I followed approximately half an hour later with radiogold. The various possible combinations of results and their interpretation are shown in Table 16-1.

Rose bengal [131]*I.* Another test for evaluation of parenchymal cell function depends on estimation of the amount of rose bengal ^{131}I accumulating in the liver per unit of time and expressing it as a fraction of the hepatic blood pool. The hepatic blood pool (not blood flow) is estimated by recording the counting rate over the liver by means of a strip chart recorder after the intravenous injection of 10 μCi of radioiodinated serum albumin. This is followed by the intravenous administration of an exactly equal dose (10 μCi) of radioactive rose bengal; the hepatic counting rate is recorded with respect to time. This enables calculation of the amount of activity caused by radioactive rose bengal accumulating in the liver per unit of time. This is then expressed as percentage of the counting rate caused by the hepatic blood pool.

The sensitivity of this test can be enhanced by the simultaneous injection of BSP (2.5 mg per kilogram) with the radioactive rose bengal. The BSP acts as a stress to the liver cells and thus helps to differentiate borderline normal and abnormal cases.

Under these specifications, the lowest value for normal is 10.5%. Lower values are indicative of impaired parenchymal cell function.

These radioactive liver function tests have the advantage of demonstrating the functional capacity of the parenchymal cells without being affected by the state of the liver blood flow. In contrast, the result of the chemical BSP test (the most commonly used liver function test in cases without jaundice) is affected by both the liver blood flow and the parenchymal cell function. Consequently, an abnormal

BSP test does not necessarily indicate impaired parenchymal cell function as is usually thought.

Patency of the biliary system. Normally rose bengal is extracted from the blood by the hepatic parenchymal cells, where it stays for a short time before being secreted with the bile into the duodenum. Therefore, after the intravenous injection of a tracer dose of rose bengal ^{131}I, radioactivity should be detectable by a collimated scintillation detector centered over the intestine. (Care should be taken to avoid having the liver in the field of the detector.) In cases of biliary obstruction, there is no significant rise above background radioactivity in 1 hour after the injection. More valuable information can be obtained if this test is performed concomitantly with radionuclide photoscanning of the liver.

Clinical applications

The previously described radionuclide techniques are indicated in the evaluation of hepatic disorders irrespective of the presence or absence of jaundice. They are most commonly used in the study of hepatic cirrhosis, parasitic affection of the liver, jaundice, postnecrotic scarring, or any diffuse affection of the liver.

RADIONUCLIDE SCANNING OF THE LIVER

Since successful visualization of an organ depends on the selective deposition of a gamma-emitting radionuclide in that organ, any of the previously mentioned labeled colloids or dyes can be used for radionuclide scanning of the liver. However, each one has advantages and drawbacks.

Rose bengal [131]I. Radioiodinated rose bengal is extracted from the blood by the hepatic parenchymal cells and rapidly secreted with the bile. This particular behavior is the source of both its advantages and its disadvantages.

Because of its rapid secretion with the bile, the biologic half-life of rose bengal ^{131}I is very short, resulting in marked diminution of the radiation dose delivered to the liver and to the patient as a whole. In addition, the appearance of radioactivity in the region of the bowel can be taken as an indication of biliary patency.

On the other hand, the secretion of radioiodinated rose bengal with the bile into the gallbladder might mask any lesion in the area of the bed of the gallbladder. Furthermore, the level of hepatic radioactivity changes over the period of scanning; this definitely affects the quality of the scan picture obtained.

In an attempt to solve the difficulties outlined in the previous paragraph, scanning is started from below in order to hit the area of the gallbladder before the radioactivity-containing bile reaches this region. Another method is to inject some nonradioactive rose bengal with the tagged material in order to slow down its excretion and stabilize the counting rate. There is still one main problem without solution. It depends upon the fact that rose bengal ^{131}I is extracted from the circulation by the hepatic parenchymal cells. When there is parenchymal cell dysfunction, the hepatic counting rate is low, with wide statistical fluctuations, resulting in a poor scan picture. Allowing more time for the hepatic uptake process to increase the counting rate does not overcome this difficulty, since it is counteracted by the occurrence of secretion, which tends to decrease the level of radioactivity over the liver.

Usually 150 µCi of rose bengal ^{131}I is used. At least two views, anterior and right lateral, are obtained. Then the area to the left of the umbilicus is scanned. A normal abdominal scan picture indicates biliary patency. If patency is not verified, scanning is repeated after 24 hours. Absence of radioactivity in the bowel without significant change in the hepatic counting rate indicates complete biliary obstruction. With partial biliary obstruction, there is progressive diminution in the hepatic counting rate, accompanied by increased visualization of radioactivity in the region of the intestine.

Accordingly, the main indication for hepatic scanning with rose bengal ^{131}I is the study of cases with possible biliary obstruction.

Colloidal gold ([198]Au). Colloidal gold particles are picked up by the phagocytic Kupffer cells, where they stay until they are discharged with the cells. Therefore, the biologic half-life of radiogold depends mainly on its physical half-life, which is 2.7 days. This makes the radiation dose delivered by radiogold administration for hepatic scanning higher than that caused by radioiodinated rose bengal. Nevertheless, it is definitely much lower than the permissible levels. The persistence of radiogold particles in the Kupffer cells can be considered, from another point of view, an advantage. Thus in cases where the uptake of radiogold is impaired by vascular affections leading to a low hepatic counting rate, the level of radioactivity can be increased simply by allowing a longer time interval between the injection of the radiogold particles and the scanning procedure. In this connection it should be remembered that in contrast to labeled dyes, the hepatic uptake of radiocolloids is not affected by the functional capacity of the parenchymal cells of the liver. Therefore, a reasonable hepatic uptake of the radiogold colloid can be obtained even with marked hepatic parenchymal cell dysfunction. Further advantages of radiogold are its easy preparation and its widespread commercial availability.

Scanning of the liver is performed after the intravenous injection of about 150 µCi of colloidal gold [198]Au. It is preferable to start the scanning procedure 2 to 4 hours after injection in order to allow enough time for the hepatic counting rate to be reasonable and stable, especially in patients with hepatovascular impairment. At least two views, anterior and right lateral, should be obtained.

[99m]Tc-labeled sulfur colloid. As is true of radiogold, the biologic half-life of technetium sulfur colloid depends mainly on its physical half-life, which is short (6 hours); the radiation dose is therefore rather low. For this reason, and because technetium is low in energy, a relatively large dose (2 mCi) can be used, with the production of a higher counting rate and good counting statistics. Consequently, the time needed for scanning of the liver is shortened. However, because of the low energy of technetium and its short penetration, deep-seated lesions are easily missed. To overcome this difficulty, more views are performed; this undoubtedly involves more time. Furthermore, because of its short shelf half-life, technetium sulfur colloid shipments should be frequent; otherwise, the colloid has to be prepared on location. This fact limits the widespread use of technetium sulfur colloid for radionuclide scanning of the liver.

Denatured human serum albumin and microaggregated albumin colloid tagged with [131]I. Particles of denatured human serum albumin and microaggregated al-

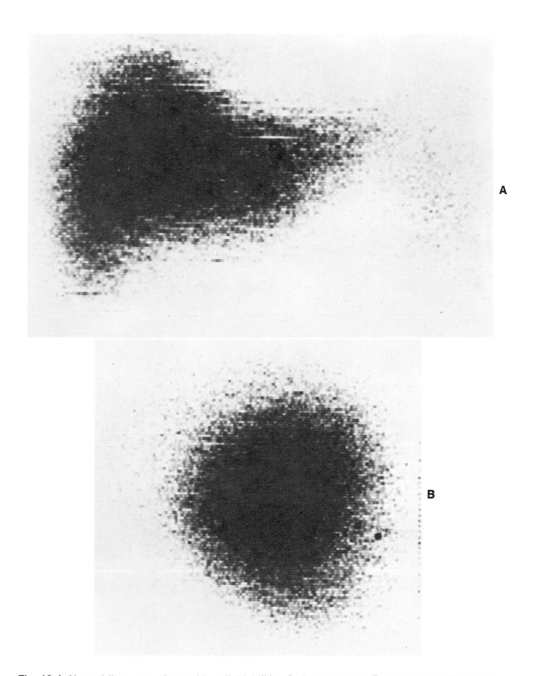

A

B

Fig. 16-4. Normal liver scan done with colloidal ^{198}Au. **A,** Anterior view; **B,** right lateral view. Note the rather even distribution of radioactivity in the right lobe with less radiogold in the thinner left lobe. The spleen is barely visible.

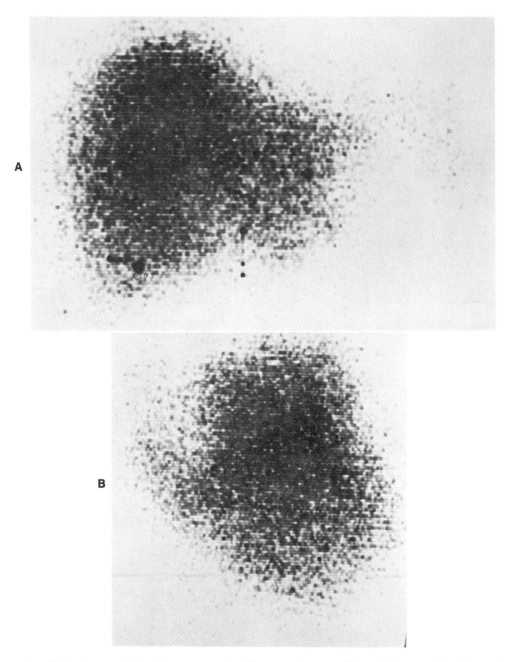

Fig. 16-5. Abnormal ¹⁹⁸Au liver scan series. The anterior scan **(A)** could be considered normal. The right lateral scan **(B)** shows a very large metastatic site in the posterior portion of the right lobe, which is confirmed decisively on the posterior scan **(C).**

bumin tagged with ^{131}I differ from those of other colloids in being metabolized after their capture by the phagocytic Kupffer cells. This behavior makes the radiation dose delivered to the liver lower than that caused by the other radio-colloids. However, the preparation of such particles with uniform size has not yet become standardized on a commercial basis.

Usually 500 μCi of the radioactive material are used and two views are obtained.

Interpretation of hepatic scans

In the interpretation of the scan pictures obtained, the size, site, and shape of the liver are to be considered. This is facilitated by the application of some fixed reference points on the scan picture. The reference points suggested are the xiphisternum in the midline, the fifth intercostal space, and the costal margin in the midclavicular planes of both sides. Further help is achieved by the super-imposition of the scan picture on a plain x-ray film of the abdomen. Normally the liver lies immediately underneath the diaphragm and extends slightly below the costal margin in the right midclavicular plane. The other points to be considered are the distribution of radioactivity all over the liver and the visualization of the spleen. Usually the distribution of radioactivity is more or less homogeneous (Fig. 16-4), with density maximal in the center of the right lobe and decreasing gradually towards the periphery. Sometimes, the extreme lateral end of the left lobe and the lower part of the right lobe are not quite apparent. Furthermore, because of their relative thinness, they may manifest areas of diminished concentration of radioactivity. Minor defects and irregularities along the margins are

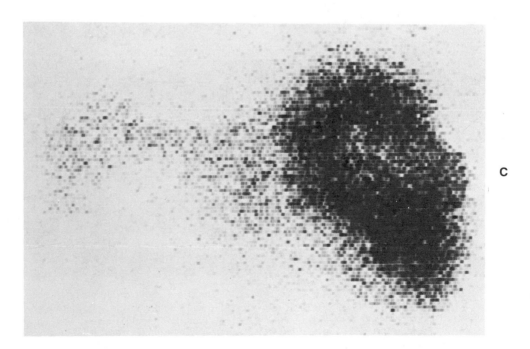

C

Fig. 16-5, cont'd. For legend see opposite page.

occasionally seen and explained by movements of the liver during respiration. Apart from these, diminished concentration of radioactivity whether localized or diffuse should be considered abnormal. In this connection, it should be always remembered that radionuclide scans are diagnostic of morphology rather than pathology. Thus, a localized area of diminished or absent concentration of radioactivity is diagnostic of a space-occupying lesion and can be due to a variety of causes, such as tumor (whether primary or metastatic), abscess, or cyst (Figs. 16-5 and 16-6). Similarly, diffuse irregular deposition of radioactivity or mottling is seen with metastatic disease as well as with diffuse parenchymatous hepatic involvement as in cirrhosis (Fig. 16-7).

Visualization of the spleen is a remote possibility in radiogold scans of the liver, normally due to the low splenic uptake of colloidal gold particles. However, in cases of cirrhosis, where the hepatic uptake is slow and diminished, the splenic

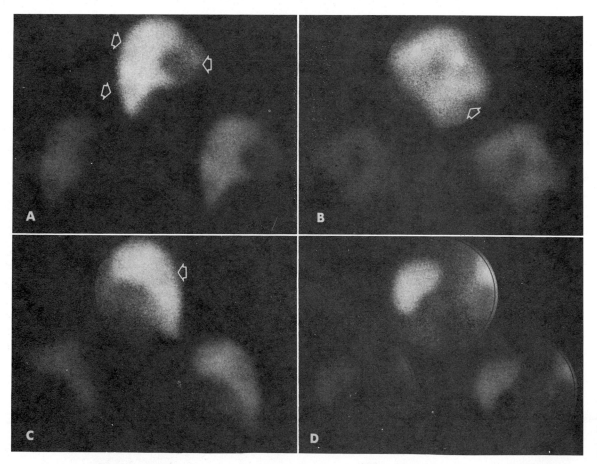

Fig. 16-6. Abnormal ¹⁹⁸Au liver study. **A,** There are multiple decreases in concentration in both lobes with a very large lesion involving the left lobe and extending into the porta hepatis. There are other smaller areas seen in the right lobe. **B,** The right lateral view shows the lesions as being in the lateral right lobe. **C,** Posterior view confirms the previous two views. **D,** A view of an enlarged spleen. Enlargement is probably caused by portal hypertension secondary to the metastatic disease.

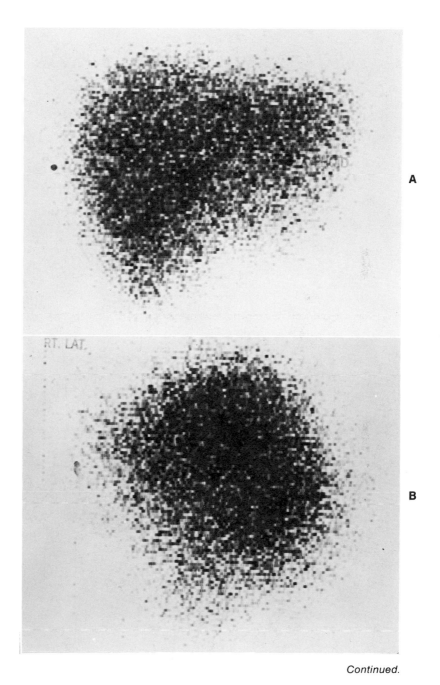

Continued.

Fig. 16-7. Abnormal [198]Au liver scan series. **A** and **B,** Initial liver scans done in January, 1967, with colloidal gold could be read as within normal limits or as a borderline abnormal scan. **C,** The scan obtained 3 weeks after the second series does not even appear related to the earlier scans. There is gross infiltration in apparent hepatic enlargement caused by an infiltrating tumor. The spleen can be visualized without difficulty.

297

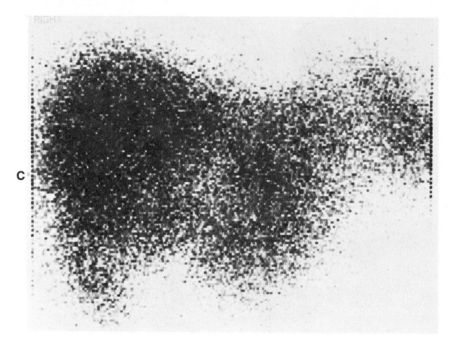

Fig. 16-7, cont'd. For legend see page 297.

uptake of radiogold is high enough to permit its visualization. In more advanced cases of cirrhosis the radioactivity is also seen in the bone marrow, especially that of the vertebral column.

The main indication for radionuclide scanning of the liver is the demonstration of space-occupying lesions, especially metastatic deposits. In addition, accurate information about the size, shape, and site of the liver is obtained. This information may prove very helpful in the detection of subdiaphragmatic abscess as well as in the differential diagnosis of pain or mass in the right upper quadrant of the abdomen. Furthermore, hepatic scanning can be used for the evaluation of diffuse parenchymal disease of the liver without any danger or discomfort to the patient. Similarly, a follow-up of patients suffering from hepatic disorders can be obtained by a nontraumatic technique.

17 *Spleen*

ANATOMY AND PHYSIOLOGY

The spleen is a soft, friable, highly vascular organ situated principally in the left hypochondrium behind the stomach and in close relation with the left leaflet of the diaphragm. It lies in the shelter of the ninth, tenth, and eleventh ribs, with its long axis parallel to them. Its medial end is approximately 2 inches from the midline in the back at the level of the eleventh dorsal vertebra, whereas its lateral end reaches the midaxillary line in the ninth intercostal space (see Figs. 15-1, *A* and *C*; 16-1, *A* and *B*).

In normal adults, the spleen measures nearly 5 inches in length, 3 inches in breadth, and 1.5 inches in thickness.

The blood vessels and nerves supplying the spleen enter and leave the organ along a fissure on its visceral surface, called the hilum. At the hilum, the fibroelastic capsule that covers the spleen is prolonged inward around the vessels in the form of sheaths. From these sheaths and, to a lesser extent, from the capsule, small fibrous bands or trabeculae are given off and constitute the framework of the spleen. The arteries branch repeatedly with the trabeculae and ultimately give off branches that leave the trabeculae to enter the pulp of the organ. As a support, these arterial branches are ensheathed with condensed reticular tissue that is heavily infiltrated with lymphocytes. From time to time, this sheath with its lymphocytic infiltration expands to form lymph nodules or follicles. These nodules represent the white pulp and appear as islands of irregular gray areas scattered throughout the red pulp, which constitutes the remainder of the organ. The red pulp is made of a framework of reticular fibers accompanied by fixed macrophages and reticular cells. This framework is permeated by passways termed venous sinusoids. In the meshes of the reticular framework, lymphocytes, free macrophages, and elements from the circulating blood are encountered. The arteries that emerge from the lymph nodules (white pulp) into the surrounding red pulp ultimately terminate in tufts or penicilli of minute arteries. According to the closed theory of intrasplenic circulation, these arterioles open directly into the venous sinusoids. According to the open theory, the arterioles open into the meshes between the venous sinusoids and blood returns to the sinusoids by way of apertures in their walls. Having reached the sinusoids by whichever route, the blood is drained by the red pulp veins, which coalesce to form veins of the trabeculae. These latter unite to give approximately six branches that emerge at the hilum and ultimately form the splenic vein, which is the largest radicle of the portal vein.

299

Functions of the spleen

As a blood-forming organ, the normal adult spleen is chiefly involved in the production of lymphocytes and monocytes. However, under certain conditions of bone marrow stress or disease, the spleen can become the site of extensive extramedullary erythropoiesis.

On the other hand, because of its unique type of circulation, the spleen functions as an organ of red blood cell destruction. The intrasplenic circulation permits separation of plasma from cells and allows stasis in either the sinusoids or pulp spaces. This arrangement enables phagocytosis and lytic factors to work more effectively on the senescent and abnormal red cells, leading ultimately to their destruction.

The iron derived from the destruction of aged erythrocytes, as well as from those cells that did not meet the minimum body standards, is conserved and made available by the splenic macrophages for further erythropoiesis.

Because of its large content of lymphoid and reticuloendothelial cells, the spleen plays a major role in the immunologic reactions and defense mechanisms of the body.

RADIONUCLIDE SCANNING OF THE SPLEEN

There is no doubt that successful visualization of an organ by radionuclide scanning depends on the selective deposition of a gamma-emitting radionuclide in that organ, which produces a higher concentration of radioactivity relative to the surrounding structures. Consequently, splenic scanning can be achieved by the use of radioactively tagged erythrocytes that have been treated or altered in order to promote their rapid and selective trapping by the functioning splenic tissue.

Alteration of the red cells can be induced by physical factors, chemical agents, or by the application of antibodies.

Coating with incomplete anti-D antibodies

Although this was the method used to obtain the first clinically usable scans for the human spleen, this technique cannot be applied in patients with D negative blood grouping, and it necessitates serologic typing of the patient's blood. In this technique the red cells are labeled with radiochromate.

Heat treated ^{51}Cr-tagged red cells

The red cells are tagged with 200 to 300 μCi of ^{51}Cr-labeled sodium chromate. If the anticoagulant used is ACD (acid citrate dextrose solution) care should be taken not to exceed a 1:5 ratio of ACD to whole blood; otherwise excessive damage to the red cells might occur during heating. After tagging, either the cells are washed or ascorbic acid is added, and the mixture heated in a drying oven or water bath at 50° C for 60 minutes. This step is critical, since raising the temperature or increasing the duration of heating results in fewer cells accumulating in the spleen and more appearing in the liver. The heated cells are left to cool to room temperature prior to their reinjection into the patient from whom they have been withdrawn. Scanning is performed at least 4 hours later.

Additional information about the spleen can be obtained by studying the disappearance of the heat treated ^{51}Cr-tagged red cells from the circulation. For this purpose, serial blood samples are withdrawn from the patient's other arm at 15 minute intervals over a period of 90 minutes. Radioactivity per unit volume from each sample is determined and plotted against time on semilogarithmic paper in order to calculate the disappearance half-time of radioactivity from the circulation. In order to identify the abnormals, the range for normal subjects should be determined for each laboratory. The same steps involved in tagging and alteration of the red cells should be used each time, since there is a wide variability in the results reported by various groups of workers. Disappearance half-times that are shorter than normal are identified and studied further in order to determine whether this abnormally rapid disappearance of the altered red cells is caused by an abnormality in the cells or by extracorpuscular factors. This can be achieved by repeating the test using homologous heat treated erythrocytes obtained from a known normal subject.

The main disadvantages of this technique of splenic scanning are the extreme care needed in the control of the degree of heat applied and the time consumed in the preparation of the altered erythrocytes.

Application of chemical agents

N-ethyl-maleimide. N-ethyl-maleimide can be used for alteration of the red cells to promote their sequestration by the spleen. However, since it is a sulfhydryl inhibitor, the degree of damage to the erythrocytes cannot be controlled because of the variability in the concentration of the sulfhydryl-containing enzymes in the red cells of different individuals.

MPH ^{197}Hg. MPH ^{197}Hg (I-mercuri-2-hydroxypropane labeled with ^{197}Hg) is able to tag red cells and it causes only moderate damage to the cells.

Three-hundred microcuries of MPH ^{197}Hg are placed in a sterile Vacutainer. Since the specific activity is known, the weight of the stable MPH present in this amount of radionuclide is calculated. A sufficient volume of blood is withdrawn from the patient and added to the MPH ^{197}Hg in the vacutainer to provide 1 ml of packed red cells for each microgram of MPH. The contents are allowed to mix well for a few minutes, then the labeled blood is reinjected into the patient; scanning is performed after 1 hour.

• • •

The main advantages of this technique are its simplicity and the shorter time involved to complete the test. The use of a radioactive compound with high specific activity and accurate calculations are essential in order to avoid any possibility of toxic reactions. However, because of the renal accumulation of radioactivity in the absence of a spleen, this method cannot be used in the search for accessory spleens, since they can be hidden by radioactivity in the left kidney.

Splenic scanning can be performed from either the anterior or posterior approach. An added lateral view can sometimes be of great value. In the accurate interpretation of the obtained picture, the scan is superimposed on a plain x-ray film of

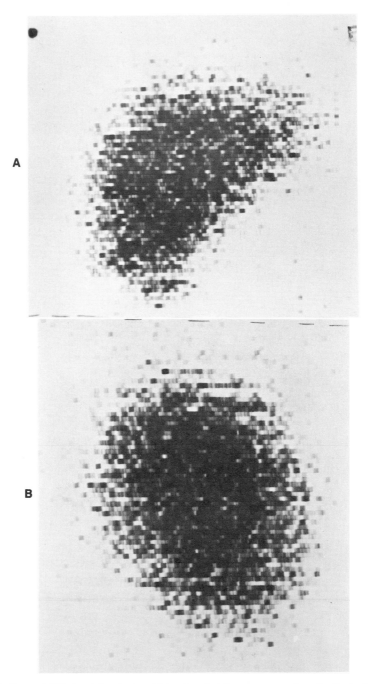

Fig. 17-1. Normal ^{51}Cr heat treated red blood cell spleen scan series. **A,** Posterior view of the spleen; **B,** lateral view of the spleen. These two views are necessary to correctly estimate the size of the spleen.

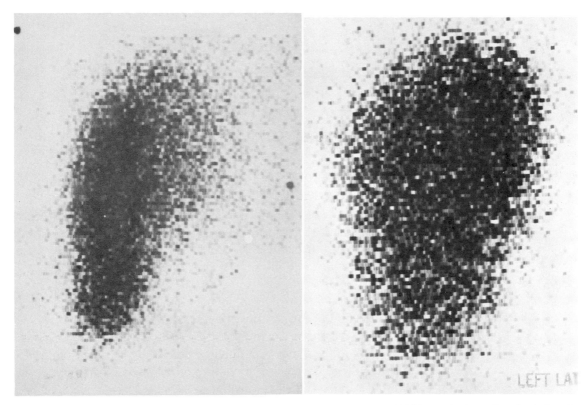

Fig. 17-2. Abnormal ⁵¹Cr spleen scan. The spleen is enlarged. This particular patient had chronic lymphatic leukemia; however, an enlarged spleen can be found in any patient with leukemia, lymphoma, or any condition that causes portal hypertension.

the left half of the abdomen. Proper superimposition is obtained through the use of fixed landmarks, such as the left fifth intercostal space in the midclavicular plane, xiphisternum, and the top of the iliac crest.

In interpretation, the first points to be checked are the site, size, and shape of the organ. The spleen is normally oval and lies immediately underneath the diaphragm. The distribution of radioactivity throughout the spleen is almost homogeneous. Since the distribution of radioactivity represents the functioning splenic tissue, areas of destroyed function such as tumors, cysts, abscesses, and infarcts, should appear as regions with little or no radioactivity (Figs. 17-1 and 17-2).

The main clinical indication for splenic scanning is to detect the presence of functioning splenic tissue and provide information about its quantitative assessment. This would be of great help in the differential diagnosis of a shadow or mass in the left upper abdomen. Furthermore, the presence of accessory spleens could be detected and intrasplenic space occupying lesions delineated.

18 *Gastrointestinal system*

Foods, minerals, vitamins, and fluids enter the body by mouth. Chewing breaks down the large food particles and mixes the food with the secretions of the three pairs of salivary glands (parotid, submaxillary, and sublingual) that open into the oral cavity. By virtue of its lubricating action, the saliva facilitates swallowing and keeps the mouth moist and clean. The salivary enzyme, ptyalin, begins the process of starch digestion. The lubricated food is then propelled through the pharynx, down the esophagus, and into the stomach.

In the stomach, food is stored and mixed with the gastric secretions that contain hydrochloric acid, mucus, pepsin, lipase, and intrinsic factor. In the presence of acidity, pepsin breaks down the proteins into polypeptides. The gastric lipase plays a minor role in the digestion of fats. Intrinsic factor is needed for the absorption of dietary vitamin B_{12}. The partially digested food is released from the stomach at a controlled steady rate into the duodenum, the first portion of the small intestine. The rate of gastric emptying depends on the nature of the stomach contents. It is most rapid with carbohydrates and slowest with fats.

The small intestine measures about 3 yards and can be divided into the duodenum, jejunum, and ileum. In the lumen of the small intestine, the contents are mixed with the intestinal secretions, pancreatic juice, and bile. The pancreatic and intestinal enzymes complete the breakdown of the partially digested food stuffs. The proteins are ultimately broken down into amino acids, carbohydrates into simple sugars, and fats into glycerides and fatty acids. These final products of digestion are then absorbed from the small intestine into the blood and lymph. The proper absorption of fats and fat-soluble substances requires the presence of bile. What remains after the process of absorption is driven from the ileum into the large intestine or colon.

In the colon, absorption of water and minerals converts the contents into semisolid feces. The colonic contents are propelled from the ascending colon through the transverse, descending, and sigmoid colons into the rectum. The colon normally contains large numbers of bacteria. Some of these are beneficial, while others are possibly harmful.

ASSESSMENT OF GASTROINTESTINAL BLOOD LOSS

The presence of blood in the stool indicates a break somewhere in the gastrointestinal mucosa. With relatively large amounts of blood, the color of the stools is changed. Red blood is almost always caused by bleeding from the lower large bowel; blood that has passed through the intestine becomes darker and gives the stools a tarry color. If the amount of blood is insufficient to cause a change in fecal color, certain tests must be applied for the detection of this occult blood. In this respect, microscopic examination of the stools is not very helpful. The chemical methods (guiac, benzidine) are much more adequate. They depend on color change of an indicator in the presence of an added source of oxygen and a peroxidase catalyst. What makes these tests positive in the presence of blood is the peroxidase found in the heme portion of the hemoglobin. However, the fact that other fecal constituents such as meat fibers, pus, and plants contain peroxidase, makes these chemical tests nonspecific. In contrast, the radionuclide techniques are more specific and offer an accurate estimate of the amount of blood loss.

Radiochromium method. An anticoagulated blood sample is withdrawn from the patient and the red cells are tagged with sodium chromate ^{51}Cr as described on p. 208. Following the reinjection of the labeled erythrocytes into the patient, the stools are collected for the next 72 hours. Blood samples are obtained 15 minutes after the injection of the tagged cells and at the end of the test period. Radioactivity in the stools is measured on top of a scintillation counter. Using identical geometry and equal counting time, radioactivity in the blood samples is measured in order to calculate the average net counting rate per milliliter of blood. The amount of gastrointestinal blood loss is determined by dividing the net counting rate of the collected stools by that present in 1 ml of blood.

Normally, the amount of blood lost in the stools never exceeds 3 ml per day.

The main use of this test is the detection and estimation of blood loss through the gastrointestinal tract, which has been known to be the underlying cause in some cases of unexplained anemia.

ASSESSMENT OF PROTEIN LOSS
THROUGH THE GASTROINTESTINAL TRACT

Under normal circumstances, a significant proportion of the daily breakdown (catabolism) of plasma albumin and probably other plasma proteins occurs by exudation into the gastrointestinal tract, where they are subsequently digested and reabsorbed. In order to maintain a state of equilibrium, albumin is manufactured by the liver at a rate equal to its catabolism. With the exudation of abnormally large amounts of proteins into the gastrointestinal tract, the ability of the liver to synthesize albumin is exceeded. This results in diminution of the concentration of the plasma proteins with the production of generalized or localized edema.

Excessive loss of albumin has been shown to occur in the stomach in giant hypertrophic gastritis, diffuse ulceration of the stomach, and gastric carcinoma. An increased loss of albumin from the intestine has been observed in regional enteritis, ulcerative colitis, celiac disease, intestinal lymphangiectasia, and carcinoma. Extraintestinal disorders, such as nephrosis, hepatic cirrhosis, constrictive pericarditis, and congestive heart failure can also lead to excessive protein loss through the gastrointestinal tract.

Since the protein leaking through the gastrointestinal tract is liable to digestion by the proteolytic enzymes and reabsorption, the level of fecal nitrogen is not affected. Consequently, chemical methods would not be suitable for the detection of these cases of protein-losing gastroenteropathy. However, the diagnosis of this phenomenon can be easily and accurately done by means of radionuclide techniques.

Radioiodinated human serum albumin. The earliest evidence for excessive protein loss through the gastrointestinal tract was obtained by recovering injected ^{131}I-labeled human serum albumin from gastric aspirates in patients with giant hypertrophic gastritis. However, because of the technical difficulties of intubation, this approach cannot be applied for the detection of enteric protein loss in routine clinical practice. Furthermore, the leaking protein is liable to digestion by the proteolytic enzymes with the production of amino acids and ^{131}I, both of which are reabsorbed. Also, ^{131}I is secreted in the saliva and gastric juice, leading to false elevation in the fecal radioactivity.

In order to prevent iodine reabsorption, an ion exchange resin (Amberlite IRA 400) is given orally (5 gm every 4 to 6 hours) to bind the radioiodine freed during the breakdown of the leaking labeled albumin. The radioactivity thus bound is excreted with the resin in the stools. However, the problem of secretion of ^{131}I in the salivary and gastric secretions has not been solved.

Another source of error is that a fraction of the radioiodine might be reabsorbed before being bound by the resin. Furthermore, part of the ^{131}I originally bound to the resin might be lost during its passage through the intestine.

The most accepted method utilizing radioiodinated albumin depends on following the daily levels of plasma, urinary, and fecal radioactivity over a period of at least 2 weeks after the intravenous injection of 30 to 100 μCi of ^{131}I-labeled human serum albumin. From the obtained values, the plasma volume, total exchangeable body albumin, half-life of ^{131}I-labeled albumin, and albumin turnover are calculated. Lugol's solution is administered in order to block the uptake of ^{131}I by the thyroid gland, whereas radioiodine reabsorption is prevented by the resin. The information obtained about the protein metabolism by means of this technique is extensive and very valuable. However, collection of the stools and urine over such a prolonged period, together with the tedious calculations involved, makes the application of this technique for clinical use impractical.

Radioiodinated polyvinylpyrrolidone (PVP). The patient's stools are collected for 96 hours following intravenous injection of 10 to 25 μCi of ^{131}I-labeled PVP. Fecal radioactivity is measured and expressed as percentage of the administered dose, and care is taken to use identical geometry during counting. Normally, the level of radioactivity in the 96 hour stool does not exceed 1.5% of the injected dose.

The main advantages of PVP are its resistance to proteolytic enzymes and its relatively poor absorption. However, this substance is not a natural plasma constituent, but is a synthetic polymer with a spectrum of different molecular weights. Therefore, it cannot reflect the true picture of protein metabolism. The survival of PVP in the blood is shorter than that of plasma proteins. It is rapidly cleared by the reticuloendothelial system and excreted by the kidneys. Consequently, the fecal excretion of radioiodinated PVP cannot be used as a quantitative measure of protein loss through the gastrointestinal tract, but is a very useful simple screening test.

Radiochromium human serum albumin. The dose applied is 30 to 50 μCi of

^{51}Cr-labeled albumin. Normal subjects excrete less than 0.7% of the intravenously administered dose in stools collected over a period of 96 hours.

In this technique, there is neither salivary secretion nor intestinal reabsorption of radioactivity. However, since ^{51}Cr is gradually eluted from the albumin, this technique cannot be used for determination of albumin turnover.

In order to quantitate the gastrointestinal protein loss, fecal radioactivity is expressed as number of milliliters of plasma lost through the intestine per day. This is obtained by dividing radioactivity in the 24 hour stool by the counting rate of 1 ml of plasma of the same day. Normally, 5 to 25 ml of plasma are cleared from their albumin into the gastrointestinal tract on each day.

This technique not only detects protein leakage through the gastrointestinal tract, but also offers a quantitative measure of the amount lost.

Chapter
19 *Pancreas*

ANATOMY AND PHYSIOLOGY

The pancreas has both an exocrine (external) and endocrine (internal) function. It is approximately 5 to 6 inches in length, and it extends obliquely upward from the duodenum behind the stomach and across the posterior abdominal wall to the spleen at the level of the first and second lumbar vertebrae. The pancreas lies within the concavity of the duodenum to which it is attached by blood vessels, pancreatic ducts, and loose connective tissue. The adult pancreas is divided into a head, neck, body, and tail. The head is flattened dorsally and ventrally. The body of the pancreas is extremely thin; the tail thickens out slightly and is the pointed tonguelike left end of the gland which lies in contact with the spleen.

The primary exocrine function of the pancreas is mediated through the acinar cell where the pancreatic enzymes are manufactured. The pancreatic enzymes and juices are carried through a ductal system, which empties into the duodenum through a primary duct and an accessory duct. The endocrine function of the pancreas is the manufacture of insulin in the islets of Langerhans found throughout the pancreas.

The pancreas is made up of alveoli, which resemble the salivary gland in their general arrangement and design. The part of the pancreas involved in its exocrine function is made up chiefly of groups of cells forming acini, which tend to be spherical. Groups of acini form primary lobules, and numerous adjacent primary lobules form a secondary lobule. Therefore, the pancreatic tissue proper is composed of acinar cells, islet cells, and ductal cells. The acinar cells are large, have well-developed nuclei, and abundant grandular cytoplasm. The granules, called zymogen granules, vary in number and position in the cell depending on the state of activity of the gland.

The pancreas receives an abundant nerve supply from both the vagi and splanchnic nerves. The pancreas secretes a colorless, odorless, alkaline fluid of low viscosity through its ductal system. The pancreatic juice has a high bicarbonate content. Secretin is an endogenous hormone secreted by the duodenal mucosa. This hormone has a direct effect on the ductal cell and does not alter the output of enzymes from the gland. Pancreozymin, which is also an endogenous hormone secreted by the duodenal mucosa, does not stimulate the flow of juice, but sharply increases enzyme concentration. Vagal stimulation, when superimposed on secretin-stimulated flow, also increases enzyme output. The protein content or the enzyme content of pancreatic juice varies between 0.1 and 0.3%. The enzymes of the pancreas are capable of digesting all three types of food stuff; therefore, pancreatic juice is proteolytic, amylolytic, and lipolytic. The main proteolytic enzymes secreted from the pancreas are trypsinogen, chymotrypsinogen, peptidase, and carboxypeptidase. The lipolytic enzymes are lipase, phospholipase A, and phospholipase B. The amylolytic enzyme is pancreatic amylase.

Amino acid requirements for enzyme synthesis

It has been found that ten amino acids are required for maximum exocrine enzyme synthesis. These amino acids are tryptophan, arginine, threonine, valine, tyrosine, lysine, leucine, histadine, isoleucine, and phenylalanine. The only essential amino acid present in the crystalline enzymes which is not required for maximum synthesis is methionine. This amino acid is present in smaller amounts in the enzymes than any of the other amino acids. Presumably, the levels of free methionine in the tissue can satisfy the small demands for this amino acid for protein synthesis.

Pancreatic enzyme synthesis

Pancreatic enzymes removed from their site of synthesis in the pancreatic acinar cell are transported through a series of cell compartments and finally stored intracellularly in the zymogen granules. This transport has been studied, and has been found to take approximately 45 minutes to 1 hour. The enzymes remain in storage in the zymogen granule. There is still controversy as to whether there is intermittent or continuous pancreatic secretion in humans.

SPECIAL PROCEDURES IN THE STUDY OF PANCREATIC FUNCTION
In vitro testing

Nonradioactive tests. Pancreatic exocrine insufficiency may be caused by a number of diseases. Since the pancreas is the principal source of lipase used for the digestion of fats, any decrease in the amount of lipase secreted will result in maldigestion of fats and will cause steatorrhea. Digestion is not affected as seriously as it would be if there were a defect in the output of proteolytic enzymes of the pancreas, since there are other proteolytic enzymes found in the intestine. However, one of the clinical manifestations of pancreatic insufficiency is an excess of fat excreted in the feces.

Fecal fat excretion. Fecal fat excretion may be chemically measured. Normal individuals on an average diet seldom excrete more than 6 to 7 gm of fat in the feces in a 24 hour period.

Secretin and pancreozymin tests of function. Secretin, pancreozymin, or the combination may be injected into patients. The secretion of the pancreatic tree is collected by intubation. A double lumen tube is passed through the patient's nose or mouth into the stomach and duodenum, one lumen opening into the stomach for draining gastric juice and the other into the duodenum for collection of the pancreatic and duodenal secretions. Samples from the duodenum are collected every 10 to 20 minutes. Depending on the type of study performed, secretin or pancreozymin is injected, and the duodenal contents are collected over a period

309

of time. Volume, pH, bicarbonate, and enzyme determinations are then made on the collected samples.

In diseases of the pancreas associated with destruction of the secreting parenchyma, the flow rate of the pancreas is decreased below 1 to 2 ml per kilogram of body weight for a 30 minute period. The bicarbonate content is decreased in inflammatory disease of the pancreas below 90 mEq. per liter. It has been found that the addition of pancreozymin to the standard secretion test does not significantly improve the diagnostic accuracy of the procedure. The secretin test has been found to be of limited usefulness in the diagnosis of acute pancreatitis, and its chief usefulness has been in the determination of chronic pancreatitis. In pancreatic carcinoma, there is a depression of the volume flow if the carcinoma is in the head. The amount of depression depends upon the size and extent of the pancreatic duct obstruction. The secretin test has limited usefulness in patients with carcinoma of the body or tail of the pancreas. However, many of the pancreatic carcinomas of the head may be inferred by a carefully performed secretin test.

Radionuclide pancreatic studies. Fecal fat may be quantitated chemically; however, the fecal measurement is somewhat tedious. In 1949 it was found that following the ingestion of ^{131}I triolein, there was a characteristic fat tolerance blood curve, as well as a fecal excretion of the labeled fat in 72 to 96 hours. The latter was found to be a more reliable indicator of the total absorption of the labeled fat.

The normal blood values were 10% or more of the administered dose of the radioactive material in the average of the fourth, fifth, and sixth hour blood samples (or a peak blood radioactivity of 9% or more using a total blood volume radioactivity based on the anticipated volume of 3,000 ml per square meter of body surface). The fecal fat results are usually interpreted over the 72 to 96 hour period; the upper limit of normal is 7% of the ingested dose. Obviously, any disease that would lower the lipase content of the pancreatic secretion should give an abnormal result.

However, the triolein test has been found to be most unreliable as a predictor of malabsorption. In 1963, it was found that the commercially available radio-iodinated triolein was contaminated with many free fatty acids and other substances. However, even with purified ^{131}I triolein, the most reliable test (the 96 hour stool collection) still does not exclude the presence of steatorrhea.

Iodine 131-labeled oleic acid test. By the combined use of a neutral fat, ^{131}I triolein, and a radioiodinated fatty acid (^{131}I oleic acid), early studies indicated that in pancreatic insufficiency the radioiodinated fatty acid was absorbed normally, while the labeled neutral fat was absorbed poorly. Of course, in malabsorption, it was found that the absorption of both substances was depressed. However, through the years it has been shown that the ^{131}I oleic acid absorption is extremely unpredictable.

Carbon 14-labeled fats. Recently ^{14}C-labeled fats have been introduced into medicine to help estimate pancreatic insufficiency or malabsorption of the small bowel. The ^{14}C-labeled fat on absorption is monitored as the ^{14}C is expired as labeled carbon dioxide. These studies are still in the experimental stage at the present time.

PANCREATIC IMAGING WITH ^{75}SE SELENOMETHIONINE

In 1949 it was found that tagged methionine localized within the pancreas. In 1962 Blau and Bender reestablished this fact when they employed ^{75}Se selenomethionine for visualization of the pancreas. Of all the organs that have been imaged successfully utilizing a gamma ray imaging device, the pancreas is undoubtedly one of the hardest organs to picture successfully.

If the reader will review the transverse section anatomic drawings (Fig. 16-1) he will notice that the pancreas is a deep-seated organ, normally 5 inches or more away from the abdominal wall. This 3½ oz organ is also surrounded by a number of large organs of the abdomen. These points will be stressed in the following discussion.

Physiopharmacology

The physiopharmacology of ^{75}Se selenomethionine is quite complicated. Methionine is a basic amino acid important to all organ metabolism. The normal circulating volume of methionine is approximately 100 μg. Approximately 50% of the methionine is taken up by muscle, and the remainder of the methionine is distributed in the other large organs. Approximately 4% of the injected ^{75}Se selenomethionine is found in the pancreas 1 hour after injection. Twelve percent is found in the liver, 2.5% in the lung, and 1.5% in the kidney. On a per gram basis, the intestine has one-tenth as much selenomethionine per gram as the pancreas. Obviously, the amount of radioactivity found in the organs surrounding the pancreas makes the imaging of this organ more difficult, for example, than the imaging of the thyroid gland with ^{131}I. It has been found that none of the proposed procedures to increase the amount of ^{75}Se selenomethionine in the pancreas was useful in our investigations on animals.

Clinical considerations

Position of the patient. If the reader will refer to Fig. 16-1, *B*, it will be noted that in the anterior view the left lobe of the liver overshadows the tail of the pancreas; with slight enlargement of the right lobe of the liver, the head of the pancreas will be overshadowed. It will also be noted that if the left side of the patient is elevated, the liver is thrown upward and the pancreas may be visualized from the anterior view. This is the pancreatic scanning position.

Rectilinear scanning. Since by animal investigation it has been shown that the peak uptake of ^{75}Se selenomethionine is between 30 minutes and 2 hours, the rectilinear scan is begun immediately after the dose is given and the abdomen is searched for the 15 to 30 minutes while the selenomethionine is being concentrated by the pancreatic tissue. The head of the pancreas is always found below the porta hepatis; therefore, if the rectilinear crystal is placed over the umbilicus and moved diagonally toward the porta hepatis, the first organ that the crystal will pass over is the head of the pancreas. Since the head of the pancreas measures about 2 cm in diameter, there will be a slight counting drop as the probe passes over the head and into the edge of the right lobe of the liver. Thus, the pancreas may be localized without difficulty. In rectilinear scanning a crystal larger than the 3 by 2 inches

311

must be used, since the pancreas is usually more than 5 inches away from the abdominal wall. Therefore, the collimator focal depth must be 5 inches or more to put the pancreas into the correct focal plane. Other rectilinear techniques include the use of twin 5 inch probes and recently subtraction techniques.

Camera imaging techniques. Recently, the camera has been utilized successfully to image the pancreas (Figs. 19-1 to 19-3). Compared to rectilinear scans of the pancreas, the imaging studies of the camera have proved successful, and patient time has been saved. Almost immediately after injection of selenomethionine the pancreas can be visualized, and following a short positioning view of approximately

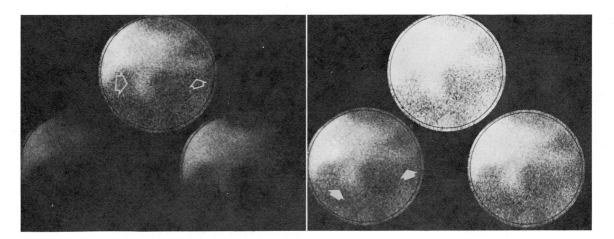

Fig. 19-1. Normal ⁷⁵Se selenomethionine pancreatic image series. It takes approximately 15 minutes to accumulate 120,000 counts in the field of view of the camera. By shielding the liver with lead, we have ascertained that 20,000 counts of the 120,000 counts are coming from the area of the pancreas.

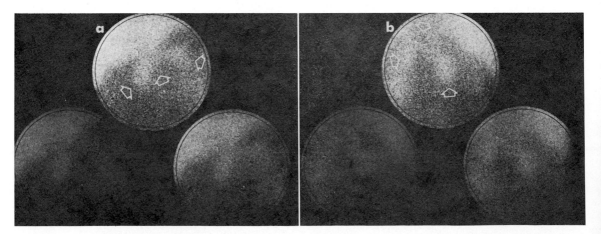

Fig. 19-2. Normal ⁷⁵Se selenomethionine pancreatic image series. **a,** Anterior image of the pancreas; **b,** posterior image of the pancreas. Notice that the pancreatic tail abuts the spleen and lies on top of the left kidney, which is visualized in the posterior image.

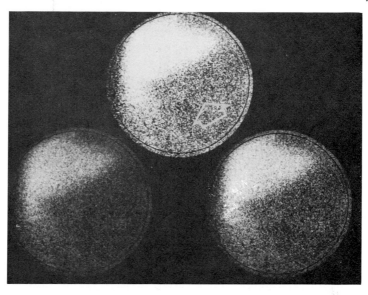

Fig. 19-3. Abnormal ⁷⁵Se selenomethionine pancreatic scan. Pancreatic carcinoma had been previously inferred from the scan, and the impression was confirmed at surgery. This image of the pancreatic area was obtained approximately 6 months later; almost the entire pancreas has been destroyed by tumor.

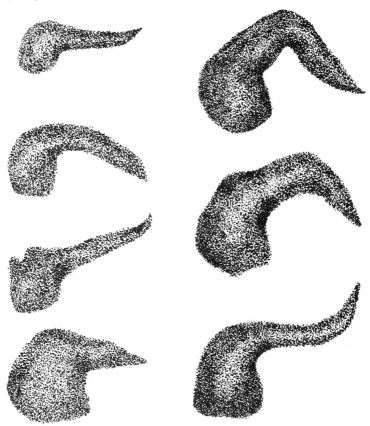

Fig. 19-4. Normal pancreatic images.

5 minutes, consecutive 15 minute views of the pancreas are made. We have found through experimentation that approximately 15% of the count rate obtained from the imaging area is from the pancreas; therefore, we collect approximately 120,000 counts to make a statistically good image. By slight rotation of the camera head we have approximated the pancreatic scanning position of rectilinear scanning.

CLINICAL RESULTS OF PANCREATIC IMAGING

The pancreas in the human has many different shapes as illustrated in Fig. 19-4. As will be understood by a review of the anatomy of the pancreas, the head of the pancreas will have greater activity than the tail; the body is very thin and is visualized very poorly in pancreatic imaging.

The normal pancreas is obviously the easiest to visualize and once the normal variants of pancreatic shape are understood, the imaging and interpretation of the normal pancreas may be done without difficulty (Figs. 19-5 and 19-6).

Inflammatory disease of the pancreas, such as pancreatitis, is difficult to infer with pancreating imaging because even with inflammatory disease there may be a normal counting rate over the pancreas. Conversely, a decreased counting rate from the pancreatic bed may be caused by many technical factors, such as tissue absorption, scatter, or positioning of the focusing collimator at the wrong focal depth.

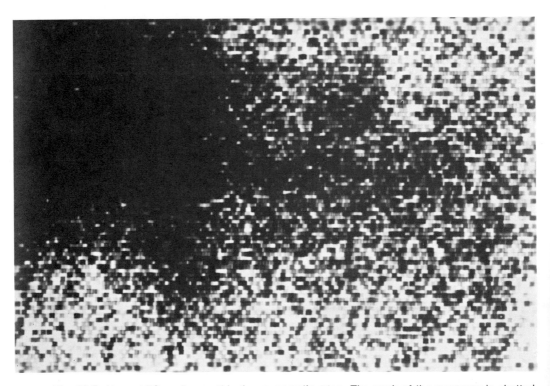

Fig. 19-5. Normal ^{75}Se selenomethionine pancreatic scan. The neck of the pancreas is abutted near the right lobe of the liver; however, a well-defined round head, body, and tail can be seen on this scan. The patient is in an oblique position with the left side elevated to separate the pancreas from the liver image.

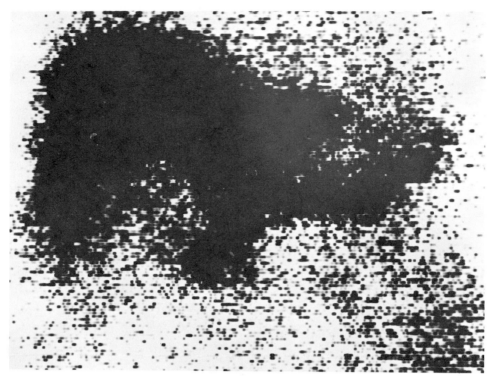

Fig. 19-6. Normal ^{75}Se selenomethionine pancreatic scan.

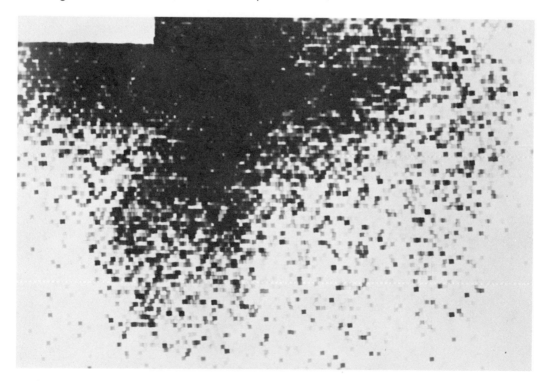

Fig. 19-7. Abnormal ^{75}Se selenomethionine pancreatic scan. Large infiltrating defect in the head of the pancreas.

In carcinoma of the pancreas there is decreased metabolism of methionine by the carcinoma (Fig. 19-7). Therefore, pancreatic carcinoma may be inferred by pancreatic imaging. Again, correct differentiation of a small area of abnormality can only be done using the rectilinear scanner only if the focusing collimator is focused at the correct depth. In studying abnormalities in pancreatic imaging, it has been found that taking two or three pancreatic rectilinear scans, although an investment of 2 to 3 hours of technical as well as patient time, enhances the diagnostic quality of the procedure tremendously. Camera studies appear to equal the rectilinear studies of the pancreas with a saving of patient study time.

Based on clinical experience with pancreatic imaging, patients suspected of having pancreatic carcinoma should undergo this procedure.

Chapter
20 *Bone*

ANATOMY AND PHYSIOLOGY

Inorganic materials make up 45% of the constituents of bone. These materials include calcium, phosphate, and magnesium. Organic materials make up 30% and water constitutes 25% of bone weight. Calcium makes up about 15% of the weight of fresh osseous tissue. Bone calcium exists in two forms, calcium carbonate and tricalcium phosphate; the ratio of calcium to phosphate is approximately 2.2:1.

There are two types of ossification—intramembranous and intracartilaginous (endochondral). The cranial vault, maxilla, and mandible are formed through ossification of membranes. The bones of the limbs, trunk, and the base of the skull are transformed from cartilage to bone by both forms of ossification. It has been shown that calcium and phosphorus are first laid down in the epiphysis of developing bone and later move to the shaft, or diaphysis. Growth occurs at both ends of the bone. The cells involved in ossification are called osteoblasts; cells which deossify bone are called osteoclasts. Through the combined action of the osteoblasts and osteoclasts, complete replacement of calcified cartilage results in adult bone.

There is hormonal control of bone formation and bone breakdown. Both parathormone, which is related to the parathyroid gland, and thyrocalcitonin, which is produced by the thyroid gland, have primary roles in bone formation and destruction. The gross anatomy of the bony skeleton will not be considered here as this is covered in any textbook of anatomy.

USE OF RADIONUCLIDES IN THE STUDY OF BONE

For many years the metabolism of bone has been studied by the use of radioisotopes of calcium. Calcium 47, which is a gamma emitter, has been used in the study of bone metabolism; however, the high energy of its gamma ray requires extremely heavy shielding. Therefore, the use of this radionuclide is limited.

More recently, the radioisotopes of strontium, which mimic calcium metabolism, have been used. The useful isotopes of strontium are ^{85}Sr and ^{87m}Sr. These radionuclides have come into extensive use because bone has to be decalcified by approximately 50% before decreased density can be visualized on radiographs. Therefore, lesions have usually been existent for sometime and have destroyed a great deal of bone before standard radiographs become positive. In abnormalities of bone, it has been found that the radionuclides ^{85}Sr and ^{87m}Sr may be statistically counted with any standard detector or may be imaged at a very early stage of the disease process. The increased deposition of these radionuclides is strongly linked to osteoblastic activity and new bone formation.

Since these radionuclides are found in areas of new bone formation, there is increased strontium deposition in the normal areas of new bone growth (the epiphyseal ends of the long bones).

The clinical injected dose of ^{85}Sr is usually between 50 and 100 μCi and the amount of ^{85}Sr deposited in any unit area of bone is extremely minute. Therefore, minor changes in deposition of ^{85}Sr can only be discerned by the use of static counting techniques over long periods of time. Static counting is still utilized by many investigators and the statistical validity of this method cannot be argued. Many investigators, however, at present are using scanning or imaging equipment to picture the localization of radiostrontium in abnormal bony tissue. It must be understood that, in this particular study, statistical validity is difficult to attain because of the small quantity of ^{85}Sr deposited in bone. It was hoped that the other radionuclide of strontium, ^{87m}Sr, would aid in bone counting and imaging, as this radionuclide has a short half-life (2.83 hours) and is available from a generator. The cost of the radionuclide and the lesions missed in ^{85}Sr and ^{87m}Sr studies have limited the use of ^{87m}Sr.

One hour after the injection of radioactive strontium most of the strontium deposition has taken place in bone. Strontium is excreted both by the kidney and the large bowel; therefore, these two organ systems will interfere with bone counting and imaging for a period of time. Most of extraskeletal strontium has been excreted from the body within 72 hours. This is usually aided somewhat by the clinician by giving the patient cleansing enemas for several days after the administration of strontium.

The clinical use of strontium bone scanning is strongly related to metastatic bone disease. It has been shown that metastatic bone disease can be suspected on the basis of bone counting and imaging at a much earlier stage than by roentgenographic studies. In clinical bone counting and scanning about half of the amount of strontium is deposited per unit volume in the long bones as in the vertebral column. The amount of strontium deposited in normal bone is about the same for all patients. Since fracture, primary or metastatic disease, osteomyelitis, active osteoarthritis, rheumatoid arthritis, and Paget's disease of bone all have increased osteoblastic activity and new bone formation, the presence of these diseases must be suspected in all patients who have abnormal bone counts or images. An accompanying radiograph may aid in the diagnosis of abnormal strontium deposition. As a general rule, metastatic or primary cancer of bone usually increases the deposition of strontium in relation to the deposition of strontium in the normal bone surrounding the tumor by a factor of 2 or more.

Further investigation of strontium bone counting and imaging is strongly warranted. Surgical intervention of primary cancer and a radiotherapeutic approach to metastatic cancer may be aided greatly if the physician knows of existent sites and spread of metastatic disease. Therefore, there will be increasing interest in this particular study and stress will be placed on discovering other bone-seeking radionuclides.

Chapter

21 *Urinary system*

KIDNEY

The functional portion of the urinary system is composed of two kidneys, whose primary function is to produce urine. The urine is conveyed from the kidneys via the ureters into the urinary bladder, where it is temporarily stored before being discharged to the outside through the urethra.

The kidneys are a pair of highly vascular, retroperitoneal, elastic organs situated in the posterior part of the abdomen. They are located mainly in the lumbar regions and are imbedded in a considerable mass of fatty tissue termed the renal fat (see Figs. 15-1, *A*; 16-1, *A* and *C*). Their long axes are directed downward and laterally; their upper poles are nearer to the median plane than their lower poles. The right kidney is slightly lower than the left, possibly because of its relationship to the liver. Normally, the kidneys measure 4 to 5 inches in length, 2.5 inches in width, and 1 inch in thickness.

The outline of the kidneys can be mapped out on the patient's back within a pair of rectangles included between two horizontal lines drawn through the eleventh thoracic and third lumbar spines and two vertical lines drawn at 1 and 4 inches from the middle line.

In shape, the kidneys resemble a bean and have an ovoid outline. The lateral border is convex; the medial border is concave in the center and convex at each end. In the central part of the medial border there is a deep vertical fissure (hilum) and it transmits the renal vessels and nerves, together with the funnel-shaped upper end, or pelvis, of the ureter. This hilum leads into a central recess or cavity, called the renal sinus, and is almost entirely filled by the ureteral pelvis and renal vessels. Within the sinus, the pelvis of the ureter is formed by the union of two or, less commonly, three major calyces. Each major calyx is formed by the union of several minor calyces that embrace the renal papillae and receive the urine.

The renal arteries are wide vessels that take origin from the sides of the aorta opposite the second lumbar vertebra. Before entering the kidney, each artery divides into four or five branches. Blood returns from the kidneys by way of the renal veins, which join the sides of the inferior vena cava; the left vein is longer than the right.

Structure

The kidney is enclosed by a fibrous capsule that is prolonged around the lips of the hilum into the renal sinus to become continuous with the outer coat of the calyces and ureteral pelvis. The kidney is made up of two main parts: an inner

319

medulla and an outer cortex. The medulla consists of a series of conical masses (the renal pyramids) the bases of which face outward. They are separated by extensions from the cortex, called cortical columns. The apices of the pyramids converge toward the renal sinus, where they project into the interior of the calyces as small nipples or papillae. The cortical substance is more vascular and uniformly granular. It arches over the bases of the pyramids and dips in between them.

In the renal sinus, the branches of the renal artery divide into lobar arteries, one for each papilla. Each lobar artery divides into two interlobar arteries that proceed outward along the sides of the pyramids. At the junction between the medulla and cortex, the interlobar arteries divide into branches, called the arcuate arteries, that run at right angles to the parent stem. These give off a large number of vertically arranged branches, termed the straight or interlobular arteries, from which arise a number of lateral branches, called the afferent arterioles. Each afferent arteriole divides into about fifty capillaries that stay together to form a glomerulus. The blood leaves this glomerulus in a smaller efferent arteriole that divides to form a second capillary network around the tubules of its nephron (glomerulus and tubule). These capillaries finally converge to form venules that drain into the interlobular veins. The medulla receives its relatively scanty blood supply through branches from the efferent arterioles.

Each capillary tuft, or glomerulus, is surrounded by the expanded blind end of a renal tubule. This capsule consists of a basement membrane lined by a single layer of flattened epithelium and is called the glomerular or Bowman's capsule. This, together with its glomerulus, consititutes the Malpighian or renal corpuscle. The rest of the renal tubule runs a long tortuous course and consists of various parts, the most important of which are the first convoluted tubule, the loop of Henle (descending and ascending limbs), and the second convoluted tubule. This latter opens into a collecting tubule. The collecting tubules converge to form the ducts of Bellini that finally open on the summit of a papilla. The loops of Henle, the collecting tubules, and ducts of Bellini lie in the medulla; the rest of the renal tubules, as well as the renal corpuscles, are found in the cortex.

Functions

The main function of the kidney is to maintain the constancy of the osmotic pressure, volume, reaction, and composition of the extracellular fluid. This is achieved through urine secretion and elimination from the plasma of water and various nonvolatile solutes at rates and ratios that counterbalance the effects of the forces which tend to alter the composition of the internal medium. In addition, the kidney has certain functions that are unrelated to urine secretion. For example, through renin formation it may help in maintenance of normal blood pressure. Furthermore, the renal tubular epithelium carries out certain chemical transformations, including some detoxicating reactions.

Urine formation

The first step involved in the formation of urine is the maintenance of a large renal blood flow that amounts to 25% of the cardiac output (or roughly 1,250 ml blood per minute), containing approximately 700 ml plasma. This step is followed by ultrafiltration from the plasma through the walls of the glomerular tuft of capillaries into Bowman's capsule of a large volume of fluid containing the small molecules of the plasma in unchanged concentrations. The glomerular filtrate thus formed resembles the plasma except for the absence of plasma proteins and lipids; it amounts to 120 ml per minute or 170 liters per day. As it passes along the tubule, the filtrate is concentrated and the essential substances are conserved. Most of the water is reabsorbed, so that only 1 ml per minute passes into the collecting ducts to produce approximately 1.5 liters of urine per day. High threshold substances, such as glucose, sodium chloride, vitamin C, and amino acids, are nearly completely reabsorbed into the bloodstream. In contradistinction, only small amounts of the low threshold substances such as urea, phosphates, and uric acid are reabsorbed. Practically all of substances such as creatinine and sulfates are excreted. Apart from reabsorption, the renal tubules have the power to excrete certain substances such as iodopyracet (Diodrast), organic iodine compounds, sodium para-amino-hippurate, and penicillin.

After the urine is formed it passes via the ureters into the urinary bladder where it is temporarily stored. When empty, the urinary bladder lies in the lower and anterior part of the pelvis behind the pubic bones. As it fills, it balloons upward, and rises gradually into the abdominal cavity.

DETERMINATION OF RENAL BLOOD FLOW

According to the Fick principle, if a substance is consumed solely by one organ, the blood flow to this organ can be determined by dividing the amount consumed per unit time by the arteriovenous difference in the concentration of this material. This means that the concentration of this particular substance must be determined both in the arterial blood going to this organ and in the venous blood coming out of this organ. However, if this substance is totally consumed or excreted during a single passage through the organ, the concentration in the venous outflow will be zero. Accordingly, the arteriovenous difference is going to be equal to the arterial concentration of this material. Consequently, the blood flow to this organ can be estimated by dividing the amount consumed per unit time by the arterial concentration of this material.

In the case of the kidney, the criterion of almost complete removal from the plasma during a single passage is fulfilled by sodium para-amino-hippurate (PAH). Following the intravenous injection of a loading dose, PAH is administered in the form of a continuous infusion at a rate to maintain a steady blood level. So long as the PAH blood level is constant, the rate of infusion should be equal to the rate of excretion. Therefore, the renal plasma flow can be determined by dividing the amount infused or its equivalent (the amount excreted per unit time) by the plasma PAH concentration. However, maintenance of a steady blood level of PAH is not easy. Furthermore, accurate estimation of PAH urinary output per unit time necessitates the application of a urethral catheter and bladder washes.

These drawbacks were partly resolved by the application of the single injection technique with subsequent analysis of the disappearance curve of PAH from the

321

blood. However, since the diminution in the plasma PAH concentration is not only caused by its removal by the kidneys but also by its diffusion to equilibrate in a hippuran space, recording of the data should be extended for more than an hour to solve for the two components according to the two compartmental system. A further disadvantage is the estimation of the rather low concentrations of PAH in the collected plasma samples.

This difficulty was overcome by the introduction of ^{131}I-tagged sodium ortho-iodohippurate (radiohippuran). Using radiohippuran, the disappearance curve is recorded either by plasma sampling or by external monitoring. The obtained curve is then analyzed according to the two compartmental system. This is both time consuming and inconvenient to the patient.

To simplify matters, a segment from the disappearance curve is selected on condition that during this period the disappearance is mainly due to its removal by the kidney. Accordingly, the disappearance curve can be analyzed on the basis of a single compartment system. Under such circumstances, the renal blood flow is equal to the radiohippuran disappearance rate constant times its volume of distribution. The suggested segment is that between 8 and 18 minutes after injection. The effect of radiohippuran diffusion on the disappearance curve during this segment is counterbalanced by the incomplete removal of radiohippuran during its passage through the kidney. This is partly caused by the use of whole blood samples instead of plasma, taking into consideration that the intracorpuscular radiohippuran is not as available for removal as that present in the plasma. The

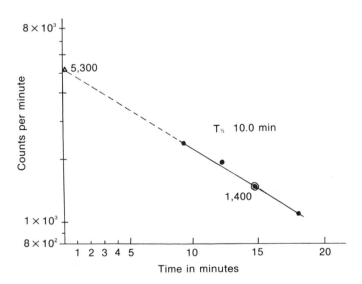

Fig. 21-1. Determination of the disappearance half-time of radiohippuran from the circulation by serial blood sampling.

$T_{1/2}$ = 10.0 minutes
λ = 0.693 ÷ 10.0 = 0.0693 (6.93% per minute)
DV = injected dose ÷ intercept at zero time
   = injected dose ÷ 5,300

disappearance curve can be recorded either by serial blood sampling or by external monitoring.

Procedure

Following the intravenous injection of 60 to 80 μCi of radiohippuran, four blood samples are obtained at 3 minute intervals starting at 9 minutes after injection. Radioactivity in 2 ml from each of these whole blood samples, as well as the standard for dose calibration, is assayed in a scintillation well counter. Radioactivity per milliliter in the serial blood samples is plotted on semilogarithmic paper as a function of time. The disappearance half-time of radiohippuran ($T_{1/2}$) is estimated, and the disappearance rate constant (λ) is calculated $\frac{0.693}{T_{1/2}}$. The volume of distribution (DV) is obtained by dividing the injected dose by the radiohippuran concentration at zero time as derived by backward extrapolation of the exponential curve (Fig. 21-1). The renal blood flow is calculated as $\lambda \times DV$.

By external monitoring, radiohippuran disappearance is measured by a collimated scintillation detector placed over the manubrium sterni at the level of the

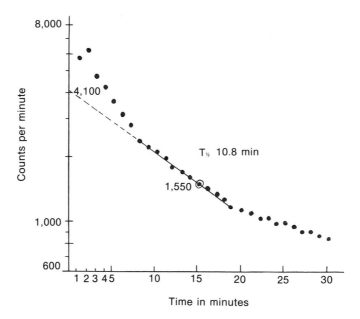

Fig. 21-2. Determination of the disappearance half-time of radiohippuran by external monitoring.

$T_{1/2}$ = 10.8 minutes
λ = 0.693 ÷ 10.8 = 0.0642 or 6.42% per minute
External counting at 15 minutes = 1,550 cpm
Blood activity at 15 minutes (Fig. 21-1) = 1,400 cpm
Calibration factor = 1,400/1,550
Intercept at zero time = 4,100 cpm by external monitoring which
        corresponds to blood activity of
        $4,100 \times \dfrac{1,400}{1,550}$
    = 3,700 cpm
  DV = injected dose ÷ 3,700

323

second rib. Recording is performed by a rate meter and stripchart recorder or by a printing scaler. Recording is continued for about 30 minutes. Fifteen minutes after injection, a blood sample is withdrawn and the radioactivity in 2 ml from this sample is assayed. From the record curve $T_{1/2}$ and λ are estimated. The volume of distribution is calculated as with the serial blood sampling with the application of a calibration factor to relate the external counting rate to the level of blood radioactivity at 15 minutes. Then the renal blood flow is calculated from λ and DV (Fig. 21-2).

Using these techniques, the renal blood flow in normal subjects proved to be 630 ± 70 ml/minute/meter squared or $1,100 \pm 120$ ml/min/1.73 meter squared surface area (mean $\pm$ SD).

RADIONUCLIDE RENOGRAPHY

Although the radionuclide renogram has been in use for almost 15 years, there is no agreement regarding the radiopharmaceutical to be used, the technical details of the procedure, or the interpretation of the obtained tracing. Of the various radionuclides used, only sodium orthoiodohippurate ^{131}I and chlormerodrin [197]Hg or chlormerodrin [203]Hg have stood the test of time. In this respect, radiohippuran is much more widely used than labeled chlormerodrin.

Radiohippuran renogram

Following the intravenous injection of 50 to 100 μCi of radiohippuran, the time course of radioactivity over both kidneys is measured by a pair of well-matched collimated scintillation detectors. The information collected is counted by two rate meters with a time constant of 3 to 10 seconds; it is subsequently recorded on a dual stripchart recorder moving at a rate of 0.75 inches per minute over a period of 30 minutes. Recording can be also done by means of a pair of printing scalers activated at 15 second intervals. The obtained data is plotted to illustrate radioactivity as a function of time.

Although it has been shown that the shape of the renographic curve is affected to a great extent by the degree of hydration of the patient, there is disagreement as to what is the optimum state of hydration required. With hydration, the tracing is more smooth, which makes calculations easier. In addition, in normal subjects the level of peak radioactivity attained by both kidneys is more or less equal, whereas in the dehydrated state the levels are not equal. Therefore, it is felt that hydration is better, and this can be achieved by asking the patient to drink about 600 ml of fluids during the hour preceding the test.

In regard to the position of the patient during performance of the test, some investigators prefer the sitting position in order to help urine drainage by gravity. Others keep the patient supine or prone to limit movements. A combination of these benefits can be achieved by performing the renogram with the patient prone and the head of the table raised 30 degrees.

Since accurate placement of the detectors is critical, the kidneys are localized either by radiography (in the same position of renography) or by moving the detectors over the patient's back after intravenous injection of 5 μCi of chlormerodrin [197]Hg to mark the site showing the highest counting rate.

There has been much controversy concerning the choice of collimators and depth of crystal. Wide apertures minimize the effects of errors in detector placement at the expense of including more extrarenal radioactivity. Similarly, increasing the depth of the crystal in the collimator minimizes the effect of variability in the distance at which the kidney is situated underneath the skin, but the count rate is diminished. As a compromise, a collimator with an aperture diameter of 1.5 inches is used and the crystal is recessed 3 inches from the surface.

The obtained tracing starts with an abrupt initial rise in radioactivity because of its arrival in the field monitored by the detector. At least part of this radioactivity is extrarenal, since it can be demonstrated even after removal of the kidney. This segment is followed by a slower increase in radioactivity to reach a peak value (ascending limb). The rate of rise is affected by changes in the renal blood flow and cellular function. In addition, the rate of rise and the time necessary to reach the peak depend on the state of hydration of the patient. With hydration, the time required is shorter and the slope of this limb is steeper. The last segment of the renogram (descending limb) represents removal of the radioactivity from underneath the detector. The rate of fall is influenced by the rate of removal of radioactivity from the renal pelvis as well as the disappearance of radioactivity from the blood. With hydration, the fall in radioactivity is initially faster and then becomes slower because of the appearance of bladder radioactivity in the field monitored by the detector (Fig. 21-3).

For the proper interpretation of the radiohippuran renogram, several methods

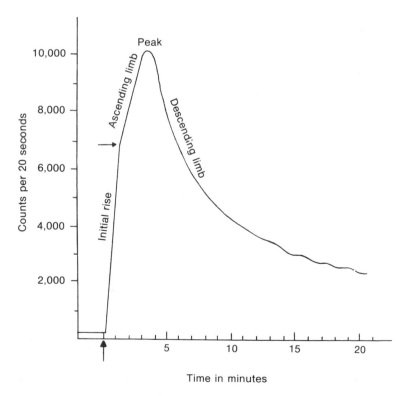

Fig. 21-3. Radiohippuran renogram of a normal subject after hydration with 600 ml of water.

have been suggested for analysis of the obtained tracing. The easiest and quickest method is visual comparison of height and shape of the curve of both sides. However, this method of analysis cannot be applied after nephrectomy or in patients having bilateral renal affection. Therefore, it was proposed that the tracings should be compared with an envelope drawn to include a group of curves from normal subjects using exactly the same procedure and equipment. However, this needs standardization of the curves to a certain height and does not allow any quantitation of the abnormality. For quantitation, various criteria were suggested, such as the time to reach peak radioactivity, the ratio of the peak values, the slope of the ascending limb, and the rate of decrease of radioactivity on the descending limb. The normal values for the suggested criteria should be determined in each laboratory using the same procedure and equipment every time.

A completely different approach in the analysis is based on the fact that radiohippuran renograms represent an integrated response to changing radioactivity levels within the kidneys, as well as different levels of activity within the blood perfusing these organs and other tissues within the area monitored by the detector. Therefore, accurate correction for the external factors must be applied. This is achieved by the application of a third detector centered over the manubrium sterni and then subtraction of the obtained curve representing extrarenal radioactivity from the simultaneously recorded renograms. The resultant curve can be called the derived renogram and consists of the ascending and descending limbs. It can be analyzed by calculation of the rates of ascent and descent, respectively. A further advantage of this method of analysis is that the renal blood flow can

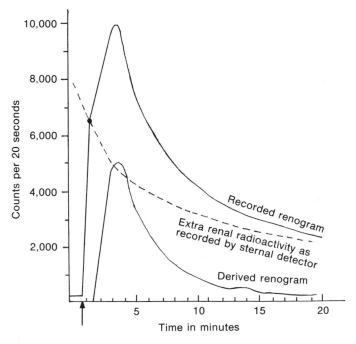

Fig. 21-4. Analysis of radiohippuran renogram by subtraction of the extrarenal radioactivity as recorded by a sternal detector from the recorded renographic tracing.

be estimated from the tracing recorded by the sternal detector, as explained earlier (Fig. 21-4).

Clinical applications

It must be made clear that abnormal renogram tracings are not diagnostic of any specific disease. Renography has its greatest value in screening patients for a suspected abnormality and in the follow-up of such abnormality when present.

Abnormal tracings are seen with decreased kidney function and diminished blood supply, as well as with urinary obstruction whether caused by stones, tumors, or otherwise.

Special indications for renography include the follow-up after renal artery reconstruction or kidney transplantation. Another indication is screening patients for cases of unilateral renal hypertension. An abnormal tracing on one side favors this possibility and is an indication for the application of further investigations by means of the more difficult and traumatic techniques, such as arteriography and differential urethral catheterization in an effort to reach a definite diagnosis.

Mercury renogram

Following the intravenous injection of 30 to 300 μCi of chlormerodrin ^{197}Hg, the rate of accumulation of radiomercury is measured by a pair of well-matched collimated scintillation detectors placed opposite the previously determined renal sites. The collected information is recorded by a pair of rate meters attached to a dual stripchart recorder. The result is calculated by comparison of the count rates at 30 and 60 minutes to that at 5 minutes after injection. The ratio of the rate of accumulation on the right side to that of the left is then computed. This value normally ranges from 0.85:1 to 1.05:1.

Since chlormerodrin is temporarily bound in the renal tubules, the described accumulation test is less influenced by the rate of urine flow or the state of hydration of the patient than is the case of radiohippuran renography. Furthermore, mixing does not affect the tracing because of the slow rate of accumulation together with the long time of observation. This leaves the chlormerodrin accumulation test to be affected mainly by the renal blood flow and the renal tubular efficiency. A further advantage is the possibility of obtaining a scan picture for the kidney with the same dose of radiomercury used for the functional study. However, since the result is expressed in the form of a ratio between both sides, bilateral functional renal impairment of an equal degree would give a normal result. In addition, this test does not lead to any information about the potency of the urinary passages.

RADIONUCLIDE SCANNING OF THE KIDNEYS

Since chlormerodrin accumulates in the renal tubular cells at a rate that greatly exceeds its excretion, this radiopharmaceutical can be used for the visualization of viable renal tissue. Usually, 300 μCi are injected intravenously and scanning is started at least 1 hour later, through the posterior approach. It must be remembered that some of the radiomercury appears in the liver (more so with depressed renal function), which could cause some confusion concerning the size of the right kidney under such circumstances.

Renal scanning is indicated for the accurate determination of the size, site, and shape of the kidney, together with the detection of any space occupying lesions. The suggested reference points to be marked on the scan picture are the midline, and the last rib and iliac crest on both sides. Normally, the renal picture measures 5 by 2.5 inches (Fig. 21-5).

Scanning is diagnostic of morphology and not pathology. A space-occupying lesion in a scan picture might be caused by a tumor, cyst, abscess, or infarct (Figs. 21-6 and 21-7).

A special indication for radionuclide scanning of the kidneys is the detection of tumors that do not cause distortion of the calyceal system and consequently would be missed by intravenous pyelography. In addition, in the presence of moderate renal failure, scanning usually succeeds in visualization of the kidneys, whereas pyelography fails. Another indication for renal scanning is the investigation of patients who are allergic to iodine-containing contrast media.

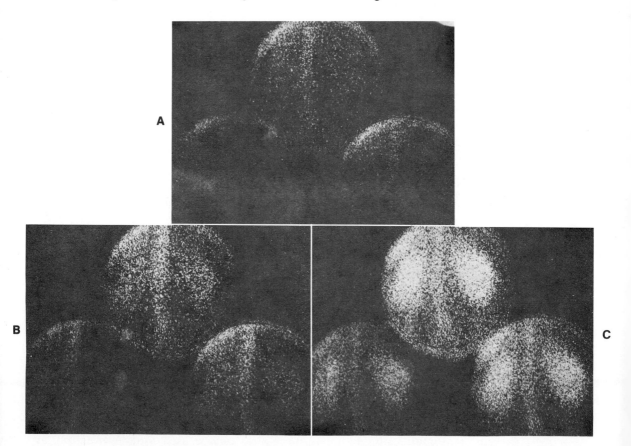

Fig. 21-5. Renal perfusion study following the intravenous injection of 10 mCi pertechnetate. **A,** Aorta just becoming visible; **B,** early renal perfusion bolus has reached the common iliacs; **C,** normal renal image. (Courtesy, Laurence B. Rentschler, M.D.; Memorial Hospital, Roxborough, Philadelphia.)

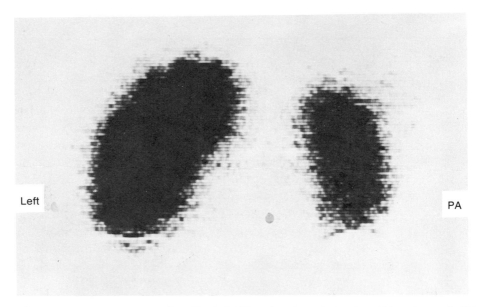

Fig. 21-6. Abnormal ¹⁹⁷Hg renal scan. The left kidney is enlarged, the right kidney Is small. This type of scan can be caused by a multitude of diffuse disease states; however, it is most commonly linked with hypertensive unilateral renal disease.

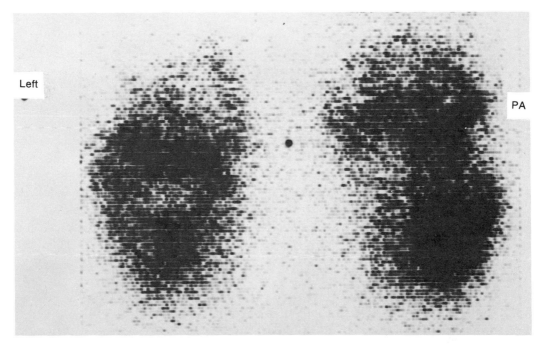

Fig. 21-7. Abnormal ¹⁹⁷Hg renal scan. Both kidneys are enlarged. There are multiple round cold areas bilaterally. This is a typical scan of multicystic (polycystic) renal disease.

22 *Cardiovascular system*

The cardiovascular, or circulatory, system is the chief transport system in the body. It delivers oxygen and nutrients to the tissues, and carries carbon dioxide and other waste products to the lungs and kidneys for elimination from the body. It carries the protective substances that can help in the combat of noxious agents, and distributes chemicals and hormones to regulate cell function.

The cardiovascular system consists of the heart, blood, and blood vessels. The vessels are differentiated into arteries (which carry the blood from the heart to the different tissues of the body), capillaries (where the interchange of gases, food, and waste occurs), and veins (which return the blood from the tissues back to the heart).

The heart is a hollow, muscular organ that lies between the lungs behind the body of the sternum and the adjoining parts of the rib cage, projecting farther to the left than to the right of the median plane. Normally, it measures about 5 inches from base to apex and roughly 3.5 inches traversely at its broadest part. When projected on the anterior chest wall, the outline of the normal heart can be simulated by an irregular quadrangular area. Its upper border, or base, corresponds to a line drawn from the lower border of the second left costal cartilage 1.5 inches from the median plane to the upper border of the third right costal cartilage an inch from the middle line. From there, the right border extends down to the sixth right cartilage 0.5 inch from its junction with the sternum. The lower border is represented by a line drawn from the last point to the apex beat, which normally lies in the fifth left intercostal space 3.5 inches from the median plane. A line joining the cardiac apex with the left end of the upper border represents the left border of the heart.

The heart, together with the roots of the great vessels, is enclosed in a fibroserous sac called the pericardium. The external layer is fibrous, whereas the internal is a closed, invaginated, two-layered serous sac. The serous pericardium is made of an inner visceral layer and an outer parietal layer separated by a thin film of fluid to lessen the friction between these two surfaces as they move during the cardiac cycle of contraction (systole) and relaxation (diastole). Under abnormal conditions, excess fluid accumulates in the serous pericardial sac and is called pericardial effusion.

The heart itself is divided into four chambers, which are lined with endothelium or endocardium. Two of these chambers—the right and left atria—receive blood from the great veins and expel it into the distributing chambers, called the right and left ventricles. Since they have to pump the blood for a short distance in the face of minor resistance, the artia have thin walls of cardiac muscle or myocardium. The distributing chambers, or ventricles, have thicker walls of myocardium; the thickness being more marked in the left ventricle. Each atrium communicates freely with its corresponding ventricle, whereas the right and left chambers are completely separated from one another by partitions called interatrial and interventricular septa. In order to prevent the backflow of blood, each atrioventricular communication is guarded by a valve (the tricuspid on the right, and mitral on the left). Similarly, the backflow from the great vessels into the corresponding ventricles is prevented by the presence of the semilunar valves on the origins of the pulmonary artery and aorta.

With each heartbeat, blood is pumped by the left ventricle into a large artery (the aorta) and is distributed via its numerous branches to all tissues and organs of the body with the exception of the lungs. The deoxygenated blood carrying the waste products returns to the right atrium by means of the superior vena cava from the head, neck, and upper limbs and by the inferior vena cava from the trunk and lower limbs. This constitutes the greater or systemic circulation.

The deoxygenated blood passes from the right atrium into the right ventricle, which expels it through the pulmonary artery to the lungs for its fresh supply of oxygen. The oxygenated blood, which has lost some of its carbon dioxide, returns via the pulmonary veins to the left atrium and on to the left ventricle. The passage of blood from the right ventricle through the lungs to the left atrium is called the lesser, or pulmonary, circulation.

The rhythmic contraction of the heart is called heartbeat. Normally, the heart beats 70 to 80 times per minute. The heartbeat originates in a specialized tissue in the wall of the right atrium called the sinoauricular node (SA node). From there, the wave of excitation spreads throughout the muscles of both atria, which respond by contraction. The impulse is picked up by another mass of nodal tissue, called the auriculoventricular node (AV node), and is relayed by a specialized conducting bundle to the ventricles, which respond and contract. During ventricular contractions, blood is forced into the aorta. The amount of blood pumped per unit time is designated as cardiac output. The expelled blood moves the blood in the vessels forward and sets a pressure wave that travels down the arteries. The pressure wave expands the arterial wall as it travels and is felt as the pulse. It must be noted that the rate at which the pulse wave travels is completely independent of the velocity of the blood flow.

After the onset of ventricular systole, the aortic semilunar valve opens. Blood passes into the aorta and the large arteries. The pressure rises smoothly to a maximum (systolic blood pressure) and normally measures 120 mm Hg. As the blood passes onward into the arterioles and the ventricles relax during ventricular diastole, the pressure drops to a minimum (diastolic pressure). This usually amounts to 80 mm Hg. The arterial pressure is usually written as systolic over diastolic (120/80 mm Hg). Down the arterial tree, the vessels decrease in caliber and the blood pressure falls, with diminution in the difference between systolic and diastolic levels. In the arterioles the average pressure is approximately 40 mm Hg.

By a process of repeated divisions and ramifications, the arterioles open into a closely meshed network of microscopic vessels (capillaries) that have semipermeable walls, which allow movement of water and solutes. This movement is governed by diffusion and filtration. because they are in higher concentration in the blood, oxygen and glucose diffuse outward into the tissue spaces. Carbon dioxide, because it is in higher concentration in the tissues, moves inward. The rate and direction of filtration depend on the net result of the intracapillary pressure driving outward and the osmotic pressure of the plasma proteins and the pressure in the tissue spaces working in the opposite direction. With a more or less steady osmotic pressure of plasma proteins (25 mm Hg) and an interstitial pressure of 1 to 2 mm Hg, the main determining factor in filtration is the capillary pressure. At the arteriolar end, the capillary pressure is 35 mm Hg. Therefore, the net result is a driving force that moves the fluid and electrolytes outward into the tissue spaces. At the venular end where the capillary pressure averages 15 mm Hg, the net result is a pulling force that draws water and electrolytes from the tissue fluids back into the bloodstream. The excess fluid that does not return by this route is drained by the lymphatics and is carried back into the blood. The exchange that takes place across the capillary membrane results in a continuous turnover and removal of tissue fluids.

After passing through the capillaries, blood is collected by a series of minute vessels called venules. These unite with one another to form veins that ultimately form two main venous trunks (the superior and inferior venae cavae), which open in the right atrium. Toward the heart, the caliber of the vessels increases and the pressure diminishes. In the venules the pressure is about 15 mm Hg, whereas in the large veins outside the chest it averages 5 mm Hg or 6 cm water. The pressure in the great veins at the entrance in the right atrium amounts to 4 cm water and fluctuates with respiration and cardiac contractions. In this connection, it should be noted that the negative intrathoracic pressure with its fluctuations during respiration aids the venous return to a great extent. This return is further aided by contractions of the skeletal muscles, which squeeze the veins and move the blood toward the heart.

DETERMINATION OF THE CARDIAC OUTPUT

Cardiac output can be defined as the effective volume of blood expelled by either ventricle per unit time. It is usually expressed as milliliters or liters per minute. The output of either ventricle per beat is called the stroke volume. Consequently, the cardiac output would be equal to the stroke volume times the heart rate.

If the concentration of oxygen in the blood going to the lungs is 14% and that in the outflowing blood is 19%, then each 100 ml blood has gained 5 ml oxygen (or each liter of blood has absorbed 50 ml oxygen) as it passed through the lungs. If the individual has consumed 250 ml of oxygen from the alveolar air per minute, then the amount of blood that has passed across the alveoli during this minute in order to absorb this amount of oxygen should be 250/50, or 5 liters. This is actually the pulmonary blood flow or the right ventricular output; or simply, the cardiac output, according to the Fick principle.

The oxygen consumption can be estimated by a spirometer. The oxygen concentration should be determined in an arterial blood sample as well as in venous blood. The arterial blood is obtained by arterial puncture, whereas the venous

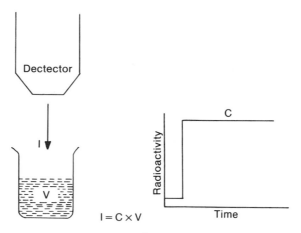

Fig. 22-1. Indicator dilution in a static system: *I*, indicator; *C*, concentration; *V*, volume.

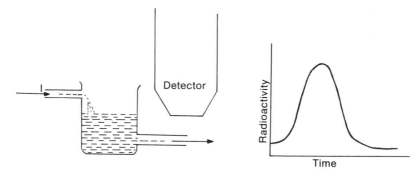

Fig. 22-2. Radionuclide dilution in a dynamic system with an inlet and an outlet.

sample is collected through cardiac catheterization from the right ventricle or pulmonary artery. Although this method is accurate, the technical requirements make it impractical for routine clinical use.

A completely different approach for this problem of the determination of the cardiac output depends on the application of the indicator dilution principles. In a static system (Fig. 22-1) in which an indicator is mixed with a certain volume of fluid, the relationship between the amount of indicator (1), its concentration (C), and the volume of the fluid present (V) is exemplified by the equation:

$$I = C \times V$$

In a dynamic system represented by a receptacle having an inlet and an outlet (Fig. 22-2), in which the indicator is injected as a bolus of highly concentrated material through the inlet, application of the principle of dilution implies certain changes. With sampling along the outlet, the volume of dilution (V), or the amount of fluid flowing during the time interval taken by the dilution process, can be calculated from the flow rate (F) and the time for dilution (T)

$$V = F \times T$$

333

Therefore the primary equation becomes:

$$I = C \times F \times T$$

However with sampling along the outlet in a dynamic system, the concentration is going to be changing. It begins from zero, rises to a maximum, and then diminishes. Therefore, the average concentration (C_{av}) must be used during the time of dilution, rather than using an absolute concentration. Consequently, the equation becomes:

$$I = C_{av} \times F \times T$$
$$F = \frac{I}{C_{av} \times T}$$

In a similar system, but one in which the outflow pours back into the inflow, some of the indicator will circulate back to the site of sampling before completion of the dilution process, causing a rise in the concentration (Fig. 22-3). This would definitely affect the estimation of the average concentration. However, this diminution in concentration is an exponential function of time. Therefore, if this segment is plotted on a semilogarithmic scale, the expected behavior of the concentration curve can be derived by extrapolation, and the average concentration can be calculated.

The latter system simulates the heart to a great extent. If a known amount of indicator (I) is injected, the flow rate (F) or cardiac output (CO) can be estimated from the average concentration (C_{av}) and the time of dilution (T) according to the above equation. The indicators used are usually dyes, such as Evans blue, indigo carmine, or cardiogreen. The average concentration of the dye is obtained from serial blood samples collected at 1 to 3 second intervals by arterial puncture. To simplify matters, blood is led from an indwelling arterial needle through a

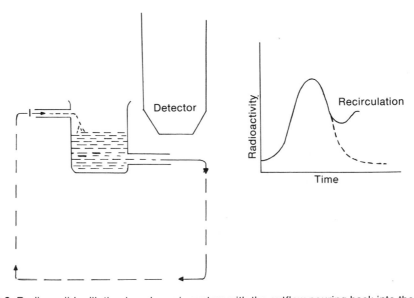

Fig. 22-3. Radionuclide dilution in a dynamic system with the outflow pouring back into the inflow.

constant flow cuvette with an automatic recording device to give a continuous record of the dye concentration. The concentration curve thus obtained is corrected for the effect of recirculation in order to determine the average dye concentration and the time of dilution, since both are needed for cardiac output determination. To obviate the need for arterial punctures, the dye concentration curve can be recorded externally by a photoelectric densitometer that measures changes in the optical density of the ear lobe following the intravenous injection of the dye. The optical density curve is obtained with the application of a calibration factor relating external recording to dye concentration.

As indicators, radionuclides have the advantage of easy and accurate quantitation even at low concentrations. In addition, gamma emitters have the unique qualification for external detection. The radionuclides used are ^{32}P-tagged red cells, ^{85}Kr, and ^{131}I-labeled human serum albumin (RISA); the latter is most commonly used. After injecting a known amount of the radionuclide, the average concentration of radioactivity during the period of observation is determined by the assay of serial arterial blood samples or from a continuous recording of radioactivity in the blood led by external tubing through a scintillation detector. This necessitates the application of a calibration factor relating the counting rate to its equivalence in concentration. This is obtained by estimating the counting rate of a known concentration of radioactivity led through the tubing.

In order to obviate these technical difficulties, the nuclide dilution curve is recorded by means of an external detector focused over the heart. The same principles that have been described are applicable and the cardiac output (CO) is calculated from the equation:

$$CO = \frac{I}{C_{av} \times T}$$

However, since the tracer concentration is not measured directly, but by external monitoring, it becomes necessary to apply a factor of proportionality relating the external rate and the tracer concentration in the blood. This is achieved by recording the external counting rate (C_f) at the same time of withdrawing a venous blood sample in order to estimate the blood tracer concentration (C_b) by the in vitro assay of radioactivity in this sample. This proportionality factor is applied to the previous equation:

$$CO = \frac{I}{\dfrac{C_{av} \times C_b \times T}{C_f}}$$

$$= \frac{C_f \times I}{C_{av} \times T \times C_b}$$

However, the fraction $\frac{1}{C_b}$ represents the diluting volume of the tracer (DV), which approximates the blood volume (BV) if enough time is allowed for the tracer to attain uniform concentration and the radionuclide does not diffuse outside the vascular system. Substituting for this fraction, the equation becomes:

$$CO = \frac{C_f \times DV}{C_{av} \times T}$$

Clinical nuclear medicine

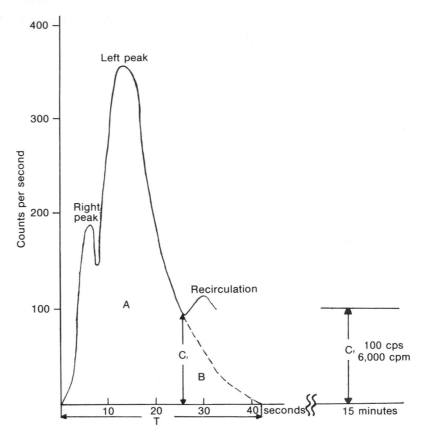

Fig. 22-4. Determination of cardiac output. A = area prior to recirculation. T = time of primary circulation. C_f = final counting rate by external monitoring. C_r = counting rate just prior to recirculation by external counting. B = extrapolated area.

The denominator in this equation is equivalent to the area under the primary dilution curve expressed in counts. Therefore, the equation will read

$$CO = \frac{C_f \times DV}{area}$$

This area consists of the area until recirculation (A), together with the extrapolated area (B) (Fig. 22-4). This gives the final equation:

$$CO = \frac{C_f \times DV}{(A+B)}$$

Therefore, it becomes quite evident that for the determination of the cardiac output, all that is needed is an estimation of the final counting rate by the external detector (C_f), the diluting volume (DV), and the total area under the primary dilution curve (A+B).

Procedure using radioiodinated human serum albumin

The patient lies comfortably in bed and a collimated scintillation detector is placed over one side of the heart. Usually the left side is chosen and the detector

336

is focused over a point 1.5 inches medial and 1 inch upward from the site of the maximal apical impulse. The collimator used has a straight bore, with an aperture 1.5 inches wide; the crystal is recessed 3 inches from the surface. The information to be collected is counted through a count rate meter with a time constant of 0.5 seconds and is recorded on a stripchart recorder moving at a rate of 12 inches per minute. After the background counting rate has been recorded, 20 to 40 μCi of radioiodinated human serum albumin in a volume not exceeding 2 ml are rapidly injected as a bolus in an antecubital vein, followed by a flushing dose of normal saline. After the passage of the radioactive bolus through the heart and the re-circulation have been recorded, the time constant of the rate meter is switched to 5 to 10 seconds, and the rate of the stripchart recorder is changed to 12 inches per hour. After 10 to 15 minutes a venous blood sample is withdrawn from the opposite arm and its timing is marked on the stripchart.

Radioactivity in 1 ml from the blood sample, as well as from the standard for dose calculation, is assayed in a scintillation well counter. Dividing the dose injected by the concentration of radioactivity in the blood (C_b) gives the diluting volume (DV), which, under the circumstances described, approximates the blood volume.

The final counting rate (C_f) in counts per minute is obtained from the strip-chart recording at the time marked simultaneously with the blood sampling.

For calculation of the area under the primary dilution curve, the net counting rate recorded on the stripchart is replotted against time. Recirculation is identified by a sudden change in the trailing edge of the concentration curve. The count rate on the trailing edge is plotted as a function of time on semilogarithmic paper. This enables calculation of the clearance half-time ($T_{1/2}$) of RISA from the heart. By extrapolation to zero, the duration of the primary dilution curve is estimated, and the area under the curve can be completed. The whole area under the primary circulation curve is measured in cm^2 by a planimeter, and is converted to its equivalent in counts by the application of the scaling factors used in plotting the data. These factors relate counts per minute per centimeter on one axis and minutes per centimeter on the other. As an alternative, the area under the primary curve until recirculation (A) is measured by planimetry, whereas the extrapolated area (B) is calculated using the following equation:

Area B $= C_r \times T_{1/2} \times 1.443 \times$ scaling factor
C_r = Net counting rate at the last point before the occurrence of recirculation
$T_{1/2}$ = Clearance half-time of RISA in seconds
Scaling factor = The one used for drawing and relates centimeters to time in seconds

If a planimeter is not available, the net counting rate as recorded on the strip-chart is tabulated to give the counting rate for every 1 second interval. The area under the curve until recirculation (A) equals the sum of the products of each counting rate multiplied by the period of counting (1 second). The extrapolated area (B) is calculated from the net counting rate per second at the point prior to recirculation multiplied by 1.443 times the clearance half-time ($T_{1/2}$) in seconds. The clearance half-time is obtained as usual by plotting the trailing edge of the curve on semilogarithmic paper. The whole area under the primary curve (A + B) expressed in counts is obtained by summation of area A and area B.

337

A much easier and more rapid method to estimate the area under the primary circulation curve is achieved through the use of a pair of printing scalers activated at 1 second intervals. The first scaler records the counting rate at increments of 1 second, whereas the second continuously integrates the isotope dilution curve. The count rate of the trailing edge of the curve as recorded by the first scaler is plotted on semilogarithmic paper against time. This yields the clearance half-time of RISA in seconds as well as the counting rate and time prior to recirculation. From these data, the extrapolated area (B) is calculated in counts as previously described. The rest of the area (A) is obtained in counts by reading the value recorded at the point prior to recirculation by the integrating scaler. The total area under the primary circulation curve expressed in counts is computed by summation of the values obtained for both areas (A and B).

The total area under the primary circulation curve (A + B) in counts, the diluting volume (DV) in liters, and the final counting rate (C_f) are determined in counts per minute by external counting. The cardiac output (CO) is then calculated using the following equation:

$$CO = \frac{C_f \times DV}{(A + B)}$$

In normal individuals using the external radionuclide technique, the cardiac output averages 6.13 ± 0.73 liters per minute (mean $\pm$ 1 standard deviation), with a range of 4.93 to 7.25 liters per minute. The cardiac index or cardiac output/m^2 surface area ranges from 2.75 to 4.10 liters/minute/m^2 with a mean of 3.36 ± 0.35 liters/minute/m^2. The stroke volume or cardiac output per beat averages 92 ± 14 ml per beat; the range is from 70 to 120 ml per beat. The stroke index, which represents the stroke volume/m^2 of surface area amounts to 50 ± 7 ml/beat/m^2.

Measurement of the cardiac output is indicated for the evaluation of patients with coronary disease and cardiac disease of other etiology, and for the follow-up of patients submitted to cardiac surgery.

CIRCULATION TIME

The circulation time represents the shortest interval between the intravenous injection of a substance and its arrival at some distant site in sufficient concentration to produce a recognizable end point.

The methods of calculating circulation time in common use depend on the application of chemicals (decholin, calcium gluconate) or volatile substances (ether) in order to determine the arm-to-tongue and arm-to-lung circulation times. However, these methods suffer from the disadvantage of having a subjective end point which depends on the patient's reaction and cooperation.

Radionuclides, however, produce a sharp, well-defined end point that is identifiable objectively by specialized sensitive equipment. In this connection, the most commonly used nuclide is ^{131}I-labeled human serum albumin. By the use of collimated scintillation detectors connected through count rate meters to synchronized stripchart recorders, various circulation times can be measured and the velocity of flow calculated.

For the determination of the velocity of flow along the veins of the lower limbs,

10 to 20 μCi of **RISA** are injected into a vein of the dorsum of the foot. A record is obtained of the appearance of radioactivity at two points along the femoral vein by a pair of collimated scintillation detectors. From this record, the transit time of radioactivity from one detector to the other is estimated. Since the distance between the points examined is known, the velocity of the venous flow can be calculated according to the equation:

$$\text{Velocity} = \frac{\text{Distance}}{\text{Transit time}}$$

On the arterial side, the same principle applies. The radionuclide is injected through an antecubital vein, and the velocity is calculated.

In cases of arterial obstruction, the application of a set of detectors enables identification of the site of obstruction. The detector proximal to the obstruction shows the arrival of radioactivity, whereas the distal detector does not.

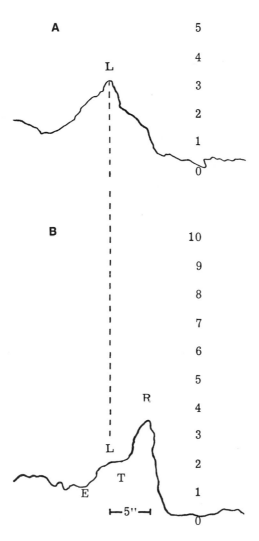

Fig. 22-5. A, The radioactivity build-up curve as recorded by a detector placed over the left side of the heart. **B,** Build-up curve as recorded by a detector focused over the right side of the heart. The pulmonary circulation time is represented by the time interval between *R* and *L* in the two recorded tracings.

Measurement of the pulmonary circulation time can be achieved by the use of two synchronized sets of recording equipment. One detector is focused over the right side of the heart and the other placed over the left side. Following the rapid intravenous injection of 20 μCi of RISA, the arrival of radioactivity in the field of each detector is recorded (Fig. 22-5). The time interval between these two events roughly represents the pulmonary circulation time (PCT). The same result can be obtained by means of one detector placed over the heart to record events occurring in both sides. The obtained tracing is called a radiocardiogram (Fig. 22-6). It is a double peaked curve, consisting of R and L waves, which represent the right and left sides of the heart respectively. The transitional zone between the two waves (T) is caused by the passage of radioactivity from the field of the detector into the lesser circulation. Thus, the pulmonary circulation time can be roughly estimated by measuring the time interval between the peaks of the R and L waves. This is called the peak-to-peak pulmonary circulation time.

A more accurate estimation can be obtained by correcting the peak of L for any possible lateral displacement by overlap from the terminal portion of the R wave. This is called the corrected pulmonary circulation time. The mean pulmonary circulation time can be estimated by measuring the time interval between the mean times for R and L waves.

In normal subjects, the peak-to-peak pulmonary circulation time ranges from 2.6 to 6.1 seconds, with a mean of 4.4 ± 0.9 seconds. The mean pulmonary circulation time averages 5.7 ± 1.1 seconds, with a range of 2.8 to 8.5 seconds.

Diminution of the pulmonary circulation time is observed with tachycardia, severe anemia, and thyrotoxicosis. Prolongation of the pulmonary circulation time is seen with heart failure, heart block, myxedema, pulmonary hypertension, and old age.

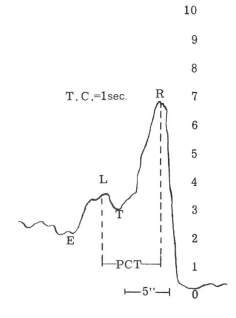

Fig. 22-6. A normal radiocardiogram. *R* represents arrival of radioactivity to the right side of the heart; *L* represents radioactivity to the left side. *T* (decrease in counting rate) is caused by passage of radioactivity from the field of the detector into the pulmonary circulation. *E* is the end of the radiocardiogram before the recirculation. The *PCT* equals the time interval between *R* and *L*. The time constant (T.C.) of the rate meter used in this tracing was 1 second.

Measurement of the circulation times is used as an aid to proper diagnosis of cardiovascular disorders and to determine the velocity of blood flow.

PERIPHERAL CIRCULATION

The nonradioactive techniques, such as colorimetry, oscillemetry, and plethysmography, used to evaluate the state of the peripheral circulation are indirect and liable to technical errors and variations because of physiologic and environmental factors that are difficult to control and interpret. Procedures that utilize radioactive materials have the advantage of being ways to directly obtain data representing the peripheral circulation (Fig. 22-7).

Although diffusion or disappearance of a freely diffusible substance injected directly into a muscle has been a satisfactory index of the vascular flow, this technique is dependent on the site, volume, and depth of injection.

A better approach depends on measurement of the uptake curves of both feet of the patient following the intravenous injection of a radionuclide. The collimated scintillation detectors used are placed in close contact with the balls of both feet. The information collected is counted by a pair of count rate meters with a time constant of 3 seconds and is recorded by a dual stripchart recorder moving at a rate of 0.75 inches per minute. Labeled electrolytes were first used. However, in interpretation, the diffusion gradient of the radionuclide has to be considered together with the degree of vascularity. Therefore, these tracers were replaced by

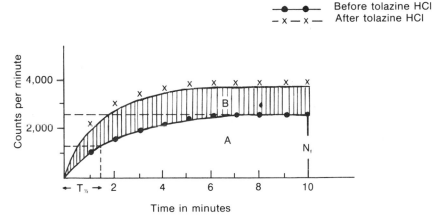

Fig. 22-7. Radioactivity build-up curve before and after the administration of tolazoline hydrochloride to demonstrate the method of calculation of the result of a test to evaluate the peripheral circulation.

A   = original build-up curve
B   = increase in build-up curve after administration of tolazine HCl
$T_{1/2}$ = time to reach 50% of plateau activity
t   = 10 minutes
N_f = level of activity at 10 minutes
Area = $N_f[t - (T_{1/2} \times 1.443)]$
Final result = $\dfrac{B}{A} \times 100$

radioactive materials that remain in the vessels and consequently reflect only the intravascular radioactivity. These criteria are met by the use of labeled human serum albumin.

The test should be performed in a quiet room that is free from draft and has a relatively constant temperature. The patient is given an intravenous injection of 20 μCi of RISA, and the radioactivity build-up curves are monitored by a pair of identical, collimated scintillation detectors. The slope of the segment of the radioactivity build-up curve from the time of arrival until plateau indicates the rate of mixing of RISA with normal plasma in the capillary bed surveyed by the detector. The height of the plateau represents the size of the vascular bed in the field of the detector. In order to gain more information, the ability of the vessels to dilate is tested. This is done by repetition of the test, using an exactly equal amount of RISA after the application of external heat to the legs or after an intravenous administration of a vasodilator as 10 mg tolazoline hydrochloride (Priscol). External heating can be performed by applying an electric blanket to the feet for 30 minutes. If tolazoline hydrochloride is used, it is necessary to wait only 3 minutes before beginning the second test.

The result is either expressed qualitatively by visual comparison of the tracings obtained before and after the induction of vascular dilatation or quantitatively by estimating the differences between the build-up curves and expressing this difference as percentage from the original curve ($\frac{B}{A} \times 100$). The areas are either measured by planimetry or calculated according to the equation:

Area $= N_t[t - (1.443 \times T_{1/2})]$
$N_t =$ Level of activity at 10 minutes
$T_{1/2} =$ Time to reach 50% of plateau activity
$t = 10$ minutes (which is more than enough time to reach plateau)

Normally, under the effect of heat or tolazoline hydrochloride the vessels dilate. Consequently, the size of the vascular bed surveyed by the detector is increased, causing a higher level of plateau. Therefore, in normal individuals there should be a difference between the radioactivity build-up curves recorded before and after the induction of vasodilatation. Quantitatively, the lowest figure representing the difference between the two normal tracings expressed as percentage of the original is 27%. However, it would be better to define the limits of normality by the apparatus used in each laboratory.

This test is generally used for patients who have manifestations suggestive of peripheral vascular affections, such as changes in the temperature and/or color of a limb, trophic ulcers, intermittent claudication, and absent pulse.

DELINEATION OF THE CARDIAC BLOOD POOL

If a radiopharmaceutical that remains within the cardiovascular system for a reasonable time is injected intravenously, the configuration of the cardiac blood pool can be obtained by the determination of the spatial distribution of radioactivity by radionuclide scanning (Fig. 22-8). Various radiopharmaceuticals are used such as ^{131}I human serum albumin (150 μCi), 99m Tc (5-10 mCi), ^{131}I cholegrafin (300 μCi), ^{99m}Tc serum albumin (2 mCi), and stabilized [113]In (2 mCi).

Because of the better counting statistics achieved by the use of large doses allowable of short-lived radionuclides, ^{99m}Tc and ^{113}In preparations are preferred. However, they have to be prepared and sterilized at the time of the test.

Following the intravenous injection of the radiopharmaceutical, scanning is begun from the root of the neck downward. Certain fixed reference points are marked on the scan picture to help in its accurate superimposition on the x-ray film. The suggested reference points are the suprasternal notch and the middle of the clavicles on both sides.

Since proper interpretation of the scan depends on its superimposition on a radiograph of the chest showing the exact size of the heart, the roentgenogram is either obtained through the anteroposterior approach at a distance of 6 feet or is taken in two halves to lessen the magnification of the radiographic image of the cardiac silhouette.

Normally, the cardiac scan picture shows no separation from the hepatic and

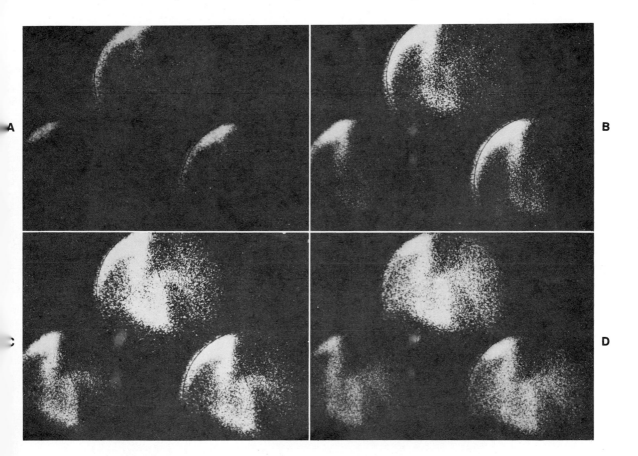

Continued.

Fig. 22-8. Dynamic cardiac study following the injection of a bolus of 10 mCi pertechnetate. **A,** Bolus entering superior vena cava; **B,** bolus has reached the level of the pulmonary outflow tract; **C** and **D,** bolus in pulmonary vasculature; **E,** bolus in left heart; **F,** arch of the aorta visualized; **G,** descending aorta visualized.

343

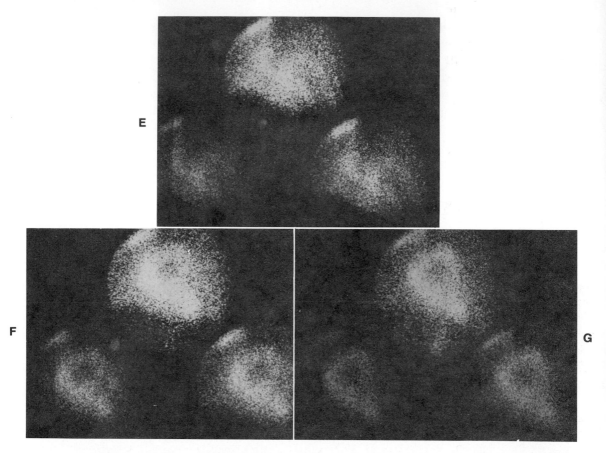

E

F

G

Fig. 22-8, cont'd. For legend see page 343.

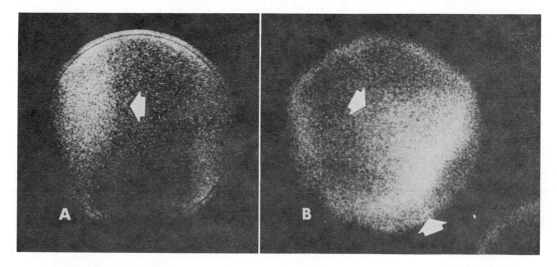

A

B

Fig. 22-9. A, Normal placental scan done shortly following the injection of 1 mCi ^{99m}Tc-labeled albumin. **B,** Abnormal placental scan. The placenta is in the lower left quadrant of the uterus covering the cervical os. (Courtesy, August Miale, Jr., M.D. and Glen A. Landis, M.D.; Radio-isotope Unit, Georgetown University, Washington, D.C.)

A

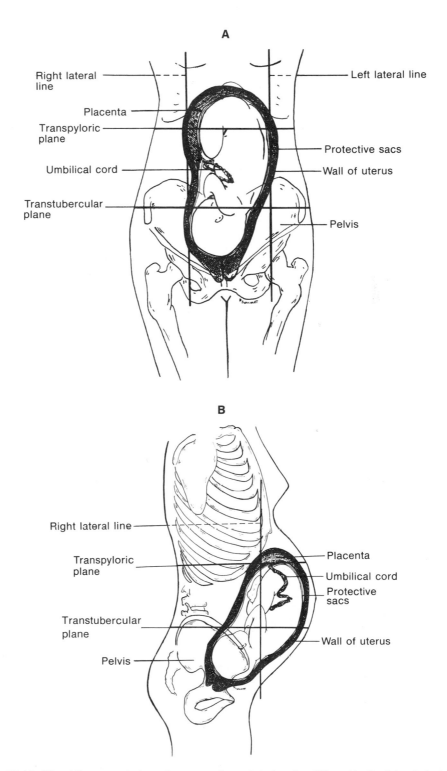

Right lateral line

Placenta

Transpyloric plane

Umbilical cord

Transtubercular plane

Left lateral line

Protective sacs

Wall of uterus

Pelvis

B

Right lateral line

Transpyloric plane

Transtubercular plane

Pelvis

Placenta

Umbilical cord

Protective sacs

Wall of uterus

Fig. 22-10. Site of the normal placenta as seen in an anterior view **(A)** and in the lateral view **(B).**

pulmonary blood pools, and corresponds to the radiographic cardiac silhouette, which has normal dimensions. In the presence of cardiac hypertrophy or dilatation, the cardiac blood pool in the scan corresponds to the enlarged radiographic picture of the heart. With pericardial effusion, the cardiac scan measures less than 80% of the enlarged radiographic image of the heart. In addition, there is a zone of diminished radioactivity separating the cardiac from the hepatic and pulmonary blood pools. The least amount of pericardial effusion to be diagnosed by this technique is 200 ml.

On the same principles, a mediastinal shadow in which the photoscan coincides with the plain x-ray picture is diagnostic of vascular dilatation or aneurysm. On the other hand, if the shadow is caused by a mediastinal mass (glands or tumor), the cardiovascular scan is going to be smaller than the shadow observed on the x-ray film of the chest.

Cardiac photoscanning is a simple, harmless procedure that can be used to differentiate pericardial effusion from cardiac hypertrophy and/or dilatation. Furthermore, it can be applied for the differential diagnosis of cardiovascular from nonvascular shadows in the mediastinum.

PLACENTAL LOCALIZATION

Because of its accuracy, safety, and relative simplicity, radionuclide placentography has gained wide acceptance over the older nonradioactive techniques (Fig. 22-9). Because it is a pool of maternal blood in the gravid uterus, the placenta can be delineated by the use of radionuclides that do not leave the vascular compartment. Such nuclides include ^{131}I human serum albumin (5 μCi), ^{51}Cr-tagged red cells (10 to 20 μCi), ^{99m}Tc-labeled serum albumin (1 mCi), and ^{113}In transferrin (1 mCi). Because of their physical characteristics, the latter two compounds are preferred. However, the excretion of ^{99m}Tc into the urinary bladder might be the cause for some confusion. The radiation dose delivered to both the mother and fetus is well below the permissible levels; much less than that used in plain radiography.

An intravenous injection of the radiopharmaceutical is given to the mother, and the placenta is localized either by point counting or by photoscanning. For point counting, the abdominal surface of the uterus is divided into nine to twelve areas and counting is done by a collimated scintillation detector. The obtained counts are expressed as percentage of the counting rate over the xiphoid.

The main indication for placental localization is differentiating placenta praevia from other causes of vaginal bleeding in the third trimester of pregnancy.

23 *Radionuclide therapy*

RADIOACTIVE PHOSPHORUS

^{32}P (soluble radioactive phosphorus) is used in medicine in the therapy of polycythemia vera, a disease characterized by an increased circulating red cell mass. It is also used in the treatment of chronic leukemia, primary hemorrhagic thrombocythemia (a disease where there is an increased number of circulating platelets), and in the treatment of some of the malignant lymphomas and multiple myelomas.

^{32}P is a pure beta emitter with maximum energy of 1.7 mev and a half-life of 14.3 days. The average distance its beta particle travels in tissue is approximately 2 mm. ^{32}P will accumulate in tissues where there is a rapid metabolic turnover of phosphate. The tissues primarily involved are the hematopoietic tissues and bone. Therefore, the student will find the physician primarily using radioactive phosphorus in therapy of polycythemia. Radioactive phosphorus is also utilized in the therapy of metastatic disease to the bone where there is a need for palliation. Radioactive phosphorus will accumulate in the area of most metastatic tumors in bone, as there is an attempt of bone to form new bone in place of the bone destroyed by the metastatic carcinoma. Radioactive phosphorus would then be deposited in the area of the tumor and with its pure beta radiation would limit the growth of the tumor and possibly destroy a portion of the tumor.

Because there has been suggestive evidence of a causal relationship between ^{32}P therapy and the development of acute leukemia, ^{32}P therapy for polycythemia is not used as frequently now as it was in the past.

RADIOACTIVE COLLOIDS

Radioactive colloidal suspensions of gold or phosphorus (as chromic phosphate, ^{32}P) are being used today in therapy of metastatic malignancy. These colloidal suspensions are usually instilled into the cavities of the body to limit the growth of metastatic disease. They are also used to halt fluid collection, which is secondary to tumor invasion of the intracavitary spaces, pleural space, pericardial space, or the peritoneal space. With radioactive gold the beta ray penetrates less than 4 mm and, therefore, the therapy is very localized. The gamma ray of gold contributes only about 10% of the total dose.

The pure beta emission of ^{32}P localizes the radiation dose. Both colloidal ^{198}Au and colloidal ^{32}P when instilled into the cavitary spaces stay localized in the spaces. Only a small percent of the total dose is found in the excreta of the patient over a period of days. At the present time there is a preference for colloidal chromic phosphate (^{32}P) as the pure beta emissions are easier to handle than all the mixed gamma and beta radiations of ^{198}Au. The student will find, however, that in therapy centers there are many forms of ehcmotherapy used in the therapy of intracavitary tumor other than radiocolloid therapy.

STRONTIUM 90

Strontium 90 in a sealed source applicator is used in the therapy of superficial malignancies as well as in ophthalmology. Its primary use is in the therapy of superficial lesions of the eye.

THERAPY OF HYPERTHYROIDISM

As mentioned in Chapter 13 there are two distinct forms of hyperthyroidism, and different therapy is indicated for each form.

Graves' disease

There are three separate approaches to the therapy of hyperthyroidism associated with Graves' disease—medical, surgical, and radioiodine therapy.

Medical therapy with thyroid blocking agents, such as propylthiouracil or tapazole. These antithyroid drugs block iodide organification and, therefore, inhibit thyroid hormone production by the thyroid. By clinical management, as well as laboratory follow-up, the hyperthyroid patient with Graves' disease can be maintained in a euthyroid state on these antithyroid drugs. In a very small portion of patients the antithyroid drugs have adverse effects, primarily on the hemopoietic system. Therefore, patients must have clinical and laboratory follow-up, usually at weekly or bimonthly intervals.

Approximately 50% of the patients with Graves' disease will go into a remission after a period of 1 to 2 years. Therefore, the medical antithyroid therapy must be continued for this period of time.

Surgical therapy of thyrotoxicosis is becoming less popular, since complications are frequent and may be serious.

Radioiodine therapy is the preferred way to treat hyperthyroidism. There is a scientific approach to the radioiodine therapy of this disease; however, the student will find that medical judgment is utilized in establishing the amount of radioiodine to administer to a patient with Graves' disease. There are no particular side effects of this form of therapy. However, hypothyroidism may be induced by radioiodine as well as by surgery, and this should be taken into consideration when the patient is chosen for therapy.

Plummer's disease (nodular goiterous hyperthyroidism)

In Plummer's disease, the individual nodules or multiple nodules are autonomous, and the patient becomes hyperthyroid because of overproduction of thyroid hormone. Medical therapy is not predictable in this group of patients; surgical therapy is predictable if the individual nodules are removed.

There is, and will always be, controversy about the correct form of therapy of hyperthyroidism. The student should understand that this almost always is the case when the etiology of the disease is unknown. As more basic information of the etiology is discovered, the therapy of this disease will become more scientific.

THYROID CARCINOMA

Iodine 131 has been utilized since its introduction in the diagnosis, follow-up and palliation of thyroid carcinoma. Since follicular function is necessary for the concentration of ^{131}I, clinical results utilizing this radionuclide in thyroid carcinoma have been variable. Thyroid carcinoma can be made up of any of the epithelial cellular components of the thyroid; therefore, there is usually a mixture of papillary, follicular and/or connective tissue elements in thyroid carcinoma.

There have been reported cures of thyroid carcinoma with ^{131}I, however, these are rare. Its use in the palliation of and inference with metastatic thyroid carcinoma is highly recommended. Recently, technetium 99m has been found to be localized in the cellular component of thyroid carcinoma. Its usefulness in the diagnosis of this disease is still under investigation.

CONCLUSION

Therapy procedures with internally administered radionuclides is now a small segment of nuclear medicine. As more is learned of radiation biology's relationship to tumor growth and other disease states, there will be more specific applications of therapeutic nuclear medicine.

Bibliography

Astwood, E., and Cassidy, C.: Clinical endocrinology, vol. 2, New York, 1968, Grune & Stratton, Inc.

Beeson, P. B., and McDermott, W.: Cecil-Loeb textbook of medicine, ed. 12, Philadelphia, 1967, W. B. Saunders Company.

Best, C., and Taylor, N. B.: Physiological basis of medical practice, ed. 6, Baltimore, The Williams & Wilkins Co.

Blahd, W. H.: Nuclear medicine, New York, 1965, McGraw-Hill Book Company.

Charkes, N. D.: Some differences between bone scans made with ^{87m}Sr and ^{85}Sr., J. Nucl. Med., **10** (7): 491, 1969.

Copenhaver, W. M.: Bailey's textbook of histology, ed. 15, Baltimore, 1968, The Williams & Wilkins Co.

Goss, C. M.: Gray's anatomy of the human body, ed. 28, Philadelphia, 1966, Lea & Febiger.

Grant, J. C. B., and Basmajiam, J. V.: A method of anatomy, ed, 7, Baltimore, 1965, The Williams & Wilkins Co.

Guyton, A. C.: Textbook of medical physiology, ed. 3, Philadelphia, 1966, W. B. Saunders Company.

Jacobi, C. A.: Textbook of anatomy and physiology in radiologic technology, St. Louis, 1968, The C. V. Mosby Co.

de Reuck, A. V. S., and Cameron, M. P.: The exocrine pancreas—normal and abnormal functions, Boston, 1961, Little, Brown and Company.

Silver, S.: Radioactive nuclides in medicine and biology, ed. 3, Philadelphia, 1968, Lea and Febiger.

Tepperman, J.: Metabolic and endocrine physiology, ed. 2, Chicago, 1967, Year Book Medical Publishers, Inc.

Tow, D. E., and Wagner, H.: Management of pulmonary embolism, New Eng. J. Med., **278:** 339, 1968.

Wagner, H. N.: Principles of nuclear medicine, Philadelphia, 1968, W. B. Saunders Company.

Williams, R. H.: Textbook of endocrinology, ed. 4, Philadelphia, 1968, W. B. Saunders Company.

Annual review of physiology, Volume 30, 1968, Palo Alto, California, Annual Reviews, Inc.

Annual review of medicine, Volume 19, 1968, Palo Alto, California, Annual Reviews, Inc.

Glossary

Acinus: A saccular terminal division of a compound gland having a narrow lumen, as contrasted with an alveolus. Several acini combine to form a lobule.

Agglutination: A mass formed by the joining together or aggregation of suspended particles.

Allergy: Altered reaction capacity to a specified substance; Acquired sensitivities to drugs and biologics.

Antecubital vein: The vein located in front of the elbow in each arm.

Blood pigments: Pigments normally found in blood, such as hemoglobin and bilirubin.

Carcinoma: A malignant epithelial tumor.

Catabolism: Destructive phase of metabolism in which complex compounds are broken down by the cells of the body, often with the liberation of energy; the opposite of anabolism.

Cirrhosis: A chronic, progressive disease of the liver, essentially inflammatory; characterized by proliferation of connective tissue, degeneration of parenchymal cells, and distortion of architectural pattern. The liver may be either enlarged or reduced in size.

Clot retraction: The contraction or shrinkage of a blood clot resulting in the extrusion of serum.

Coagulation: The formation of a coagulum or clot, as in blood or in milk.

Corpuscle: 1. An encapulated sensory nerve end—organ. 2. Old term for cell, especially a blood cell.

Cytoplasm: The protoplasm of a cell other than that of the nucleus, as opposed to nucleoplasm.

Detoxify: The process, usually consisting of a series of reactions, by which a substance foreign to the body is changed to a compound or compounds more readily excretable.

Electrolyte: A substance which in solution is capable of conducting an electric current, and is decomposed by it.

Electrophoresis: The migration of charged colloidal particles through the medium in which they are dispersed, when placed under the influence of an applied electric potential.

Elution: The process for the extraction of the adsorbed substance from the solid adsorbing medium in chromatography.

Endocrine: Internal secretion; pertaining to ductless glands that secrete substances directly into the bloodstream.

Endogenous: Produced within or due to internal causes; applied to the formation of cells or of spores within the parent cell.

Endothelium: The mesodermally derived, simple, squamous epithelium lining any closed cavity in the body.

Enzyme: A substance formed by living cells having the capacity to facilitate a chemical reaction.

Exocrine: Pertaining to glands which deliver their secretion or excretion to an epithelial surface, either directly or by means of ducts.

Extracellular: Occurring outside the cell.

Exudation: The passage of various constituents of blood through the walls of vessels into adjacent tissues or spaces in inflammation.

Hemolysis: The destruction of red cells and the resultant escape of hemoglobin.

Hemopoiesis: Formation of blood cells.

Interstitial: 1. Situated between important parts; occupying the interspaces or interstices of a part. 2. Pertaining to the finest connective tissue of organs.

Intrathecal: Within a sheath, particularly within the meninges into the subarachnoid space.

Intrinsic factor: Substance produced by the stomach which combines with extrinsic factor (vitamin B_{12}) to yield an antianemic factor.

Kinetic: Pertaining to motion; producing motion.

Lobule: A small lobe or a subdivision of a lobe.

Macrophage: A phagocytic cell (not a leukocyte) belonging to the reticuloendothelial system. It has the capacity for storing certain aniline dyes in its cytoplasm in the form of granules.

Maturation: The process of coming to full development.

Occult: Hidden; concealed; not evident, as occult blood—the blood in excrement or secretion not clearly evident to the naked eye.

Osmotic pressure: The pressure developed when a solution and its solvent component are separated by a membrane permeable to the solvent only, or when two solutions of different concentration of the same solute are similarly separated.

Pancreozymin: A crude extract of the intestinal mucosa which stimulates the secretion of pancreatic enzymes.

Pernicious anemia: Anemia that results from defects of the bone marrow, such as hypoplasia, euplasia, and degenerative changes. It is caused by a deficiency of red cells, hemoglobin and granular cells, and a predominance of lymphocytes.

Phagocytosis: Ingestion of foreign or other particles, principally bacteria, by certain cells.

Pinocytosis: Absorption of liquids by cells.

Precordium: The area of the chest overlying the heart.

Proteolysis: The enzymatic or hydrolytic conversion of proteins into simple substances.

Secretin: A hormone produced in the epithelial cells of the duodenum by the contact of acid. It is absorbed from the cells by the blood and excites the pancreas to activity; it has been isolated as secretin picrotonate.

Sequestration: Separation.

Somatic: 1. Pertaining to the body. 2. Pertaining to the framework of the body and not to the viscera, as the somatic musculature (the muscles of the body wall or somatopleure), as distinguished from those of the splanchnopleure (the splanchnic musculature).

Specific gravity: The measured mass of a substance with that of an equal volume of another taken as a standard. For gases, hydrogen of air may be the standard; for liquids and solids, distilled water at a specified temperature is the standard.

Steatorrhea: 1. An increased flow of the secretion of the sebaceous follicles. 2. Fatty stools.

Threshold: 1. The lower limit of stimulus capable of producing an impression upon consciousness or of evoking a response in an irritable tissue. 2. The entrance of a canal.

Transferrin: Siderophilin; a pseudoglobulin of blood, having a molecular weight of about 90,000. It is capable of combining with 2 atoms of ferric iron to form a compound which serves as a transport form of iron in blood.

Vagus nerve: The parasympathetic pneumogastric nerve; the tenth cranial nerve, composed of both motor and sensory fibers. It has a wide distribution in the neck, thorax, and abdomen, and sends important branches to the heart, lungs, stomach, and so on.

Vitamin B$_{12}$: An essential vitamin needed for the normal maturation of cells of the erythrocytic series, and for normal neurologic function. When given parenterally it corrects both the hematologic and neurologic symptoms of pernicious anemia.

Viscus: Any one of the organs enclosed within one of the four great cavities, the cranium, thorax, abdomen, or pelvis; especially an organ within the abdominal cavity.

Zymogen: The inactive precursor of an enzyme which, on reaction with an appropriate kinase or other chemical agent, liberates the enzyme in active form.

Appendixes

Appendix A   *Physical data for radionuclides used in nuclear medicine*

Element	Chemical symbol (X)	Atomic number (Z)	Mass number (A)	Half-life	Radiation	Principal gamma energy (mev)
Arsenic	As	33	74	17.9d	EC, β^+, β^-, γ	0.596
Calcium	Ca	20	47	4.5d	β^-, γ	1.308
Carbon	C	6	11	20.3m	β^+	none
Cesium (^{137m}Ba)	Cs	55	137	30y	β^-, γ	0.662
Chromium	Cr	24	51	27.8d	EC, γ	0.320
Cobalt	Co	27	57	270d	EC	0.122
			58	71.3d	EC, β^+, γ	0.810
			60	5.26y	β^-, γ	1.17, 1.33
Gold	Au	79	198	2.7d	β^-, γ	0.412
Iodine	I	53	125	60d	EC, γ	0.035
			131	8.1d	β^-, γ	0.364
Iron	Fe	26	59	45d	β^-, γ	1.1, 1.3
Indium	In	49	113m	1.7h	IT, γ	0.393
Krypton	Kr	36	79	1.45d	EC, γ	0.398, 0.606
Mercury	Hg	80	197	2.7d	EC, γ	0.077
			203	46.9d	β^-, γ	0.279
Molybdenum	Mo	42	99	2.78d	β^-, γ	0.740
Oxygen	O	8	15	2.1m	β^+	none
Phosphorus	P	15	32	14.3d	β^-	none
Rubidium	Rb	37	86	18.7d	β^-, γ	1.078
Selenium	Se	34	75	120d	EC, γ	0.265
Strontium	Sr	38	85	64d	EC, γ	0.514
			87m	2.83h	IT, γ	0.388
			90	27.7y	β^-	none
Technetium	Tc	43	99	6h	IT, γ	0.140
Tin	Sn	50	113	115d	EC, γ	0.255
Xenon	Xe	54	133	5.27d	β^-, γ	0.08

B Universal decay table

Activity remaining for t÷T½ from 0.001 to 1.00

	.000	.001	.002	.003	.004	.005	.006	.007	.008	.009
.000	.00000	.99969	.99862	.99793	.99723	.99645	.99586	.99516	.99446	.99379
.010	.99309	.99238	.99172	.99103	.99034	.98966	.98898	.98828	.98759	.98693
.020	.98623	.98554	.98487	.98419	.98350	.98243	.98214	.98146	.98076	.98010
.030	.97942	.97874	.97807	.97740	.97671	.97603	.97517	.97446	.97399	.97333
.040	.97262	.97299	.97132	.97065	.96997	.96930	.96880	.96795	.96726	.96662
.050	.96594	.96527	.96461	.96393	.96326	.96260	.96190	.96125	.96058	.95994
.060	.95928	.95862	.95795	.95728	.95661	.95596	.95529	.95452	.95395	.95331
.070	.95264	.95199	.95133	.95067	.95000	.94936	.94870	.94800	.94738	.94673
.080	.94587	.94522	.94457	.94392	.94326	.94261	.94196	.94130	.94063	.94000
.090	.93926	.93888	.93833	.93759	.93693	.93628	.93564	.93499	.93434	.93370
.100	.93304	.93240	.93175	.93112	.93046	.92982	.92906	.92853	.92887	.92725
.110	.92660	.92596	.92532	.92468	.92403	.92340	.92276	.92216	.92152	.92085
.120	.92020	.91956	.91893	.91785	.91766	.91702	.91639	.91575	.91511	.91448
.130	.91339	.91321	.91265	.91196	.91132	.91069	.91008	.90939	.90841	.90817
.140	.90747	.90691	.90629	.90566	.90502	.90440	.90378	.90314	.90250	.90190
.150	.90127	.90064	.90002	.89931	.89840	.89816	.89754	.89690	.89627	.89566
.160	.89504	.89442	.89381	.89319	.89257	.89195	.89133	.89071	.89008	.88949
.170	.88888	.88825	.88763	.88702	.88650	.88579	.88518	.88456	.88393	.88334
.180	.88272	.88211	.88150	.88098	.88030	.87967	.87905	.87885	.87852	.87724
.190	.87663	.87602	.87542	.87481	.87420	.87320	.87300	.87216	.87178	.87118
.200	.87057	.86997	.86937	.86877	.86816	.86756	.86697	.86636	.86576	.86517
.210	.86456	.86396	.86337	.86277	.86217	.86157	.86082	.86037	.85978	.85919
.220	.85859	.85800	.85741	.85681	.85621	.85579	.85503	.85443	.85384	.85326
.230	.85266	.85207	.85148	.85097	.85030	.84975	.84914	.84853	.84794	.84736
.240	.84677	.84619	.84561	.84502	.84443	.84384	.84326	.84268	.84210	.84152
.250	.84092	.84034	.83976	.83918	.83860	.83802	.83744	.83685	.83628	.83570
.260	.83511	.83454	.83396	.83339	.83283	.83223	.83208	.83166	.83050	.82993
.270	.82935	.82875	.82820	.82763	.82705	.82648	.82591	.82533	.82476	.82419
.280	.82362	.82313	.82248	.82191	.82136	.82077	.82021	.81962	.81907	.81850
.290	.81792	.81736	.81681	.81624	.81567	.81511	.81454	.81397	.81341	.81300
.300	.81228	.81172	.81116	.81060	.81004	.80948	.80892	.80819	.80779	.80702
.310	.80667	.80609	.80556	.80500	.80444	.80489	.80333	.80277	.80222	.80166
.320	.80110	.80055	.80000	.79944	.79888	.79834	.79779	.79731	.79668	.79613
.330	.79557	.79502	.79447	.79392	.79337	.79282	.79227	.79172	.79118	.79063

Activity remaining for t÷T½ from 0.001 to 1.00—cont'd

	.000	.001	.002	.003	.004	.005	.006	.007	.008	.009
.340	.79007	.78953	.78899	.78844	.78789	.78735	.78681	.78625	.78571	.78517
.350	.78462	.78408	.78354	.78300	.78245	.78191	.78137	.78082	.78028	.77974
.360	.77920	.77866	.77813	.77759	.77704	.77648	.77597	.77543	.77489	.77436
.370	.77383	.77329	.77275	.77222	.77168	.77115	.77062	.77007	.76953	.76901
.380	.76848	.76795	.76742	.76689	.76635	.76582	.76529	.76476	.76423	.76370
.390	.76317	.76272	.76212	.76159	.76106	.76053	.76001	.75948	.75895	.75843
.400	.75790	.75737	.75685	.75633	.75580	.75528	.75476	.75423	.75371	.75319
.410	.75266	.75215	.75163	.75111	.75058	.75006	.74955	.74902	.74856	.74799
.420	.74747	.74695	.74644	.74592	.74540	.74488	.74437	.74385	.74334	.74282
.430	.74231	.74179	.74128	.74077	.74025	.73974	.73923	.73871	.73820	.73762
.440	.73718	.73667	.73616	.73568	.73514	.73463	.73413	.73361	.73311	.73260
.450	.73208	.73258	.73108	.73057	.73006	.72956	.72958	.72854	.72804	.72754
.460	.72703	.72653	.72603	.72545	.72527	.72452	.72402	.72351	.72302	.72252
.470	.72201	.72151	.72102	.72052	.72001	.71952	.71902	.71852	.71802	.71753
.480	.71702	.71653	.71604	.71554	.71504	.71455	.71405	.71355	.71306	.71257
.490	.71207	.71158	.71109	.71060	.71010	.70961	.70912	.70863	.70814	.70765
.500	.70715	.70666	.70618	.70569	.70520	.70471	.70423	.70373	.70325	.70276
.510	.70227	.70179	.70130	.70082	.70033	.69984	.69936	.69887	.69839	.69791
.520	.69742	.69694	.69646	.69598	.69549	.69501	.69453	.69404	.69356	.69309
.530	.69261	.69213	.69165	.69117	.69069	.69021	.68973	.68925	.68871	.68830
.540	.68796	.68735	.86887	.68640	.68593	.68545	.68497	.68450	.68395	.68348
.550	.68307	.68260	.68213	.68166	.68118	.68071	.68024	.67976	.67913	.67882
.560	.67835	.67782	.67742	.67695	.67646	.67601	.67554	.67507	.67461	.67414
.570	.67367	.67320	.67274	.67227	.67181	.67134	.67088	.67041	.66995	.66948
.580	.66902	.66856	.66810	.66764	.66718	.66671	.66624	.66578	.66532	.66486
.590	.66440	.66394	.66348	.66302	.66256	.66210	.66164	.66118	.66053	.66027
.600	.65981	.65935	.65890	.65846	.65798	.65753	.65707	.65661	.65616	.65571
.610	.65525	.65480	.65435	.65390	.65344	.65299	.65244	.65208	.65163	.65118
.620	.65073	.65028	.64983	.64938	.64892	.64848	.64803	.64758	.64713	.64669
.630	.64623	.64598	.64534	.64489	.64448	.64400	.64356	.64310	.64273	.64222
.640	.64178	.64133	.64089	.64044	.64000	.63955	.63911	.63886	.63822	.63778
.650	.63764	.63690	.63646	.63602	.63558	.63514	.63470	.63425	.63382	.63338
.660	.63293	.63250	.63206	.63163	.63118	.63075	.63032	.62987	.62944	.62900
.670	.62856	.62813	.62770	.62727	.62683	.62639	.62588	.62552	.62509	.62466
.680	.62422	.62379	.62336	.62293	.62250	.62207	.62164	.62120	.62077	.62035
.690	.61991	.61936	.61906	.61863	.61820	.61777	.61736	.61691	.61649	.61606
.700	.61563	.61520	.61478	.61436	.61393	.61350	.61308	.61265	.61223	.61181
.710	.61138	.61096	.61054	.61012	.60969	.60927	.60885	.60842	.60800	.60758
.720	.60716	.60674	.60632	.60572	.60548	.60506	.60464	.60422	.60380	.60339
.730	.60296	.60255	.60213	.60172	.60130	.60088	.60047	.60005	.59963	.59922
.740	.59880	.59838	.59797	.59756	.59717	.59673	.59632	.59590	.59549	.59508
.750	.59466	.59426	.59385	.59344	.59302	.59261	.59220	.59179	.59144	.59097

Continued.

Activity remaining for t÷T½ from 0.001 to 1.00—cont'd

	.000	.001	.002	.003	.004	.005	.006	.007	.008	.009
.760	.59053	.59015	.58974	.58934	.58892	.58852	.58811	.58770	.58730	.58690
.770	.58648	.58608	.58567	.58527	.58485	.58447	.58405	.58364	.58324	.58271
.780	.58243	.58202	.58163	.58122	.58082	.58042	.58002	.57961	.57921	.57910
.790	.57841	.57801	.57761	.57721	.57681	.57641	.57601	.57561	.57579	.57438
.800	.57441	.57402	.59362	.57317	.57282	.57243	.57204	.57163	.57124	.57085
.810	.57045	.57005	.56966	.56904	.56886	.56847	.56808	.56768	.56729	.56690
.820	.56645	.56611	.56572	.56533	.56494	.56455	.56416	.56377	.56338	.56299
.830	.56359	.56320	.56282	.56243	.56203	.56165	.56126	.56087	.56049	.56010
.840	.55899	.55832	.55794	.55755	.55716	.55678	.55640	.55601	.55562	.55524
.850	.55485	.55447	.55408	.55370	.55328	.55293	.55255	.55217	.55179	.55140
.860	.55102	.55064	.55026	.54988	.54950	.54912	.54874	.54841	.54797	.54760
.870	.54721	.54683	.54646	.54605	.54565	.54532	.54495	.54457	.54419	.54382
.880	.54344	.54306	.54269	.54231	.54193	.54156	.54118	.54081	.54043	.54006
.890	.53968	.53931	.53894	.53856	.53819	.53782	.53745	.53702	.53670	.53633
.900	.53595	.53558	.53538	.53485	.53447	.53410	.53373	.53336	.53299	.53262
.910	.53225	.53188	.53152	.53115	.53078	.53043	.53005	.52968	.52931	.52895
.920	.52858	.52821	.52785	.52748	.52711	.52675	.52638	.52600	.52566	.52529
.930	.52493	.52456	.52420	.52384	.52347	.52311	.52275	.52239	.52203	.52168
.940	.52130	.52094	.52058	.52022	.51986	.51950	.51916	.51898	.51842	.51806
.950	.51770	.51734	.51698	.51641	.51627	.51591	.51556	.51520	.51484	.51448
.960	.51402	.51377	.51342	.51306	.51270	.51235	.51200	.51164	.51129	.51093
.970	.51057	.51027	.50987	.50952	.50918	.50881	.50846	.50810	.50775	.50740
.980	.50715	.50670	.50635	.50600	.50570	.50530	.50495	.50460	.50426	.50390
.990	.50355	.50320	.50285	.50256	.50216	.50181	.50141	.50111	.50077	.50042
1.000	.50000	.49973	.49938	.49904	.49869	.49838	.49860	.49765	.49731	.49697

(Adapted from Health physics handbook, General Dynamics, Fort Worth, Texas.)

The above table can be used to determine the fraction of activity remaining of any radionuclide, from 0.001 half-life to 1.00 half-life.

To use the table:

1. Divide elapsed time by the known physical half-life of the radionuclide under consideration ($t \div T_{1/2}$). Note: The same time unit must be used in each instance.

2. Use above answer (to three significant figures) in locating the percent of original activity remaining. The first two significant figures are listed on the vertical column at the left of the table; the third significant figure is listed on the horizontal across the top of the table.

3. Multiply original activity by this percentage figure to obtain amount remaining.

Example: What is the strength of a 10 mCi ^{131}I source after 2 days?

1. $t \div T_{1/2} = 2 \div 8.1 = 0.247$

2. Fraction remaining from decay table = .84268

3. 10 mCi × .84268 = 8.43 mCi

Table of atomic mass units

Symbol	Element	Atomic mass units (amu)
e	Electron	0.000548
n	Neutron	1.008986
p	Proton	1.007597
^1_1H	Hydrogen	1.008145
^2_1H	Heavy hydrogen	2.014740
^3_1H	Tritium	3.017005
^3_2He	Isotopes of helium	3.016986
^4_2He		4.003874
^5_2He		5.01389
^6_2He		6.02083
$^{10}_6C$	Isotopes of carbon	10.02024
$^{11}_6C$		11.014922
$^{12}_6C$		12.003803
$^{13}_6C$		13.007478
$^{14}_6C$		14.007687
$^{15}_6C$		15.01416
$^{12}_5B$	Isobars of mass 12	12.018168
$^{12}_6C$		12.003803
$^{12}_7N$		12.02278
$^{16}_8O$	Oxygen	16.00000
$^{32}_{15}P$	Isobars of mass 32	31.98403
$^{32}_{16}S$		31.98220
$^{90}_{40}Zr$	Zirconium	89.9328
$^{143}_{60}Nd$	Neodymium	142.9541
$^{235}_{92}U$	Uranium	235.11750

(Adapted from Johns, H. E.: The physics of radiology, Springfield, Illinois, 1964, Charles C Thomas, Publisher.)

Appendix
D
Four place logarithms

N	0	1	2	3	4	5	6	7	8	9
10	0000	0043	0086	0128	0170	0212	0253	0294	0334	0374
11	0414	0453	0492	0531	0569	0607	0645	0682	0719	0755
12	0792	0828	0864	0899	0934	0969	1004	1038	1072	1106
13	1139	1173	1206	1239	1271	1303	1335	1367	1399	1430
14	1461	1492	1523	1553	1584	1614	1644	1673	1703	1732
15	1761	1790	1818	1847	1875	1903	1931	1959	1987	2014
16	2041	2068	2095	2122	2148	2175	2201	2227	2253	2279
17	2304	2330	2355	2380	2405	2430	2455	2480	2504	2529
18	2553	2577	2601	2625	2648	2672	2695	2718	2742	2765
19	2788	2810	2833	2856	2878	2900	2923	2945	2967	2989
20	3010	3032	3054	3075	3096	3118	3139	3160	3181	3201
21	3222	3243	3263	3284	3304	3324	3345	3365	3385	3404
22	3424	3444	3464	3483	3502	3522	3541	3560	3579	3598
23	3617	3636	3655	3674	3692	3711	3729	3747	3766	3784
24	3802	3820	3838	3856	3874	3892	3909	3927	3945	3962
25	3979	3997	4014	4031	4048	4065	4082	4099	4116	4133
26	4150	4166	4183	4200	4216	4232	4249	4265	4281	4298
27	4314	4330	4346	4362	4378	4393	4409	4425	4440	4456
28	4472	4487	4502	4518	4533	4548	4564	4579	4594	4609
29	4624	4639	4654	4669	4683	4698	4713	4728	4742	4757
30	4771	4786	4800	4814	4829	4843	4857	4871	4886	4900
31	4914	4928	4942	4955	4969	4983	4907	5011	5024	5038
32	5051	5065	5079	5092	5105	5119	5132	5145	5159	5172
33	5185	5198	5211	5224	5237	5250	5263	5276	5289	5302
34	5315	5328	5340	5353	5366	5378	5391	5403	5416	5428
35	5441	5453	5465	5478	5490	5502	5514	5527	5539	5551
36	5563	5575	5587	5599	5611	5623	5635	5647	5658	5670
37	5682	5694	5705	5717	5729	5740	5752	5763	5775	5786
38	5798	5809	5821	5832	5843	5855	5866	5877	5888	5899
39	5911	5922	5933	5944	5955	5966	5977	5988	5999	6010

N	0	1	2	3	4	5	6	7	8	9
40	6021	6031	6042	6053	6064	6075	6085	6096	6107	6117
41	6128	6138	6149	6160	6170	6180	6191	6201	6212	6222
42	6232	6243	6253	6263	6274	6284	6294	6304	6314	6325
43	6335	6345	6355	6365	6375	6385	6395	6405	6415	6425
44	6435	6444	6454	6464	6474	6484	6493	6503	6513	6522
45	6532	6542	6551	6561	6571	6580	6590	6599	6609	6618
46	6628	6637	6646	6656	6665	6675	6684	6693	6702	6712
47	6721	6730	6739	6749	6758	6767	6776	6785	6794	6803
48	6812	6821	6830	6839	6848	6857	6866	6875	6884	6893
49	6902	6911	6920	6928	6937	6946	6955	6964	6972	6981
50	6990	6998	7007	7016	7024	7033	7042	7050	7059	7067
51	7076	7084	7093	7101	7110	7118	7126	7135	7143	7152
52	7160	7168	7177	7185	7193	7202	7210	7218	7226	7235
53	7243	7251	7259	7267	7275	7284	7292	7300	7308	7316
54	7324	7332	7340	7348	7356	7364	7372	7380	7388	7396
55	7404	7412	7419	7427	7435	7443	7451	7459	7466	7474
56	7482	7490	7497	7505	7513	7520	7528	7536	7543	7551
57	7559	7566	7574	7582	7589	7597	7604	7612	7619	7627
58	7634	7642	7649	7657	7664	7672	7679	7686	7684	7701
59	7709	7716	7723	7731	7738	7745	7752	7760	7767	7774
60	7782	7789	7796	7803	7810	7818	7825	7832	7839	7846
61	7853	7860	7868	7875	7882	7889	7896	7903	7910	7917
62	7924	7931	7938	7945	7952	7959	7966	7973	7980	7987
63	7993	8000	8007	8014	8021	8028	8035	8041	8048	8055
64	8062	8069	8075	8082	8089	8096	8102	8109	8116	8122
65	8129	8136	8142	8149	8156	8162	8169	8176	8182	8189
66	8195	8202	8209	8215	8222	8228	8235	8241	8248	8254
67	8261	8267	8274	8280	8287	8293	8299	8306	8312	8319
68	8325	8331	8338	8344	8351	8357	8363	8370	8376	8382
69	8388	8395	8401	8407	8414	8420	8426	8432	8439	8455
70	8451	8457	8463	8470	8476	8482	8488	8494	8500	8506
71	8513	8519	8525	8531	8537	8543	8549	8555	8561	8567
72	8573	8579	8585	8591	8597	8603	8609	8615	8621	8627
73	8633	8639	8645	8651	8657	8663	8669	8675	8681	8686
74	8692	8698	8704	8710	8716	8722	8727	8733	8739	8745

Continued.

N	0	1	2	3	4	5	6	7	8	9
75	8751	8756	8762	8768	8774	8779	8785	8791	8797	8802
76	8808	8814	8820	8825	8831	8837	8842	8848	8854	8859
77	8865	8871	8876	8882	8887	8893	8899	8904	8910	8915
78	8921	8927	8932	8938	8943	8949	8954	8960	8965	8971
79	8976	8982	8987	8993	8998	9004	9009	9015	9020	9025
80	9031	9036	9042	9047	9053	9058	9063	9069	9074	9079
81	9085	9090	9096	9101	9106	9112	9117	9122	9128	9133
82	9138	9143	9149	9154	9159	9165	9170	9175	9180	9186
83	9191	9196	9201	9206	9212	9217	9222	9227	9232	9238
84	9243	9248	9253	9258	9263	9269	9274	9279	9284	9289
85	9294	9299	9304	9309	9315	9320	9325	9330	9335	9340
86	9345	9350	9355	9360	9365	9370	9375	9380	9385	9390
87	9395	9400	9405	9410	9415	9420	9425	9430	9435	9440
88	9445	9450	9455	9460	9465	9469	9474	9479	9484	9489
89	9494	9499	9504	9509	9513	9518	9523	9528	9533	9538
90	9542	9547	9552	9557	9562	9566	9571	9576	9581	9586
91	9590	9595	9600	9605	9609	9614	9619	9624	9628	9633
92	9638	9643	9647	9652	9657	9661	9666	9671	9675	9680
93	9685	9689	9694	9699	9703	9708	9713	9717	9722	9727
94	9731	9736	9741	9745	9750	9754	9759	9763	9768	9773
95	9777	9782	9786	9791	9795	9800	9805	9809	9814	9818
96	9823	9827	9832	9836	9841	9845	9850	9854	9859	9863
97	9868	9872	9877	9881	9886	9890	9894	9899	9903	9908
98	9912	9917	9921	9926	9930	9934	9939	9943	9948	9952
99	9956	9961	9965	9969	9974	9978	9983	9987	9991	9996

(Adapted from Quimby, E. H., and Feitelberg, S.: Radioactive isotopes in medicine and biology, Philadelphia, 1963, Lea & Febiger.)

E *Exponentials*

X	e^{-x}	X	e^{-x}	X	e^{-x}
0.00	1.000	0.40	0.670	1.0	0.368
0.01	0.990	0.41	0.664	1.1	0.333
0.02	0.980	0.42	0.657	1.2	0.301
0.03	0.970	0.43	0.651	1.3	0.273
0.04	0.961	0.44	0.644	1.4	0.247
0.05	0.951	0.45	0.638	1.5	0.223
0.06	0.942	0.46	0.631	1.6	0.202
0.07	0.932	0.47	0.625	1.7	0.183
0.08	0.923	0.48	0.619	1.8	0.165
0.09	0.914	0.49	0.613	1.9	0.150
0.10	0.905	0.50	0.607	2.0	0.135
0.11	0.896	0.52	0.595	2.1	0.122
0.12	0.887	0.54	0.583	2.2	0.111
0.13	0.878	0.56	0.571	2.3	0.100
0.14	0.869	0.58	0.560	2.4	0.0907
0.15	0.861			2.5	0.0821
0.16	0.852	0.60	0.549	2.6	0.0743
0.17	0.844	0.62	0.538	2.7	0.0672
0.18	0.835	0.64	0.527	2.8	0.0608
0.19	0.827	0.66	0.517	2.9	0.0550
		0.68	0.507		
0.20	0.819			3.0	0.0498
0.21	0.811	0.70	0.497	3.2	0.0408
0.22	0.803	0.72	0.487	3.4	0.0334
0.23	0.795	0.74	0.477	3.6	0.0273
0.24	0.787	0.76	0.468	3.8	0.0224
0.25	0.779	0.78	0.458		
0.26	0.771			4.0	0.0183
0.27	0.763	0.80	0.449	4.2	0.0150
0.28	0.756	0.82	0.440	4.4	0.0123
0.29	0.748	0.84	0.432	4.6	0.0101
		0.86	0.423	4.8	0.0082
0.30	0.741	0.88	0.415		
0.31	0.733			5.0	0.0067
0.32	0.726	0.90	0.407	5.5	0.0041
0.33	0.749	0.92	0.399	6.0	0.0025
0.34	0.712	0.94	0.391	6.5	0.0015
0.35	0.705	0.96	0.383	7.0	0.0009
0.36	0.698	0.98	0.375	7.5	0.0006
0.37	0.691			8.0	0.0003
0.38	0.684			8.5	0.0002
0.39	0.677			9.0	0.0001

(Courtesy, Editors of Handbook of chemistry and physics, Chemical Rubber Company.)

Index